DOES MY WALL HAVE A WINDOW?

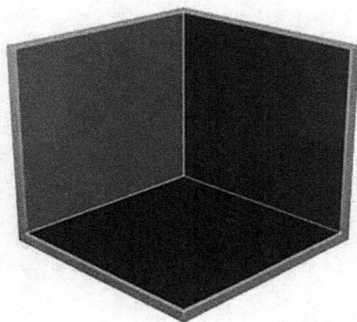

Living a Hellish Nightmare with Undiagnosed Bipolar Disorder

Rev. Dr. Wayne Driver, CD., PhD

Does My Wall Have A Window?
Copyright © 2019 by Rev. Dr. Wayne Driver, CD., PhD

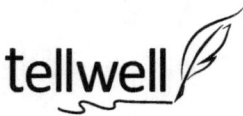

tellwell

Tellwell Talent
www.tellwell.ca

ISBN
978-0-2288-0930-2 (Hardcover)
978-0-2288-0929-6 (Paperback)
978-0-2288-0931-9 (eBook)

PREFACE

What you are about to read is a true-life story of my journey while living with an undiagnosed Bipolar Disorder and the 'living hell' it has put myself and my families through for over 50 years. I shall refer to my rollercoaster of emotional ups and down as a 'living 'hell, which are/ were like the weather. If you don't like my temperament at any particular moment in time, just wait 5 minutes because you'll either love me more… or even less… either way, I wouldn't really care nor would I know in which direction I'd be heading. I can be very unpredictable that way depending upon the people who surround me and/or the environment in which I find myself to be in. It would also depend upon how safe I feel with the people I'm with and whether or not I took my meds the night before… oh, but wait, there were no meds… I had been living a lifetime without a diagnosis. The stories and events are real as they have occurred and as I have recall of them. Unfortunately, my life events have not been placed in a time sequential order. I'm sorry [not really] to take you on a whirlwind, but welcome to my nightmare. I have written this book in an attempt to understand myself, perhaps to aide in the healing of my never-ending torment and anguish… to be somewhat educational for you and perhaps a tad humorous as well. Please keep in mind that I am neither a professional writer nor a comedian so you'll have to accept the ramblings of this maniac at face value. Thank you!

What you are about to read is really only the tip of the iceberg [and the portion of an iceberg that we see above the water is approximately 10%] of the agony to which I was subjected to, have experienced and am still attempting to figure out to this very day, which is the 4th of May, 2018 [the day I started making notes]. God forbid there should be a tomorrow without a true diagnoses and proper treatment. I really don't know how much more of this **living hellish nightmare** I am able to endure while fighting to retain some semblance of normalcy, stability and sanity. That is, if we can define each of those words. I've gone a life time of being unheard, of being misdiagnosed, while being prescribed perhaps some of the wrong medications [with minimal to no affect, which may have actually contributing to my illness while creating more insanity along the way] or having other meds abruptly ceased for no apparent reason while participating in crazy antics [if you will] because the so-called 'experts' weren't listening to my entire medical/mental/life history. Believe me, it hasn't been easy being me!

May I suggest that you look up this disorder for yourself… do the self test… have a family member answer the self testing questions on your behalf as well and then compare your answers. Should you suspect that you may be a fellow sufferer of bipolar disorder for which you have not been properly diagnosed and treated for, or you have someone that you love, who has not been diagnosed and you can identify with what you are about to read… I strongly urge you to seek help as soon as possible! Start by speaking with your medical practitioner by insisting that s/he LISTEN to your ENTIRE HISTORY before allowing her/him to jump to conclusions. Do not accept platitudes or NO, for an answer because you may regret it if you do. That is, if you aren't regretting it already. Show your doctor the results of your self test, this might be a good place to start. S/he should direct you to a mental health professional. Should they fail to do so, find the mental health unit at your nearest hospital and politely request assistance. Generally, you do not require a referral for a consultation and you may be able to refer yourself [as I had] and/or your loved one. Do not wait until the antics are out of control once again and you find your loved one being taken away in handcuffs, perhaps for the third time that year, or locked away in the mental health unit because of an attempted suicide. I referred myself after being mishandled by a mental health professional for the last time. Someone here in St. Paul neglected to refer my case to Cold Lake Mental Health Unit as they said they would. Not surprising, when I reported to the unit to give them my new phone number only to be met with… "and, who did you say you were?" Hmmm? Needless to say, more bullshit from the so-called experts. Anyway, I'm hoping the trouble was worth while this time around. I suppose only time will tell, won't it? You just might be able to save yourself from a life time of living through **hell**. Not everyone is fortunate enough to make it through to the other side alive.

IN CASE OF AN EMERGENCY!

Should you find yourself in a real Emergency situation... **Dial 911** anywhere here in North America.

If you are in dire straights and need someone to speak with and assist you from taking your own life... Please use one of the 1-800 numbers provided here.

- Canadian National Suicide Prevention Hot Line:
  1-833-456-4566

- US National Suicide Prevention Hot Line:
  1-800-273-8257

Should you find yourself to be 'confused' or in an 'uneasy' situation or a 'moment of uncertainty,' please don't hesitate to speak with a loved one, a friend, a co-worker or a neighbour, if for no other reason than to help clear your head. Remember, there is no shame in having a mental illness, especially if you don't know that you have one. And see your doctor as soon as possible. Please do not act upon your impulses as I have. Try to fight the urges because you know as well as I do, acting upon our impulses never achieves our desired results. Perhaps some day, this doctor will take his own advice. But for now, please learn from my mistakes if not from your own and call 911 or the Hot Line Number. If for no other reason than to save yourself, because Every life is important!

DEDICATION

To Family: After a number of years of encouragement from my dear friend and loving wife, I've finally decided to take her advice and have sat down long enough to write this book. Dedication also goes out to; my late wife, my children, my step-children and all of our grandchildren. I've loved you all the only way I've known how. Let me start out by saying how terribly sorry I am for the anguish that I have unknowingly caused you while living with me as I journeyed through my hellish nightmare while dealing with my skeletons which I had brought along for the ride. Thanks for loving me and putting up with my bullshit, all of those years! May you find your reward in heaven. This book is to help you understand what it's been like for me while living this hellish nightmare of a so-called life. Please read the entire book with understanding and without judgement in your heart. Remember, no one is perfect. Especially when I thought that I was crazy but no one else was listening;

Then to: the counselor in Winnipeg, one here in Cold Lake and the Dr... you folks know who you are. Even though you missed the mark, I'm sure that it was more often than not your empathetic ear, combined with your caring, gentle guiding words which I'm sure contributed to keeping my heights from being so lofty as well as preventing my valleys from being so deep that I saw no way of crawling out of them while I was in your care. I, Thank you;

Fellow Sufferers: to those who fear they may be a fellow sufferer, but have not been properly diagnosed... start by taking inventory of your

<u>entire life</u> and should you suspect as I had… that something may be out of sorts but you're not quite sure what it is… I urge you to seek help! You may not be as crazy as I thought I was; and

Even Him: The one particular individual whose drunken mean-spirited disposition combined with physical torture/abuse and psychological torment for so many years which I'm sure has contributed to most of the crap in my life, and for which I'm sure has also aided to my having the bipolar disorder in the first place… I have no idea how it is that you've managed to stay out of jail or out of a mental institution yourself all of your life. May God forgive you, because within myself, if it were not for the Grace of God, I would not be able to.

APOLOGY

Permit me to apologize up front to my Christian Brothers and Sisters and anyone else who may be offended by foul language as this book **does** contain many colourful expletives [swear words] for the purpose of quotation, to reveal thoughts and/or emotions from that particular moment in time, along with words thought of now while thinking back to assist with the descriptions of people, places, and things. And, because I have no other words in which to describe what/how I was/am feeling as these memories continue to overwhelm me as I recall the horrors for which I have lived through.

SHAMEFUL

I wrote this book with a fair bit, okay, a lot, alright then… with a substantial amount of sarcasm… because while at that time, I thought that many of my antics are/were funny and some still are. But now that I'm in a different frame of mind, some may not be as funny as I perceived them to be. However; wait until later, they may become even funnier than I recall, one never truly knows, because I don't know myself. Some of the shit I've pulled off over the years are actually down right hilarious while some are despicable at the same time, and for that, I do apologize… But, history is just that… history. There isn't anything that I can do to change my past except to share my experiences with you and pray to God that my history does not repeat itself, and that you may learn from my mistakes. I would rather that my history not be repeated and that is why I've kicked in a few more doors this time around in anticipation of finding help. However; looking back, I haven't done anything for which I have not been forgiven by God. Man is fallible and we may not forgive each other but God always forgives. Praise the Lord! You may sit in judgment, but just remember two things… when you point a finger, in my direction, you also have three pointing back at you and by whatever measure you use to judge me, is the same measure that God will use when he casts judgement upon you. Besides, Grace and Mercy are all about the love and forgiving qualities of God demonstrated towards man through his son Christ Jesus. Not that we should knowingly continue in our sin so that grace may abound, but in a sense, I couldn't help it… I wasn't and still am not in my right frame of mind… so they tell me.

Caveat: I want to make this perfectly clear, when I say that 'NO ONE, or NO BODY WAS/IS LISTENING' I'm referring to the 'so-called experts.' You know the folks who are in the mental and/or medical health fields and should have known better along with those in the school systems whom I've spoken with over the years, or who have treated me in the past who could have done something to help me, but for whatever reason had failed me and continue to do so to this very day. To those of you who are in my inner circle… I ask that you do not take it personally, please and thank you!

Interjection: noun; an abrupt remark, made especially as an aside note or interruption or an 'injection' of thoughts. There are numerous 'interjections' as I continue to write, rewrite and edit. I inform you of things and thoughts that are happening or I am feeling at that particular moment which I feel that you should know about.

But Before we start: I feel that it is important for you to know that the man who assisted in 'raising' me, [and I do use that term extremely loosely, because even that's a stretch of my imagination] for 17 years, 8 months and 17 days… was not my biological father. He was my mother's husband… and nothing more to me. Unfortunately, I do not know who my 'biological' father is/was and therefore know nothing about him, his family nor his medical history. Therefore, I refer to the fellow whom I was forced to live with as 'step-dad', 'old man', and my favorite; 'monster', along with an assortment of other descriptive words to unveil sentiments towards this man because I refuse to call him '**dad**' or <u>**Father**</u> and I make no apologies for this. I do realize that to many of you, this may be of the utmost in disrespect which goes against the 5th Commandment of God which is found in Exodus 20:5 [which also comes with a promise] "Honour your father and your mother so that you may live long in the land that Yahweh your God is giving you." May God forgive me but you may or may not understand shortly, why that it is hard for me to respect such a person. Some would say that he technically wasn't my father and therefore I didn't have to respect him. No foul no harm, right? Then we have the other side of the coin by which people say that the 10 Commandments were given to the Tribes of Israel and therefore do not apply to the Gentiles. Food for thought for sure. Either way, this is neither the time nor the place to argue semantics, so I won't and leave it as is.

Step-dad use to tell me that I was a smart-ass [generally followed by a back-hand across the mouth or upside the back of the head, but hey] while growing up when I thought I had some witty words of wisdom to pass along, or something sarcastic to say [and I always had witty words of wisdom and/or something sarcastic to say]. Truthfully, I could never distinguish between the two. So, why should I start now? Yes, I am a bit of a smart-ass, why? "Because it went to school with the rest of me", I use to say. So, in keeping with the spirit of time-honoured traditions… this book is <u>chalk</u> <u>full</u> of what I consider to be witty words of wisdom and <u>loaded</u> with sarcasm along with smart ass comments for which I am famous for. My advice to you is… either ignore them or chuckle along with them.

<u>Dad</u>: A dad is someone that is there for his children [**in reference to this man, rarely**]. A dad watches and actively participates in their lives [**the only active participation this man took in my life was to regular beat**

me senseless]. A dad helps them grow up, raises them, nurtures them, attends dance recitals and baseball games and is present. [**My step-dad helped out from time to time with something or other with Cubs, Scouts, and Cadets… but more often than not there were many complaints about how he wasn't 'thanked' or how no one so much as offered to buy him a coffee or some crap like that**].

https://www.dadtography.com/definition-of-dad-vs-father-and-a-fathers-right-to-parent/

<u>Father</u>: noun; a male parent. A father-in-law, stepfather, or adoptive father. Any male ancestor, especially the founder of a family or line; progenitor. A man who exercises paternal care over other persons; paternal protector or provider: a father to the poor. A person who has originated or established something: the father of modern psychology; the founding fathers.

SECTION ONE

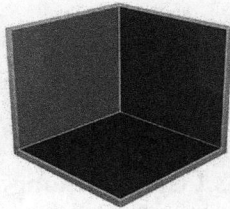

BIPOLAR DISORDER

For this first segment; my thoughts, comments, expressions, words of wisdom, sarcasm, experiences and answers to the 'so-called expert's comments and questions' are in **bold letters.**

There <u>IS</u> a fair bit of repetition here in this first section and it was done on purpose because I have gleaned information from multiple multinational sources, so please bear with me. Oh… and not to mention the inability to stay on course so try keeping up will you. Personally, I think the Americans do a better job of addressing this subject, and I thank you.

This from the Canadian Government on Mental Illnesses:

www.canada.ca/en/public-health/services/chronic-diseases/mental-illness/what-should-know-about-bipolar-disorder-manic-depression.html

What Should I Know about Bipolar Disorder (Manic-Depression)?

Everything… I want to know all that there is to know so I am able to prove that not only was I right all along… that there is something wrong with me and that I'm not really crazy as I always thought that I was/am. I've always referred to myself as being 'certifiable' but couldn't find anyone to place their stamp of approval upon me. Heck, my wife actually went and inscribed this on the inside of my wedding ring… "Certifiable, always by your side".

<u>Bipolar disorder</u> (formerly called manic-depression) is a bio-chemical condition that results in <u>an imbalance</u> of the neurotransmitters in the brain. Genetic make-up is thought to play a role but <u>so too are environmental pressures</u> such as your <u>family</u>, work and <u>social environment</u>, <u>stress</u>, <u>injury</u>, <u>illness</u> and hormone imbalances **as you will discover, the 'environment' in which I was raised may have had something to do with my being doomed right from the beginning.**

No offense to any fellow sufferer, but I prefer to refer to the 'manic' phase as they call it, to my 'maniac' phase, because I feel that I could only have been crazy to pull off some of the stunts or commit the

actions that I have over the years and have gotten away with [mostly] or so I thought! No, I haven't been arrested for them, so that would mean I've gotten away with them…

I personally think that using the word 'maniac' is more of an accurate description of what's really going on inside of my head and in the world in which I find myself to be in at any particular moment in time, as perceived by myself of course. Had I been properly diagnosed all of those years ago, it may have prevented a lot of craziness in my life over the past 50 years. Medications and therapy may have helped to stabilize my condition perhaps allowing for me to live somewhat of a 'normal' life and I would have found a different topic to write a book about. That is, if we can define what 'normal' really is. So, from hence forth, I will call their manic phase by my preferred word: MANIAC! Just for fun if for no other reason.

Bipolar disorder is characterized by mood swings that can last for days, weeks or even months. **You, don't say? Batter Up!**

Manic: adjective; If you describe someone as manic, you mean that they do things extremely quickly or energetically, often because they are very excited or anxious or these feelings may be so intense or strange as if they appear to be insane.

Maniac: noun; a raving or violently insane person, a lunatic. Any intemperate or overly zealous or enthusiastic person.

Adjective: Origin of maniac; First recorded in 1595 – 1605, maniac is from the Medieval Latin word maniacus of, pertaining to madness.

Mood swing is an extreme or rapid change in mood. Such mood swings can play a positive part in promoting problem solving and in producing flexible forward planning. However, when mood swings are so strong that they are disruptive, they may be the main part of a bipolar disorder. **Huh? You don't say.**

https://en.wikipedia.org/wiki/Mood_swing

Mood swings, that's an understatement. I think I have more swings in a year than a professional ball player does during a regular season game.

So, lets, play ball!

These swings range from <u>mild</u> to <u>severe</u>.

Severe I believe is another underestimation but I suppose they had to use some semblance of an intelligent word to describe it.

<u>Mild</u>: not severe, serious, harsh, gentle, not easily provoked.

<u>Severe</u>: of something bad or undesirable, very great or intense.

Undesirable and Intense enough to want to solve my money troubles by breaking into a bank or knocking off a liquor store one moment, thinking that I'm smart enough to get away with it, to wanting to kill someone or myself the next. So, what do I do? I try it of course… not the breaking in to commit the robberies but the killing myself… by stepping out in front of a bus, a tractor trailer, trying to outrun a freight train, trying to drown myself, slitting a wrist or two, overdosing or even praying that the old man would do the job for me and finally put me out of my misery. I hadn't tried it only once or twice mind you but several times over the course of my life time as you shall see. Perhaps one of these days I'll get my timing perfect and finally succeed! Oh, but wait… as you'll also soon find out… I'm a 'stupid-ass' who 'can't do anything right' but were my attempts seeking thrills and chills as we see upon our television? Was I just seeking much needed attention because I was an abused and neglected child or were they very real cries for help? Never Cry Wolf, unless there really is one!

The Boy Who Cried Wolf!

https://www.nursery-rhymes-fun.com/boy-who-cried-wolf.html

If it looks like a duck, swims like a duck and quacks like a duck, then damn, it probably is a duck!

The Duck Test: https://en.wikipedia.org/wiki/Duck_test

Not necessarily they say... it could have been a rabbit, but whose, hallucinating now?

The "**bi**" in <u>bi</u>polar disorder refers to the dual nature of these mood swings - from feelings of great happiness and elation to sadness and despair.

The great happiness would be the opposite of Eeyore's doom and gloom in everything where Skittles come out of a rainbow like that commercial on television. No matter what you do or say, you won't make me sad today... To feelings of being sad and despair? More like; hopeless, uselessness, even worthless while having an all around 'who cares' or a 'pessimistic' attitude of impending doom and gloom all the way down to sounding like <u>Eeyore</u>; Thanks Eeyore! To be more accurate: it is more of a '<u>fuck it all</u>' mood and I'd just go with the flow, or attempt to kill myself because if no one wants me around, why should I be here?

Sounding like Eeyore is in reference to what I shall call my 'Eeyore Complex'. He didn't care much about anything. More often than not, he'd find a rain cloud in just about everything in life and so had I while I found myself to be in a depressive state. Come to think of it... I can be like that when I'm not depressed and sort of in that 'in between' mood which will be discussed later. I think Eeyore was my favorite character in the <u>Hundred Acre Wood</u> because I could easily identify with him the most. Looking back, I really do have an Eeyore Complex when I'm in between and depressed. The Eeyore complex while Maniac would amount to having a who cared attitude and I'd just do some crazy shit and not really care what mess I'd find myself to be in to clean up later, or worse yet... do/or say something to someone and not care how they feel/felt about it. Oh well... sorry? [not really] Sorry, sometimes/most of the time, just doesn't cut it. But then if you ask me, political correctness is overrated. I suppose that's where the 'fuck it all' came from... I'd be thinking; "I'm going to get into trouble one way or another, so I may as well do or say what I'm thinking and get it over with."

I liked the Winnie The Pooh original Series so much so, that I actually went out and purchased my very own 100-acre wood in New Brunswick. Why? For no other reason then because I could, that's why. Lived on it for awhile too, until I burnt the house down, but that's another story for later on. I made the purchase I'm sure like I do every other purchase: on impulse and during a maniac phase. Shortly there after we moved and built on it during the same phase and burnt the house down during a depressive phase a few months later. Shit happens I guess. But why did/does it always have to happen to me?

Eeyore is an elderly, grey donkey, who lives by himself in a perhaps rather remote corner of the forest called Eeyore's Gloomy Place [sounds pretty good to me right about now]. His name comes from the sound that donkeys make when they are conversing (Ee-or, Ee-or). Eeyore is, to put it politely, is a bit of a pessimist. He is consistently grumpy and gloomy throughout all of the stories, although just occasionally we see that he is capable of real joy too. [**He resonates with bipolar disorder too if you ask me**]

http://www.winnie-pooh.org/eeyore.htm

Fuck it all: something said to express a vague, but intense, desperation or frustration with any or all of the following: the world, yourself, responsibilities, everything you know, a feeling, religion(s), answers without questions, questions without determination, inability it seems to start anew, fleeting, loss of faith/wonder, awareness of unawareness, unaware of self.

https://www.urbandictionary.com/define.php?term=fuck%20it%20all

In its most severe expression, bipolar disorder can result in mania which is defined as strongly held beliefs that you are a famous person, have special physical abilities or knowledge, or that you are invincible.

I never thought myself to be any particular 'famous person' because I have never idolized anyone to such heights of wanting to imitate or fantasize about being them. There are some famous people I would appreciate socializing with, but not being them. I personally wouldn't

flatter another human being in that manner because I think that people place actors/actresses, entertainers/sports players on too high of a pedestal as it is and because of this… they get a hypersensitive ego… "I'm the great so and so, and am untouchable", some even believe that they are above the law. Invincible? Often, but then again, who isn't? I didn't need psychedelic drugs to make me think that I could climb a 7-storey building for no other reason than because they built it in such a manner that it begged to be climbed. Hey, that guy is jumping lanes back and forth and has cut me off now for the third time and he's not really getting anywhere in the traffic so at the stop light I get out of my vehicle and threaten to pull him out of his and teach him some manners.

People can experience <u>mania</u> as a <u>euphoric</u> [**euphoric, now there's an interesting word**] period. Unfortunately, mania is also accompanied by unwise behaviours tied to the false beliefs [**nah, go on with you**].

These can include spending sprees…

Come on you guys, what are you waiting for? We only have 6 more hours to get this project into high gear, do I have to do it all by myself? Because I can you know and you'll find yourself in the unemployment line! Spending? Without even thinking about how much was in my bank account or that I've already maxed out three of my credit cards. They'll up my limit… go ahead, I need it or I deserve it… so, I'll purchase it without a second thought. Second thoughts… what's that? Heck, I may not have even had a first thought because I bought on impulse. Life is better than good; can it get any better? Why, yes it can… let's get this party started. So intense perhaps that I feel as though I'm on top of the world and can accomplish anything that I put my mind to? But wait, I do accomplish everything I put my mind too, don't I?

<u>Mania</u>: a state of abnormally elevated <u>arousal</u>, [sexually as well] affect, and energy level.

<u>Euphoric</u>: characterized by or feeling intense excitement and happiness which may be accompanied by risky sexual activity.

Risky sexual activity? When I was younger I always did like the sounds of that but a true gentleman never kisses and tells names and/or details that is but I suppose a one-night stand with a woman whom I just met wouldn't fit the bill because that happens all of the time, all around the world in most cultures, right? Sure, it does. How about two women and little ole me? Nah, that only happens in the movies, or in my dreams… or does it?

So, what counts then? <u>excessive drinking</u> one is often too many and ten may never be enough <u>or drug use</u>, no thank you, I've always passed on that one. I've been offered Cocaine and Heroin a few times but never wanted to get addicting, not to mention not being able to afford them, so, I've always stayed away. Not to mention already being messed up, what would I have the need for drugs? I sometimes smoked marijuana back in the day [and would often like to do so now] but nothing to excess like some people I knew/know. I was only a social smoker if you will <u>and other reckless activities</u> like smuggling marijuana in for a lawyer friend when I was on board ship out of Halifax and more often than not, payment wasn't always just in cash alone, if you get my drift? What about climbing up to the roof of the school so the bullies couldn't find me? <u>or decisions</u> who bothers making decisions, I liked my way of life which Nike stole and made it their slogan by the way… 'just do it!' [Of course, they stole it from me, those corporate guys could read my mind, couldn't they?] It worked for me, but perhaps it was not always enjoyed by all parties concerned. This one time [not necessarily at band camp], I called a buddy in Calgary, "Hey, if we move out there can you find us a place to live until I can find the family accommodations?" "Sure, come on out". We moved out to Calgary from London Ontario within a week. Maniac? Or is that 'normal' behaviour?

Bouts of mania are followed by the depths of depression where people feel worthless and hopeless [but that would never happen to little ole me, I'm always on top of the world]. This phase of bipolar disorder is excruciatingly painful. Ya! Like being awake while watching yourself living a hellish nightmare and being unable to do anything about it. Grabbing the remote to change the channel wouldn't do any good either. Oh, I've got an ever better one than that… having the dentist drill my tooth before the freezing takes affect. The mood swings of bipolar disorder deeply affect relationships, **deeply affect relationships, you don't say?** Yes, like being in the dog house on a permanent basis? But, for some reason my first wife was with me for 20 years and my current wife has been with me for 18 years now. She says that she loves me, but if that's the case… tell me why it is I feel so insulted, put down, micromanaged, and belittled? Strained relationship? Absolutely, because she my behavior doesn't make any sense. Social life; what's that? You want to go where? To see who? Why? I don't have any 'friends' that I really want to hang out with <u>and work functioning</u> I can't seem to get anything done again today because I have too much on the go. Come to think of it, I didn't want to be here yesterday, and I don't want to be here today, so, I don't think I'll be here tomorrow either… and I wouldn't be… See Ya! Or I'd walk off the job in the middle of the shift for no rhyme or reason, other than because I could and I'd never return <u>and can, in the extreme, bring people into contact with the law</u>. Cops pulling me over on the 401 because I'm going Eastbound in the Westbound lane, pulling me off of a rail on a bridge, or breaking up a fight in the downtown core of a major city in SW Ontario wouldn't be extreme, would it? I thought 'extreme' was only about Sports on television. You don't say, how can that be? Oh, please do tell me more, I'd really like to know what you have to say since you've never experienced it for yourself and I have no idea what it is that you're talking about but can read the same books for myself.

Symptoms of mania <u>can</u> include the following:

If they knew the proper definition of this word…'can' they most likely would not have used it here…'can' is a verb meaning… be able to… as if there is a possibility of doubt here. Let's look at this sentence again shall we: Symptoms of mania may 'be able to' or 'may' include the following… Nah, doesn't work here… how about '<u>does</u>' or '<u>will</u>' include the following… which presumes the high probability or the likelihood of including… Ya, that works!

+   <u>feelings of invincibility</u>

    Does jumping off a 100 ft cliff into 30' of water while passing rock climbers on my way down count or is that just me thrill

seeking again? What about running across a train trestle to see if I am able to make it to the other end before the freight train runs me over? Every 8-year-old kid tries to out run a freight train, don't they?

- more physical energy

While on a 13km rucksack march… what's the matter with you guys; why can't you keep up? We only have 10 more kms to go. Come on! We're given 2 hours and 26 minutes to accomplish this task while being weighted down with approximately 40lbs of gear. When left on my own, or permitted to go ahead… I'd often complete the march in 1 hr and 45 minutes or less. Why? Why not? Because I could I suppose. More often than not though the pansies would keep me back [while crying… "we have to stay together']. Oh, did I mention that I was in my mid 40's outdoing 20 and 30 something year old's?

- less need for sleep

Does only 3 or 4 hours [if any at all for days on end count?] I've been working on sleep deprivation again, but what else is new for me? Google search sleep deprivation sometime; it's fascinating. I have come to realize though, that I get very irritable when I'm deprived of sleep… yes, more so than usual. I was 'written-up' on one of our Military Exercises because of my conduct of 'irritability' due to sleep deprivation. More often than not, I have to really check myself on that… is it worth getting upset over? What is it going to accomplish if I verbally lash out? Okay, it's not all that bad, I do have my jovial moments. I'm currently coming down from another 3-week stint where I may have had 3 hours sleep [or less] each night. Last night I didn't sleep at all and I'm now on my 28th hour. Try it some time… it's a blast! I bet you can't stay up for 48 hrs and still function somewhat 'normally' but I can! How about for 60hrs? That's when things really start to get interesting, but I don't start to get shaky and weird until about my 80th hour. I think my record is something like 105 hrs which I think is about 4 ½ days. Use my email address on the last page and let me know how you make out with this one. Not that I'd have any advice to give you, but we could still chat about it. I personally think its awesome.

Interjection: I forgot to write the date and time… When I was finally ready to lay down last night [after being up for only 34 hrs], I self medicated with a sleeping pill that I'm sure had an expiration date of over two years ago, but, what the heck. Even with that, I still woke up several times during the night. I don't believe I slept for more than a couple of hours at a time before waking up again. I feel worse now than when I had after only having 3 straight hours of sleep. If the truth be told, I've felt better with a hangover than I did coming off of those sleeping pills so I threw them out. Why bother with sleep aides? Why bother with sleep at all actually? I'll get plenty of that when I'm dead. Sleep is highly over-rated if you ask me.

• inappropriate [not suitable or proper in the circumstances] excitement

Finding something funny at a funeral for example does not just happen in the movies for laughs, I know because I've done it… Why? I don't know why, I just started chuckling and had to leave… was it something I saw or heard? Then there are times when I start to smile or chuckle and people are asking me "what's so funny?" and I tell them that "I don't know" but they don't believe me. Why do people take it so personally? More often than not, I answer; "Nothing, nothing at all" because I really don't know and sometimes I'll break out laughing. Maybe it's something you've just said, which reminded me of something else and I've gone off in a totally inappropriate direction and I'm laughing but I don't thing you'll find it funny so I won't share. And, of course there are other expressions of 'excitement' because I've just seen someone who reminded me of someone else that I've been with and my mind instantly brings me back to that intimate moment in time. It's terrible when my mind disfunctions like that and then I have an erection to deal with… oh boy, I sure hope no one can see this, while trying to cover it up.

- <u>irritability or excessive anger</u>

Does impulsively throwing something at one of my siblings count as displaying this irritability or excessive anger? Needless to say, I became very good at throwing things. I managed to develop a fantastic arm and excellent aiming skills by doing it so often that I wanted to be a pitcher on a little league team. However, beaster had more important things to do with his time and money than to waste it on the likes of me to play baseball. Everyone throws things when they're mad… I've seen it in the movies or comedies shows at least 1000 times. How about getting angry at someone for no apparent reason or for what others would deem to be a minor infraction? Does threatening to throw someone down the stairs just because I can, and then I do… count? By the way, that's never ever a good idea, so I wouldn't recommend that one… especially while in the Military and I find myself up on charges for physical violence… etc. But what can I say? He pissed me off for the last time and I got the desired results, he stopped leaving his gear all over the room and in front of the door to our room.

<u>increased activity, talking and moving</u>

Increased activity, nah, I like staying still. Moving? Does my mother and/or my teacher having to constantly tell me to stop fidgeting, or to stay in my seat so often that both of them give up because I am unable to comply with their demands, count? How about talking for what apparently feels like a long time to someone that they are unable to get in a word to contribute to my conversation that I may as well be having with myself? I've learned to curb the talking thing though. I either really don't socialize that much anymore or I just let other people do the talking for the both of us.

- <u>increased sexual thoughts and activity, sometimes resulting in promiscuity and inappropriate or unsafe behaviour</u>

Sometimes I wonder if I'm addicted to sex, but we won't go there right now. When Kinsey researchers asked men and women how often they'd think about sex, 54% of men said they think about sex <u>several</u> times a day... they've proven the previous record of every 7 seconds to be a myth. Only several times a day? Is that all? What's the matter with these guys? Promiscuity? Okay, but only if I have to tell you... stories later but only if you promise not to judge, call me names or point fingers.

+ <u>disconnected and racing thoughts</u>

You mean like when I'm having a conversation and I switch from one idea to the next in the middle of the first one, only to leave my second thought and continue where I left off on the first perhaps jumping to a third all in the midst of the same conversation where people have no idea what it is I'm talking about? But I don't realize that I'm doing it and people come to me the next day only to ask what I was smoking or what was the matter with me? Hence the phrase, 'babbling idiot'! Comes to mind. Or thinking so fast that my fingers can't keep up on the key board so I switch to a pen or pencil thinking that would be faster only to discover that I can't write fast enough and that I am unable to read my own chicken scratches later? Is there a breaking mechanism in here somewhere? I know... what about not being able to shut my brain off so that I am able to get some much-needed sleep because I'm now working on 60 straight hours again... there has to be an off switch in here somewhere. Now, if only I could remember where I left it.

+ <u>racing speech</u>

I don't believe that I have experienced this one, not that I am aware of or that people have informed me about. So that would be a <u>NO</u>. Oh well, I can't win them all.

<u>loss of self-control and impulsive or reckless behaviour</u>

I don't think they're talking loss of Blatter control here, are they?

Well, I've already mentioned a little bit about impulsivity being my first name, and we'll cover more of that later. I don't think knocking my supervisor to the floor before quitting a job would count as losing self-control nor reckless behaviour, would it?

inappropriate spending

Everyone, at one time in their life has walked into a Toyota [or a car] Dealership and has purchased not One but Two brand new Corolla's spending something in the neighbourhood of $45,000.00 then meeting up with the Mrs. at her work place only to hand her the keys to her new car, haven't they? Oh, come on, you can't tell me I'm the only one who has done that... I wouldn't believe you.

+ Hallucinations

Perhaps seeing a little old lady sitting at the end of my brother's bed or seeing cats and/or hearing my cat beside me in bed but when I reach out to pet her she isn't there at all. What about shadows of people who aren't really there? Sometimes I see a figment or something crossing right in front of me or through my peripheral vision and when I turn to look, there isn't anyone or anything there. Heaven forbid I should ask the person who might be with me if they saw that as well... it would be time to throw away the key for sure and delusions. I believe that I can honestly say that I've never been delusional by its definition, that I know of. Huh? Maybe I'm delusional just saying that?

Delusion: is a mistaken belief that is held with strong conviction even in the presence of superior evidence to the contrary. As a pathology, it is distinct from a belief based on false or incomplete information, confabulation, dogma, illusion, or some other misleading effects of perception.

Oops, perhaps I may be delusional after all?

Some symptoms of depression may include:

I like that; '_may_' include as if it were another form of being in the slight possibility of being an improbability? How about; '_does_' include, which takes away any chance of the impossibility. Not to mention other symptoms they don't list here. Did you know that there are many different types of depressions? But we'll stick with what the 'so-called experts' have given us. They are fascinating to read about... Google them sometime, especially the one about those who suffer from bipolar disorder. They're a riot. Oh, in case you haven't noticed; I like Google for most of my research... okay, for all of my research. Fascinating tool, the internet! And I enjoy Wikipedia, marvelous, simply, marvelous.

✦ feelings of sadness and loss

We're not talking about when I have to flush my gold-fish down the toilet because I've fed him too death [again] or, that I've forgotten to feed him. We're talking about having these feelings even though family, friends, job and social life [that is, if I had a social lift] are all intact. These feelings, like everything else, just magically appear out of thin air and for no justifiable reason other than to torture me once again. Why, just this morning I heard a song on You Tube which made me cry... and I really don't know why. Sniff. Oh well. I think the power of the 'sense' of loss or loneliness is more powerful than the sense of being joyful or happy, don't you?

Sadness is an emotional pain associated with, or characterized by, feelings of disadvantage, loss, despair, grief, helplessness, disappointment and/or sorrow. **Sounds about right!**

Again, having these feelings of utter sadness and just wanting to sit down and cry and I don't know why? So, I do and that's always enjoyable. It can also be embarrassing when it happens at work and my supervisor sends me home for the rest of the day. Or? It's 23 degrees out in May, the golf course is now open and that was me faking it at 9:00am so I could have a day off? "4!" I guess we'll never know that one either, will we? And why is that we will never know? Because no one was/is listening... Tisk, tisk, tisk...

+ <u>feelings of guilt and worthlessness</u>

I thought that was just because I could hear my monster's voice in my head?

Especially after something I've done during my maniac state or for no apparent reason at all; or having thoughts that nobody cares about poor little ole me, so <u>I think I'll go eat worms</u>, that sort of thing?

Ya, it's a kid's song we use to sing back in the day...

[Verse 1]
Nobody likes me, everybody hates me
I think I'll go eat worms!
Big fat juicy ones
Eensie weensy squeensy ones
See how they wiggle and squirm!

[Verse 2]
Down goes the first one, down goes the second one
Oh how they wiggle and squirm!
Up comes the first one, up comes the second one
Oh how they wiggle and squirm!

[Verse 3]
I bite off the heads, and suck out the juice
And throw the skins away!
Nobody knows how fat I grow
On worms three times a day!

[Repeat Verse 1]

Here's Charles Van Deursen singing it on YouTube
https://www.youtube.com/watch?v=XrFViBSYPtQ

<u>Worthlessness</u>: having no real value or use.

There you go, anybody want to buy a used 'U'?

Worthlessness can also be described as a feeling of desperation and hopelessness. Individuals who feel worthless may feel insignificant, useless, or believe they have nothing valuable to offer the world. People diagnosed with depression often report these feelings, <u>and children who were **neglected** or **abused** may</u> [**will/do**] <u>carry a sense of worthlessness into adulthood</u> [**to the point where I want to kill myself**]. When worthlessness leads one to experience thoughts of suicide [**told you**] or causes other immediate crisis, it may be best to contact a crisis hotline or seek other help right away.

Hotline numbers are on Page 4!

Did you catch all of that? As it turns out; it isn't my fault after-all… and we know exactly who to blame for most of this crap, don't we? Okay, perhaps you don't as of yet, but you will. Well I'll be? I wish mom were alive today to see her dreams come true and that in spite of my terrible up bringing, I had become a 'somebody' after all, or, rather was and hopefully will be again. So, thoughts of suicide are normal when I'm feeling worthless and have nothing of value to offer to anyone. Oh, and if you do reach out, make sure you speak with a trained professional… your significant other will not always understand… trust me on this one because I speak from experience. Should there be something, anything at all wrong… why do people throw it back in your face? "Oh, you never talk to me." So, when I do… "oh, you're only making excuses for that because of this…" Why bother?

<u>feelings of extreme impatience, irritability, or a short temper</u>

Who, me? Not so much during a maniac phase except perhaps when I haven't slept for days again… let's get going already, I have places to be and people to see. The short temper though is sort of like in the cartoons when someone distinguishes a fuse on a bomb at that very last second… You don't want to be the one relighting that fuse because you wouldn't make it out alive.

But then hell, I'll do it, I'm indestructible, let's go for it… and the powder keg goes off. Especially when I have to wait for other people, like that guy in front of the line staring at a flashing green arrow, right? Or I pour the coffee cream into my cereal instead of the 2% milk because the products are both from the same dairy and the containers have similar colours and I mix the damn things up… oh, "just add water" I've been told… not bloody likely, so now I'm pissed and don't even bother to eat breakfast. I wouldn't just add water to the cream for the same reason I don't just add ice to my Scotch… give me a fucking break already.

Or… I'm dealing with people who I deem to be stupid and then I begin to tell them why I'm thinking that. That always goes over well, doesn't it? Not really but I expend the energy and really don't know why. More often than not, I don't feel better after I do that.

A great one around this town is when I have the flashing green arrow permitting me to legally make a left turn and the idiot in the on-coming traffic still has a red light but fails to come to a complete stop and cuts me off while making a right-hand turn… the biggest thing that pisses me off about that is… if I beep my horn, s/he gives me the finger as if I was in the wrong and cut them off… what the fuck? Here's your sign asshole! Am I still allowed to throw things at people at my age? Just the other day a yahoo did just that very thing and I followed them into the Shopper's parking lot. I gave him a blast of shit and warned them that I would ram them with my truck the next time we should have a similar encounter… give me the finger because you're an ass hole, will you? I'll show you what a real ass hole can look like.

But my ultimate high time <u>favorite</u> is trying to spread butter on toast even though it's 25 Degrees Celsius [77°F] in the house and the damn butter is still rock solid that it rips my toast so much so that I end up throwing it into the garbage and I want to throw the butter in after it. But I don't… butter is expensive… so, more often than not, I leave the butter on the counter and make a bee-line for the PB & J. Thanks Eeyore!

◆ <u>loss of interest or pleasure in usually-enjoyed activities</u>

What do you want to do today? Nothing! Being left a lone is a good idea, hiding in my office all day is an even better one. Did you know that they say it is mentally and physically impossible to do '<u>nothing</u>' but I beg to differ. As if doing nothing were impossible?

<u>Nothing </u>is a concept denoting the absence of something and is associated with nothingness. In non-technical uses, nothing denotes things lacking importance, interest, value, relevance, or significance, therefore; <u>it is</u> <u>possible</u> for someone to be doing nothing. **I told you!**

And I bet you thought this book wouldn't be very educational, didn't you?

How about just simply being bored and I don't know why. Or, how many projects do I have left unfinished??? Nope, it ain't going to happen today and the likelihood of accomplishing that tomorrow is looking pretty slim to nil as well. I'm not and never have been a procrastinator... If I don't want to do something, I just won't do it, there in lies the difference. Once again, the Eeyore Complex kicks in. Thanks pal! I was looking for a plush Eeyore on Amazon.ca... they range from $30.00 all the way up to $160.00... huh? How crazy is that?

<u>Interjection</u>: 1013-17-07-2018; I've been up for an hour, I want to go back to bed. I don't have any appointments today but I'm suppose to be going to the bank and running other errands, etc., weren't we just discussing 'wanting to do things?' But the probability of any thing happening is slim to nil. I'll set my sights on tomorrow. If tomorrow ever comes that is... I'm going back to bed... nighty-night! Now where's my Eeyore? Oh ya, right, the $30.00 ones were ugly and I'm not spending $160.00 for a plush Eeyore.

<u>changes in weight or appetite</u>

<u>appetite</u> is a noun which describes a <u>natural</u> desire to satisfy a bodily need especially for food.

Huh? I've always known the meaning of the word but I had to make sure I was aware of the correct definition… Natural desire? Huh? I suppose it would be right up there with being hungry which I have no comprehension of this physical concept because I don't believe I have ever experienced hunger beyond the age of 6 years of age. Explanation later. Read about the 'Corn Flakes Wars'… it's a riot, you don't want to miss that! Make sure you've popped extra corn before you begin. Have a Kleenex handy as well, you just might tear up with laughter. And then, perhaps feel sorry for this stupid little kid. And you thought your kid was stubborn… s/he's got nothing on me I guarantee you that!

Appetite? Nope, that word does not compute either, sorry.

Food is like sleep to me, it's highly over-rated. I only eat because my body requires food to stay alive. I only sleep for the same reason. If I were to go too long without food or sleep, I'm sure people would attempt to have me committed and they'd feed me through a tube or something and give me an injection of some concoction to make me sleep. Oh, the best sleep I've ever had were while under general anesthesia… got to love that stuff. The only problem with that was, the time out is/was never long enough.

How about going without food for a couple of days without intentionally fasting? I get so wrapped in a project [like this book] that I'll forget to eat, because, I'm not hungry. Come to think of it, I probably don't sleep for the same reason, I'm not tired. Now, do you see my dilemma? Have you heard that a <u>genius</u> mind is borderline insanity? But then, I've never thought to highly of myself to be considered a genius. Everyone maintains a 4.0 average through University, don't they?

<u>Genius</u>: a person who is exceptionally intelligent or creative, either generally or in some particular respect. So, we don't have to be a

'genius' in all aspects of life, but we can be in specific disciplines. Hmm?

- <u>changes in **sleep**ing patterns like insomnia</u>

Does lying in bed for hours on end watching the second-hand on the clock tick-tock away the minutes which turn into hours on end, count as being an insomniac? Well, I've been telling them for years that I can not or do not sleep, but they ain't listening.

<u>Sleep</u>: a condition of body and mind such as that which typically recurs for several hours every night, in which the nervous system is relatively inactive, the eyes closed, the postural muscles relaxed, and consciousness practically suspended.

So that's what sleep is… the consciousness practically suspended for several hours… every night… Huh? I am not capable of such activity without the assistance of sleeping aids and even then, my sleep is hit and miss to that level of unconsciousness. I've even taken sleeping aides in hope of finding this 'conscious suspension' only to miss the mark and had stayed awake all night anyway. How much sleep a night does your body generally require?

- <u>reduced ability to think clearly or make decisions</u>

One of the things my wife liked about me when we first met was the ability to make decisions… looking back, that must have been during my 'just do it' phase and to her, that was deciding… Heads I win, tails you loose kind of thing. I guess whatever works, right? Then she saw the other side of the coin. I don't know, what do you think? It doesn't matter to me; whatever you want. The blue one, no, on second thought take the green one… no wait, the blue, yes, I'm sure, take the green one and let's go before I change my mind again. It's extremely frustrating to be honest with you. Then she has the nerve to say "what's the matter with you today? You use to be able to make decisions."

- <u>difficulties in concentrating or with short-term memory loss</u>

We're not just talking about where I left my truck keys or my wallet. But I am constantly going to my truck, only having to return to the house because I've forgotten my keys in the key box [Psst, that's one of the reasons why we purchased the key box in the first place was so that I would know where my keys were]. Perhaps reading the same sentence 3 times and I still don't know what I've just read or I can't remember what I went into the other room for. So, here we were talking about making a Caesar Salad, I'm holding the Romaine Lettuce in my hand, but I could not for the life of me remember what that stuff was called... I couldn't even recall the word Lettuce... both words had been completely erased from my memory banks... it's pretty freaky when that happens. Nothing to worry about they said, it happens to everyone [with dementia, that is]

- <u>constantly feeling tired</u>

I know, we're talking about feeling naturally tired, all the time, during a depressive state... well, that does happen, but I'm still an insomniac, so of course I'm going to be tired, I haven't slept in days and even when I do sleep, I'm still tired because the sleep is never deep or long enough. There, I've answered the question, happy?

- <u>noticeable lack of motivation</u>

Nope, can't' say I recall this one, Thanks Eeyore!

A motive or motivation is what prompts the person to act in a certain way, or at least develop an inclination for specific behavior.

I 'just do it' because that's how I roll and moss don't grow on a rolling stone.

But, today, I don't want to roll, so, I won't and you can't make me.

+ <u>anxiety and restlessness,</u>

I don't know about you but there are quite a few fascinating words here to which, you've noticed that I've included their meanings for you, just in case someone isn't quite familiar with them or may be experiencing something of that nature but aren't quite sure what it is they are experiencing.

Like <u>Anxiety</u> for example is the subjectively unpleasant feelings of dread over anticipated events, such as the feeling of imminent danger or even death.

Anxiety is not the same as fear, which is a response to a real or perceived immediate threat, whereas anxiety is the 'expectation' of a future threat.

And we all know that 'fear' is false evidences appearing real… Ya, well… you grow up in a monster's lair and tell me if there is anything about false evidence seeming to be real or menacing to you, let alone appearing to be real.

Anxiety is a feeling of uneasiness and worry, usually generalized and unfocused as an overreaction [**overreaction? not bloody likely**] to a situation that is only subjectively [**nothing 'subjective' about it**] seen as menacing. **But whatever would I have to be anxious about? I've been diagnosed with having an anxiety disorder, but hey, who isn't anxious 24/7/365 about something or other these days? When is something going to happen already? Let's get this over with. Why am I not hearing from them? I just know that they're going to reject me too, so, why did I even bother applying? Am I in trouble for something? What kind of mood is he going to be in when I get home? Did I or did I not do something that I was supposed too or wasn't supposed too have done?**

sometimes leading to panic attacks, **I've only experienced this a few times that I can recall. Each time I've had slightly different symptoms but this one was really cool… I had a heaviness deep within my chest that made it almost impossible to breath and** it felt as though my heart was about to explode and my oxygen levels were so low that I passed out. Awesome! You really must try having a panic attack sometime, they're terrific!

This might help: 12 Signs of An Anxiety Attack And 6 Effective Ways to Cope with It.

https://www.calmer-you.com/12-signs-of-an-anxiety-attack-and-6-effective-ways-to-cope-with-it/

+ muscle and joint pain

Yup, sometimes I find muscles I didn't know I had without having just exercised and Tylenol, Alieve or Advil won't relieve the discomfort. I had knee pain today, I've never had pain in my knees unless I've banged them and I don't recall bumping into anything as of late.

constipation or other intestinal problems

Generally, it's the reverse situation on a regular basis. Sometimes I wonder if I have IBS as well. But then, I'm beginning to sound like my mother who I swear, had every 'unseen' ailment known to man.

+ frequent headaches

Does wanting to purchase stock options in Tylenol count? Tylenol should be covered on my medical plan but it is not. I generally just tough them out because they really are not that painful nor do they last all day.

+ lack of interest in sex

This is my favorite one! LOL!... for me, it's always been the opposite. Maybe there's something in my drinking water, or in my blood or something I'm not aware of. I can never seem to get enough no matter what cycle I find myself to be in. Sex when on a high, gets me higher. Sex when down, helps to bring me up [usually, okay… only sometimes, but sex is always good for what ever ails me]. It's also the feeling of being loved, wanted and/or appreciated by my lady. Being intimate generally helps to say; "It's Alive!", why would I, or anyone for that matter, have a lack of interest in something so wonderful as sex?

"It's alive", is a phrase used in the film Frankenstein (1931) made by Universal Pictures.

As of late however, I am finding myself having difficulties at not being able to climax. Oh dear, what is this all about and what can I do about it? I have the desire to be intimate, I'm excited to be participating in the act of intimacy, but sometimes for some unknown reason I'm unable to ejaculate, or it takes so long that I generally give up. Has anyone else experience this? If you have… apparently, it's quite normal and here is what I've found on the Mayo Clinic website…

https://www.mayoclinic.org/diseases-conditions/delayed-ejaculation/symptoms-causes/syc-20371358

Delayed ejaculation can result from medications, certain chronic health conditions and surgeries. Or it might be caused by substance misuse or a mental health concern, [that explains it right there] such as depression, anxiety or stress. In many cases, it is due to a combination of physical and psychological concerns.

So, does being 'batshit' have anything to do with it? Apparently so. It's frustrating as hell and needless to say, not at all satisfying.

recurring thoughts of suicide or self-harm

"Play it again Sam…" Is my record scratched? Yes, Record! I grew up in the age of vinyl, which is making a comeback by the way. More often than not, it would be all day and every day for a week or more. I often go as far as planning out how to take my life but found out many times that it really isn't up to me, even though I may think that it is. Just last night I thought about just stepping into the campfire and envisioned myself being immediately incinerated… but then, we all know that a campfire isn't hot enough to do that so, so I stayed on the outside looking in. Being <u>tormented</u> yet again. Just wanting the flames to leap out and engulf me.

Bar-b-que Wayne, anyone? No thanks, I've already eaten. I was so frustrated that night, that I just went off to bed at 1820hrs, now that's really early, especially for me.

"Play It Again Sam", said by Humphrey Bogart in Casablanca, 1942.

<u>Tormented</u>: causing/experiencing great mental anguish.

+   <u>withdrawal from friends and family</u>

Friends; we've already discussed this and I have more acquaintances than I do friends. To me, a friend it someone who has been there long term and would come no matter what time of day or night you would have need of them… hell, my own pastor didn't even come to my house when I called him and informed him that my son had just been killed… is that a friend? Not to me it isn't. A <u>friend</u> would also be someone who I could/would share my most 'intimate secrets' with… I don't know anyone in my life that I could/would trust to that extend so, I would venture to say that I do not have friends by its definition. I suppose I have trust issues too, but when you read about my childhood, you'll know why. In the world, I've heard it said something like this… a friend is someone who you could call to come bail you out of jail should you have done something stupid… a 'true friend', or buddy, would be right there in the cell with you.

Family can sometimes be over-rated as well, especially when they rarely contact me, or ignore me on both face-book and messenger. And no, I don't tweet… I don't even know what that is except for another social media site. Big deal, how many of these does mankind require? What about just wanting to walk away from everyone/everything/most of the time while I'm in the midst of an Eeyore Complex? Not really caring if I ever see them or anyone for that matter? I often wonder what it would be like to be a hermit in the woods somewhere. A cabin by a lake sounds nice right about now and I'd hang a sign that reads... Gone Fishing! I'm not really a fisherman, but I could become one, I suppose.

Friend: a person whom one knows and with whom one has a bond of mutual affection, typically exclusive of sexual or family relations.

Friendship: is a relationship of mutual affection between people. Friendship is a stronger form of interpersonal bond than an association. A deep friendship can last through many shifts and changes in life, as long as you write or call every now and then. When you're in a relationship, you're emotionally involved or at least connected in some way.

Nope, don't have that... No one I know of fits the bill. Why, because I don't/can't trust anyone to that level to form a bond of that nature with them, that's why. I had them once upon a time, but one abandoned me and the other two have died off without having been replaced. Well okay, I said that my wife is my 'friend' but there are somethings a guy doesn't share with his wife because she wouldn't understand.

The aftermath of a manic episode can be devastating both for individuals and for families and loved ones. They may now be dealing with financial hardship,

Does my Mrs. calling up the credit card companies to decrease my line of credit count? So, why is it than when I reach my credit limit they let me go over it but of course charge me a fee for doing so? Or, they send me letters of notification that they'll gladly increase my limit if I contact them by such 'n' such a date. I don't get it. Oops! One time, I had three times the amount of credit accessible to me than what my income was in a year, and that didn't include my mortgage. That was scary! I called the credit card companies myself at that point and cancelled a couple of them. I knew I couldn't trust myself.

the health and relational effects of risky sexual practices or the physical consequences of substance abuse

There have been many times that I have woken up not knowing who was sleeping next to me, or how it was that I got to be there in the first place, [how much did I have to drink anyway?] What do you mean you think I'm an alcoholic and should go to AA meetings? Yes, I'm taking another pain killer, and washing it down with my Scotch, what's it to you? "But you just took one two hrs ago". "I did?" "oh, well, I'm still taking another one and there isn't anything you can say or do about it. So, if you don't mind… mind your own business and I'll mind mine." And that's how I got addicted to pain killers.

or personal injury accidents I wonder if having the hospital on speed dial would mean anything? That is if we had cell phones back then that is. How many countless numbers of tetanus shots did I receive as a kid? How about spending 14 hours in a neck collar while waiting for x-rays and CT Scans, etc., because I threw myself down a flight of cement stairs? Stories later. Or assaults I've never assaulted anyone in my life who didn't have it coming to them that is, well, okay, there was that one guy in Bermuda but I was paid to do it. I only opened my car door on that cyclist because he flipped me the bird for beeping my horn at him after he cut me off when he jumped the curb without looking and flew into traffic and I hit the brakes to save his sorry ass. So, I didn't feel sorry in the least for putting him on his ass. Want to be a dick? Two can play that game. I've only put one guy in the hospital [that I know of], but no one has been laid to rest yet on account of me that may have occurred during mania.

The depressive phase can [I like their optimism] involve the risk of suicide. Nah, attempting it multiple times throughout my life has no risk factor to it at all! Bipolar disorder is a serious illness so then tell me something… if it's such a 'serious illness'; how is it that these 'so called experts' have missed all of my warning signs and symptoms all of these years? One person has attempted to offer the possibility that they may have thought that the bipolar disorder wasn't my problem, or that it may have been 'masked' by symptoms of one or more other 'similar' disorders... ya, you think? Wait, one or more? Just how many do you think I have? We'll find out later.

but with treatment, people can recover and lead fulfilling lives. I'd like to experience that. Now, who did you say that it was I needed to talk too to make that happen? Why do I ask? Because NO ONE IS LISTENING TO ME! That's why.

None of these things has Ever, and I repeat EVER happened to me. "Sure Roy?" [inside joke] If someone were to take the time and actually listen, yes... L-I-S-T-E-N to me long enough for a full history in order to make proper diagnosis, I might have received the proper treatment that I have been practically begging for all of my life!

Listen: to give one's attention to a sound! That sound would be my voice telling them what my life had been like. Synonyms: hear, pay attention, be attentive, attend, concentrate on, concentrate on hearing, give ear to, lend an ear to, hang on someone's words, keep one's ears open, prick up one's ears, be all ears, pin back one's ears, get a load of, tune in, hark, hearken too. So, what was their problem?

Oh, but wait, I have to remember... I've only been diagnosed with having Clinical Depression, at this point which might account for the suicidal thoughts and multiple attempts, which really are only a cry for attention after all. WOLF! Wolf! Where wolf? There wolf! Nah, just kidding....

Clinical Depression: ranges in seriousness from mild, temporary episodes of sadness to severe, persistent depression. Clinical depression is the more-severe form of depression, also known as major depression or major depressive disorder. It isn't the same as depression caused by a loss, such as the death of a loved one, or a medical condition, such as a thyroid disorder... but it is a major factor in... oh, let me guess... bipolar disorder! No! It can't be?

https://www.mayoclinic.org/diseases-conditions/depression/expert-answers/clinical-depression/faq-20057770

They've also hit me with 'ODD' <u>Oppositional Defiant Disorder</u>... Ya think? There's a good one for you. Google that too sometime, it's hilarious, really! Do you know any kids like that? I do, besides me that is and watching this kid in action was like a demonstration of myself but without the swearing and the name calling. Perhaps that would have been the ticket... curse at the old bat and he would have killed me for sure. May-be I'm not so smart after all?

<u>Oppositional Defiant Disorder</u>: Even the best-behaved children can be difficult and challenging at times. But if your child or teenager has a frequent and persistent pattern of <u>anger,</u> [**nope**] <u>irritability,</u> [**nope**] <u>arguing,</u> [**nope**] <u>defiance</u> [**nope, not that one either**] or <u>vindictiveness toward you</u> [**oh, come on**] and other authority figures, he or she may have oppositional defiant disorder (ODD). **And if you believe all those 'nope's' gold is going for a mere $100.00 an ounce, better get some quick. You don't say? You win a cookie... make mine a Ginger Snap please. Here's the web address to save you the trouble**

https://www.mayoclinic.org/diseases-conditions/oppositional-defiant-disorder/symptoms-causes/syc-20375831

And <u>PTSD</u> is manageable with low doses of Cymbalta and Abilify... WRONG! Someone even suggested acquiring a service dog, Hmm? Right, and who's going to pay for that? I looked into it just because I like searching the web so much and the fact that I can't sleep so I have a lot of time on my hands. I found out that a fully trained and qualified service dog here in Canada could cost as much as $8,000.00... I think I have that just laying around here somewhere, if I could only remember where I put it. Hmmm? Nope, not under the mattress. Come out, come out where ever you are. R-i-g-h-t! and how am I going to do that? My PTSD was aggravated by, but wasn't attributed to military service so, no one will help with that.

<u>Post-traumatic stress disorder</u> (PTSD) is a mental health condition that's triggered by a terrifying event [**how about a continuous series of 'terrifying' events?**] — either experiencing it or witnessing it [**yup, been there too**]. Symptoms may include flashbacks, nightmares and severe anxiety, as well as uncontrollable thoughts about the event. Most

people who go through traumatic events may have temporary difficulty adjusting and coping, but with time and good self-care, they usually get better [**bullshit!**]. If the symptoms get worse, last for months or even years, and interfere with your day-to-day functioning, you may have PTSD.

Now why on earth would I have PTSD… I've never been in a war zone, or, have I? I'll never tell.

https://www.mayoclinic.org/diseases-conditions/post-traumatic-stress-disorder/symptoms-causes/syc-20355967

I've also been diagnosed as having <u>mood and anxiety disorders</u> which may also calm down with the Cymbalta and Abilify… a little, but not enough to really make a difference, so I told them, but they weren't listening because my B-type personality traits were 'muted' as far as they could see. Oh, but that's because they had me on a couple of more drugs, which they discontinued by the way when the B-type personalities were 'muted'… oh, and if you looked up Cymbalta and Ability, they actually aggravated the symptoms of Bipolar Disorder… so ya, thanks again. Just for the hell of it, while I was on the Mayo Clinic website… in the search bar I typed 'mood disorders with anxiety disorder' and, you'll never guess what the first 'disorder' was on their hit parade that magically 'popped up'… damn, your good! Yes, you guessed it… 'bipolar disorder!' They've missed it over and over and over again! "Ah, damn you! God damn you all to hell!" Taylor on Planet of the Apes 1968, staring Charlton Heston, a must see really if you enjoy classic sci-fi.

If you have a **mood disorder**, your general emotional state or mood is distorted or inconsistent with your circumstances and interferes with your ability to function. You may be extremely sad, empty or irritable (depressed), **like having the feeling of being so 'emotionally' drained that you have nothing left for anyone?** or you may have periods of depression alternating with being excessively happy (mania). Anxiety disorders can also affect your mood and often occur along with depression. Mood disorders may increase your risk of suicide. **Gee, you think?**

Some examples of mood disorders include:

- **Major depressive disorder** — prolonged and persistent periods of extreme sadness
- **Bipolar disorder** — also called manic depression or bipolar affective disorder, depression that includes alternating times of depression and mania

And they couldn't put 2 and 2 together? I know, I'm a broken record but there's more where that came from, I promise. But the anger issues will be cleared up after I take part in Anger Management Classes and utilize the tools they give to me. I've taken so many of those I could teach them myself without my notes and in my sleep, if I ever slept that is. The suicidal tendencies will disappear they said after I experience a Suicide Prevention Seminar and utilize the tools that they give me… but then I often forget that I even have a toolbox to utilize the tools they had put in there. Then I suffer from chronic <u>insomnia</u> [yup, typed that into the Mayo Clinic search bar as well… and you'll never guess what popped up 3rd on the hit parade? I'll give you three guesses and the first two don't count] from stress at work, or things aren't moving along fast enough, or the stress of not having work, or the stresses of family or just life in general. But, how's my caffeine or alcohol intake? Stop drinking alcohol and if you can't stop drinking coffee then at least cut back or drink decafe and your symptoms should go away in a week or two. Here, take these sleeping pills in the meantime. Well, I only have 2 caffeinated coffees in the morning and will have a couple of decafe coffees later on in the day… so now what? Take a sleeping pill that doesn't work? Oh, and forget taking anything like Actifed… I get so hyper on that stuff it isn't funny.

<u>**Interjection**</u>: 1134-17-07-2018; you know… the more I do **MY** research the madder I become… in fact, I'm **<u>as mad as a hatter</u>**… again, damn them!

<u>Insomnia</u>: is a common sleep disorder that can make it hard to fall asleep, hard to stay asleep, or cause you to wake up too early and not be able to get back to sleep. You may still feel tired when you wake up. Insomnia

can sap not only your energy level and mood but also your health, work performance and quality of life.

How much sleep is enough varies from person to person, but most adults need seven to eight hours a night. At some point, many adults experience short-term (acute) insomnia, which lasts for days or weeks. It's usually the result of stress or a traumatic event. But some people have long-term (**chronic**) insomnia that lasts for a month or more [**how about, for years?**]. Insomnia may be the primary problem, or it may be associated with other medical conditions or medications.

You don't have to put up with sleepless nights. Simple changes in your daily habits can often help… **bullshit, again!**

Additional common causes of insomnia include:

+ Mental health disorders. Anxiety disorders, such as post-traumatic stress disorder, may disrupt your sleep. Awakening too early can be a sign of depression [**gee, what have I to be depressed about?**]. Insomnia often occurs with other mental health disorders as well. **There you go!**

I've also been hit with borderline personality disorder…

https://en.wikipedia.org/wiki/Type_A_and_Type_B_personality_theory

A personality disorder is a pattern of feelings and behaviors that seem appropriate and justified to the person experiencing them, even though these feelings and behaviors cause a great deal of problems in that person's life.

Borderline personality disorder (BPD) is a personality disorder that typically includes the following symptoms:

+ Inappropriate or extreme emotional reactions
+ Emotional reactions that are highly explosive
+ Highly impulsive behaviors

- A history of unstable relationships [**so, being bipolar, is apparently the least of my worries, it's just another one to add to the list. And I'm still walking around free? Ssssh! Don't tell them, they may come looking for me.**]

Intense mood swings, impulsive behaviors, and extreme reactions can make it difficult for people with borderline personality disorder to complete schooling, maintain stable jobs and have long-lasting, healthy relationships.

Who? Me? Go on with you! I quite high school, went back and finished with a grade average of 98%. I went to college, dropped out and went back to complete a different discipline. I started and quite Bible college not once but twice only to make a come back and complete a doctorate. Then there are the various jobs I've had over my lifetime not to mention being in and out of the Military. I really don't know how I managed to retire from there without being kicked out... oh, wait, I was kicked out, 'sort of' not once but twice... huh? I'll let you figure that one out.

https://www.psycom.net/depression.central.borderline.html

Give me a fucking break already! The problem is that no one has ever done the math...can they not add two plus two and with a little thinking outside of the box come up with a value of five? What's wrong with these people? Where did they go to school? They have to think 'outside' of the box! I thought that was what being an expert was all about, not knowing all of the answers but knowing where to get them. Well, apparently, they hadn't known where to get them either. Many of these people are supposed to have letters behind their names... which is supposed to mean something... so, here's a bunch of letters for you which 'they' have assigned to me... CD, ODD, AD, MD, PTSD, ST, CS, BPD, along with a couple of others... but not the Bipolar disorder. So, put them in your pipe and smoke it... Well I have a couple of titles before my name: Rev. Dr. and here are a few more letters for you behind my name: G.B.D., A.A.M., G. Th., B.A.R., M. Min., M.A.R., D. Min... Yes, that's right, those are the credentials which you'll find behind my name which have little to

do with either the medical or mental health professions. So, how is it that I can think outside of the box when the 'so-called experts' in their fields can not? I sound angry, don't I? Well, damn it, I AM! I've suffered needlessly for far too long.

"Mad as a hatter" is a colloquial English phrase used in conversation to suggest (lightheartedly) that a person is suffering from insanity. The etymology of the phrase is uncertain, with explanations both connected and unconnected to the trade of hat-making. The earliest known appearance of the phrase is in an 1829 issue of Blackwood's Edinburgh Magazine.

https://en.wikipedia.org/wiki/Mad_as_a_hatter

And yes, I also like Wikipedia... I think it's cool... back when I was in grade/high school I had to physically venture forth to the public library, find an Encyclopedia or three, to do my own research to finish projects... imagination that... I actually had to give up a Saturday afternoon or two to spend at a Library! Of all places. But I can assure you, there were times when a lot more went on than just reading books and doing research, or was it research of another nature?

If you think you or someone you know has bi-polar disorder it is **important** to get help from a mental health professional, [**seriously?**] most often a psychiatrist alone with a team of providers who have a variety of skills. Help involves a diagnosis - which can take some time while the mental health professional gets to know you or person you are concerned about and their symptoms. Next, psychiatric medication will be prescribed. Again, it may take time to get the right one at the right dosage level. You or the person you are concerned about will also learn that people with bipolar disorder do best with a combination of medication and personal therapy - which may extend to family therapy. Peer support and self-help are invaluable as nothing can substitute for the message that "**you are not alone!**"

I'm not? Then, could someone please tell me why that it is I feel so alone?

Check out the last few pages... apparently, we are not as alone as I feel! But then I only know of or about some of these people and I am not personally acquainted with any of them... so, I may as well be alone! Oh, I just remembered a long-lost friend who suffered with the same disorder that cost her, her marriage, but I haven't spoken with her in couple of years... interesting. I'd like to have a chat with her now actually.

Living with bipolar illness is not easy but full recovery is possible. **That's the second time they've said that. Ya, Right! Here's your sign, have a nice day, don't let the door hit your ass on your way out.** The first step is taking personal responsibility for your own health.

Been there, tried that, can design the t-shirt only to end up in the mental ward without the immediate help I went looking for in the first place. [Gee, how many times have I been a short-term guest at a mental ward in a hospital somewhere?] Only this time, once the 'suicide' crisis was over, they were going to keep me longer against my will, but I wanted no part of it because I wasn't getting the assistance that I thought I should be. Well, what did I expect? Oh, speaking of designer t-shirts, my sister-in-law told me about a t-shirt she saw... you're going to love this... "I hate being bipolar, It's awesome!" I have to get myself one of those. Okay, that was interesting. I just tried Amazon.ca and for some reason they can't ship the product to my address... again, another 'not deliverable' because I have a Canadian address? Go figure. It's a T-Shirt for Pete's sake. I've just recently decided to and have made an appointment to get a tattoo... which will be my first tattoo and I'm almost 60. I always said that I would get one when and if I felt the need or that the time was right. I guess that need and that time is now. It's a universal symbol for bipolar disorder... it has two eyes, a smile and two eyes... depending upon how one views it, it is either smiling or frowning, but yet both at the same time. :): which is what living with bipolar disorder is all about. I know it's supposed to be green, but I happen to like blue, so it's blue.

Some Statistics: **Oh yes, give them to me, I love Statistics...**

- 1% of Canadians aged 15 years and over reported symptoms that met the criteria for a bipolar disorder in the previous 12 months.

  But why only starting at age 15? Do they think that children are unable to articulate their feelings? If the answer is yes, well, then might I suggest that they put their education to some use and help a poor kid out and properly take care of him/her. Check out my story about the how's and why's I first tried to kill myself and tell me that a kid doesn't know shit. But, it doesn't matter anyway… No one listened to me then and no one is listening now!

- About 1 in 50 adults aged 25-44 years [**didn't listen then either, Q-Tip anyone?**] or 45-64 [**only now are they started to open their ears, story later. Perhaps they've finally invested in some hearing aides?**] years reported symptoms consistent with bipolar disorder at some point in their lifetime. **At some point? How about at <u>every</u> point, at <u>all</u> points over the past 53 years? I can't remember if I've already told you this, but did you know that a point in every direction is the same as having no point at all? That's over half a century people… time to wake up! Even Rip-VanWinkle didn't sleep that long.**

- The proportion of men and women who met the lifetime criteria for bipolar disorder decreased slightly with age. **So, what; now I'm getting too old to have the disorder? Let me know when it goes away will you, I want to see that happen. Oh, I know when that will be… when I'm dead, Ya, that'll work. I suppose my biggest problem with that is, the fact that I can arrange for that to happen.**

(2002 Mental Health and Wellbeing Survey, Statistics Canada)

- Nearly 9/10 Canadians who reported symptoms that met the 12-month criteria for bipolar disorder (86. 9%) reported that the condition interfered with their lives,

  No… come on… please do tell me why it would interfere with my life. Not being able to sleep, or when I do manage to slumber

not wanting to get out of bed, or being tired in class/work that I fall asleep during first the period, or not wanting to go to school/work at all for that matter so I don't. Or not wanting to be with family and friends or experiencing the opposite end where I lead the parade and I'm every clown in it, or I feel as though I'm in a race and the fact that I'm so far out front that I begin to wonder if I'm the only participant wouldn't have anything to do with interfering with my life? [Like the run-on sentence?] How about walking off of the job, moving again for no apparent reason, or going home with that red-head over yonder whose been looking at me? My actions don't affect other people's lives, they only affect the three of us that I'm aware of and that's the team of me, myself, and I. Team Wayne!

Go Team Wayne! See, I'm my own cheerleading squad as well.

(2002 Mental Health and Wellbeing Survey, Statistics Canada)

- While most people [I've already thought we've established the fact that I, am not 'most' people!] with bi-polar disorder (or depression) will not commit suicide, [he, he, he, okay, they do have a point, I haven't actually 'committed' suicide as of yet because I'm still alive, at least for now. But I could keep trying to end it all, if that will make them happy] the risk of suicide among those with bipolar disorder is higher than in the general population. You don't say? Does attempting suicide at least a dozen times count, or has it been more? Wouldn't happen. No, I've already established the fact that it's just an attention seeking maneuver. A Wolf crying experience… if you will.

Move along folks, go about your business, everything is fine here, nothing more to see, move along, that's it, have a nice day! Thanks for dropping by.

More information on bi-polar disorder can be found in the Public Health Agency Report: "The Human Face of Mental Health and Mental Illness in Canada 2006".

◆ <u>Mood Disorders Society of Canada</u>

Okay, I've checked out this website and it's pretty good, or you could just Google: 'Bipolar Disorder' and wade through all the wonderful information on the internet. That is if you're not too depressed already, you might be after wandering through 12,800,000 websites. I have noticed a fair bit of repetition though. Go for it, I dare you! Happy Hunting!

Here, let me save you some time and trouble: <u>The Mayo Clinic</u> is one of the better websites that I've uncovered after checking out quite a few [perhaps a hundred or so actually] I must say.

The Mayo Clinic: Bipolar Disorder; https://www.mayoclinic.org/diseases-conditions/bipolar-disorder/symptoms-causes/syc-20355955

Here is what some American experts have to say… it too is quite fascinating, crack a beer, put some cheese and Nachos into the microwave or open a bag of Doritos, or perhaps you would prefer to pop some corn and continue reading… either way, this gets good. Warning: There is some repetition, but that's okay too, because I'm use it. More wine anyone? Make mine a double Scotch with one ice cube please! Have you ever noticed that 99% of the waitresses will put ice in your drink even though you have specifically said "No Ice"! I know they're use to it and do it automatically, but they're there to take my order and I ordered my drink without ice for a specific reason… Damn. Some times I'll order water and forget to say "no ice" because I automatically assume that if I don't want ice in my soda, I'm not going to want it in my water… damn… here's my sign! I generally don't make a big deal of it and ask for an empty glass or if there's a coffee cup on the table I'll spoon the ice out into that.

<u>8 Questions</u> Therapists Ask to Diagnose Bipolar Disorder; Women's Health, 4 July 2017… Wait! Hold your horses… What? If there are only eight bloody Questions, how come no one had the forethought to ask them of me? I can answer 8-?'s with my eyes closed.

"Oh, Oh, Mr. Kotter, Mr. Kotter!" pick me, pick me! Rats, the cute blonde kid in the front row again, what does she know?

[Check out… Welcome Back Kotter sitcom, it's funny]

By Elizabeth Bacharach;

www.womenshealthsa.co.za/health/questions-diagnose-bipolar-disorder/

Up to <u>69 %</u> of patients with bipolar disorder are initially <u>mis</u>diagnosed.

69%, that's pretty high, don't you think? But did you catch that? <u>MISDIAGNOSED</u>! NO KIDDING? Here's your sign! Oh, in case you are not familiar with this saying… "here's your sign" it's referring to your mental incapacitation, which means that you are not mentally functioning in a normal way and people consider you to be stupid! Have a nice day!

Perhaps as having clinical depression, [you don't say?] or some other sort of side dish of a mood disorder or two, tossed in with perhaps… anxiety, anger issues, spending sprees, maniac episodes and a dressing of suicidal tendencies, with croutons of insomnia, but you won't find that to be a recipe for a Bipolar Salad in any of our psychological cook books. Or, just because I was in the military there is always the latest and greatest since mom's apple pie: [instead of ice cream, I'll have cheddar cheese please] I have PTSD! Okay so what of it? You're not really treating that either. The shrink finally deemed that I came in to the military with PTSD and I've been carrying it from childhood and therefore it wasn't caused by my being on tour or anything [I told him as much] but it was aggravated by military service… but how do we prove it? So, that doesn't count and Veteran's Affair won't pay out a dime… nor should they as far as I was concerned but I was coerced into applying anyway. [What was aggravated by military service was the Bipolar disorder which was never diagnosed]. Okay, I have PTSD as well but, after having grown up in hell with an evil overlord, who wouldn't? But the thing is, I wasn't nor am now, receiving counseling for that either. I've recently been made aware of the fact that the 'experts' are beginning to understand the affects on adults who have grown up in an abusive environment 'may' [and again I like their optimism here, I'll take mental disorders for $1,000, Alex] also have PTSD? You guys may interview me anytime you like, for a fee of course and I'll tell you everything you don't want to know about the horrors I went through to be awarded with such a prestigious title. Hell, you guys are 40 years behind me as far as I'm concerned, what's the matter with you? What I'm pissed about is the fact that no one arrested the bastard back in the 1960's when all of this was happening to me. Keep reading this gets even better than really good. Popcorn, peanuts, get your red hots!

Post Traumatic Stress Disorder (PTSD) is a mental disorder that can develop after a person is exposed to a traumatic event, [how about 17 years of continuously being exposed to one traumatic event after the other. And, if I wasn't the main event, I witnessed plenty more] such as sexual assault, [or being constantly sexually abused] warfare, [witnessing mom or my sibling getting the crap beat out of them only to discover that I was next wouldn't count as 'warfare'] traffic collisions, [does my face coming into contact with a gigantic fist or the refrigerator door or the nearest wall count as a collision?] or other threats on a person's life [I'm sure that would include severe beatings where I was beat so bad that I was hospitalized].

Symptoms may [we have to teach these guys to expand their vocabulary] include disturbing thoughts, feelings, or dreams related to the events [I didn't dream much as a kid because I didn't sleep much then either], mental or physical distress to trauma-related cues, attempts to avoid trauma-related cues, alterations in how a person thinks and feels, and an increase in the fight-or-flight response. These symptoms last for more than a month after the event [how about, for a lifetime?] Young children are less likely to show distress, [bullshit] but instead may express their memories through play. A person with PTSD is at a higher risk for suicide and intentional self-harm [please, do tell me more].

MAY: 1. (used to express possibility): It may rain.
2. (used to express opportunity or permission): You may enter.
3. (used to express contingency, especially in clauses indicating condition, concession, purpose, result, etc.): I may be wrong but I think you would be wise to go. Times may change but human nature stays the same.
4. (used to express wish or prayer): May you live to an old age.
5. Archaic (used to express ability or power.) **So, take your pick!**

Bipolar disorder is already confusing for those who suffer from it. The disease has **no** boundaries, affecting **all** spheres of a patient's life—home, work, social, and more. Its extreme shifts in moods can cause a patient to act <u>irrationally</u>, <u>react unpredictably</u>, <u>experience impaired judgment</u>, **and I don't have to be on any form of alcohol or chemical substance to experience any/all of these symptoms, but alcohol and other substances do add to the confusion and complicate things more and** at other times, feel so down that they can't get out of bed, **it did help though when I had a job where I couldn't hide in bed without facing dire consequences and I was required to at least report in, like being in the military for instance. I became an expert at reporting in and burying myself in my work. Sometimes I'd pull a disappearing act, so I wouldn't have to deal with other people when I knew I wasn't in an agreeable mood, was depressed or highly irritable. Overall, it managed to work out in the long run but it would appear that for every other accolade, I received a reprimand... I suppose you could say, they almost balanced out. When I was farming though, there were many days when I'd drag my sorry ass out of bed, do my chores [which were the bare minimum] go back to bed for several hours before starting the work day only to knock of early and go back to bed** reports the National Alliance on Mental Illness (NAMI). **Hey, were they spying on me? During my trucking years, it hadn't mattered if I was maniac or depressed, I'd jump in that truck and go because I would be anywhere but 'here', wherever that was and being on the move was always fine by me.**

Approximately 5.7 million adult Americans are affected by bipolar disorder every year, **you don't say? I wonder how many are walking around without a proper diagnosis… like myself for instance… oh, but wait, I'm not an American… silly me, sorry, I guess I still don't count** according to the National Institute of Mental Health (NIMH). And while the mental illness is equally common in women and men, research from the Journal of Clinical Psychiatry shows that about three times as many women as men experience four or more mood episodes of bipolar disorder in a year. A study from Psychiatry (Edgmont) shows that 69 % of patients with bipolar disorder are initially <u>misdiagnosed</u>, **haven't we seen this before? Why, Yes, yes, we have! So, if they know this for a fact, why is this 'misdiagnoses' still happening?** frequently because patients seek treatment when they're having a depressive episode. So, the challenge for health-care providers is to try to rule out whether the depression is a case of bipolar disorder or of actual clinical depression. **Again, knowing this, why wouldn't they ask the 8 questions? Why wouldn't they go over a patient's life history? Why didn't they ask ME all the right questions and check out MY personal history? Better yet, they could have asked a family member about MY behaviour over the past couple of years or decades or whatever. Damn them again. I told you… there are repeats! I like repeats. I don't know about you but the more I watch a rerun that has already been re-ran, the more I tend to learn from it.**

Dr Claudia Baldassano, director of the Bipolar Disorder Clinic at University of Pennsylvania Medical School, says the ultimate goal is to discern whether a patient has had a period of time where they've felt what Baldassano calls "**too good**," which is a sign of a manic high that involves being so emotionally elevated that the patient's movement, speech, and activity is loaded with energy and confidence (or lack of awareness). This intense mood (or mania) maniac phase is more like it. A maniac is defined as a person exhibiting extreme symptoms of wild behaviour, especially when violent and dangerous is the complete opposite of depression, and often acts as a cue for therapists that the patient might have bipolar disorder.

Here are the questions doctors typically ask to accurately diagnose bipolar disorder: First off, they never asked and second off; what's my prize if I win? So, here we go...

1. Have you ever felt that your mood was elevated or "**too good**" for a series of consecutive days?

YES!

Consecutive days? How about consecutive weeks or perhaps lasting into consecutive months? OMG, I've bounced off of so many walls that I can't keep track. Like being so happy or giddy that I can barely contain myself so much so that I feel like Scrooge who was so <u>giddy</u> near the end of '<u>A Christmas Carol</u>' when he realizes that the Spirits had transformed him in one night... and I just have to do something about it or I'll burst? Let's get this party started... never mind, I'll do it myself. Or, better yet, I am the party so what have I need of you?

To the point where there is no point in going to bed because I won't sleep anyway even though I haven't slept in 2 days as it is. This question has never been asked, but I had offered some information even before I knew what Bipolar or Manic-Depressive disorder was.

<u>A Christmas Carol</u> in Prose, being a Ghost-Story of Christmas, commonly known as A Christmas Carol, is a novella by Charles Dickens, first published in London by Chapman & Hall in 1843; the first edition was illustrated by John Leech. A Christmas Carol tells the story of Ebenezer Scrooge, an old miser who is visited by the ghost of his former business partner Jacob Marley and the Ghosts of Christmas Past, Present and Yet to Come. After their visits Scrooge is transformed into a kinder, gentler man.

https://en.wikipedia.org/wiki/A_Christmas_Carol

<u>Giddy</u>: adjective; having a sensation of whirling and a tendency to fall or stagger; dizzy.

If a patient's answer to this initial question points toward periods of mania or hypomania rather than just feeling good, therapists will proceed by asking questions that draw on manic or hypomanic symptoms of bipolar disorder, such as decreased need for sleep without feeling fatigue, increased optimism and self-confidence, reckless behaviour, and more.

2. During that period, did you find that you were sleeping less than normal but didn't feel tired or necessarily affected?

YES! What is sleep? [as previously discussed]

I would regularly function on 3 or 4 hours of sleep a day and feel as though I've had 8 or 10 hours and can continue throughout the day without feeling tired. Sometimes those periods can last for a couple of weeks before I finally crash from sleep deprivation. Even at that point, one never really catches up on loss sleep and I'll get less than 4 hours straight before waking up and I'm raring to go again. [As I'm reviewing this, I'm going on 30 hours without sleeping and I'm still feeling fine. I'm sure I can go all day and then some… I feel another marathon coming on actually]. So, if they hadn't asked question # 1, they wouldn't have known to proceed with question #2.

That's it, thanks for playing, pull their license to practice, it's game over!

Who's on first? What are you asking me for?

Here's a U-tube video of 'Who's on first?' skit by Abbott and Costello, 1953…

https://www.youtube.com/watch?v=kTcRRaXV-fg

Wait, I'm not really a baseball fan, but isn't it three strikes and the batter's out?

Oh, right… so I'll give them one more chance, but just one mind you. Okay? Okay! Let's Play Ball!

If a patient isn't sleeping or is sleeping fewer hours than usual yet feels refreshed or energized, it might be a sign that they're bipolar, says Dr Elizabeth Cohen, cognitive behavioural therapist. Changes in sleep patterns overall can be a very important signal that an episode may be starting, **what do they mean by an 'episode?' A maniac phase once again? Oh, this is encouraging, I may be on the upswing? Play it again Sam… and, Lookout world because here I come once more** says Dr Hilary P. Blumberg, director of the Mood Disorders Research Program at Yale School of Medicine. So, it's also <u>imperative</u> [**did you catch that?**] that medical providers ask this question [**but they didn't ask, even though I had offered some information to que these morons**] so they can better track if any persistent sleep abnormalities eventually lead to a switch in mood elevation or from a depressive to a manic or hypomanic episode.

I wonder where sleep walking comes into play? Oh, Ya, right… I have to be able to sleep before I can walk in my sleep, what was I thinking?

3. During that 'good mood' period, did you ever have the sense that you had a lot of ideas and that your brain felt sped up?

YES!

Does overloading the company suggestion box count? Or perhaps having a good idea and the energy to implement it without the boss's approval factored in there anywhere? I've often been told that it is generally easier to ask for forgiveness than it is to acquire permission. But some supervisors don't see it that way and I get hit with a reprimand in my file. What about racing thoughts that prevent me from turning my brain off so that I can't stay at my desk long enough to type out the suggestions in the first place? I still liked my 'Nike' attitude towards life. Then there is the constantly rehearsing conversations in my head with various scenarios attempting to figure out which is the better route to take? But, when the actual encounter takes place, I just shoot off my mouth and <u>I don't care</u> if I offend the other person? Political correctness is highly over rated, don't you think? Tell it like it is… if I want sugar in my coffee I'll ask for sugar. No thanks, I'm already sweet enough so, piss off. When the hell did everyone get so damned

sensitive? Oh, you can't tell little Johnny that he lost the soccer match because it will hurt his self-esteem and damage his ego. So, what do they do? They don't keep score because it's in how you play the game that really matters. Well really, shouldn't it be both?

Coach: "So, Johnny, did you give it 100% out there today?"

J: "Nah coach, I'm a bit off of my game today"

Coach: "Is there anything I can help you with?"

J: "No, I'll work it out."

Coach: "okay, we'll see you at practice in a couple of day, perhaps we'll get them next game... good job!"

That's all there is too it... You lost the game today for one of three reasons... you either haven't been practicing enough to hone your skills, you didn't give it your 100%. Whoever came up with this 110% bullshit? I'm not sorry, but you can't give 110% of anything because it just doesn't exist, that's why. 100% is all that there is there are only 4 parts to a whole $4 \times \frac{1}{4} = 1$ whole where did you ever go to school? Or, the other team was just better than you... we take losses in life, it's a normal fact of life and kids need to learn that concept, but they also need to learn how to deal with the losses when they come... just like Johnny can't have that ice cream sandwich half an hour before dinner... just facts of life, why protect them from it? Mind you, they also forgot about the sudden mood changes, the irritability, anger and anxiety issues which then obviously leads them to miss asking question #3 as well.

Okay, that's strike 3, are they out yet?

Yes, they are... I got them this time... go directly to jail, do not pass go, do not collect $200.00.

Next? Somebody take away the dice, they're just messing up people's life with their constant crap shoot.

By asking this question, therapists are trying to determine if a patient has another symptom of bipolar disorder: racing thoughts. But since racing thoughts can be attributed to anxiety and OCD, Baldassano says she avoids using that terminology. When in a manic or hypomanic state, patients with bipolar disorder will commonly feel that it's hard to keep up with all the thoughts that are continuing on loop in their mind and, especially in a manic state, are completely unaware that it's happening. "Some people with hypomania do not have racing thoughts," Baldassano explains. "Their thoughts are really deep, crisp, and clear. So, it's important to ask that as well to capture the milder cases."

Huh, OCD? I never thought that would be attributed to bipolar disorder. I always thought it was because the head creep ran a tight ship and everything had to be just that: 'ship-shape' to pass his inspections. There was a place for everything and everything better be in its place unless you were using it. If he went to retrieve something and you weren't using it at that particular moment... all hell broke loose believe me. But having my shirts organized by casual, semi-formal and formal wear is normal, right? But what about placing all of my short-sleeved shirts together and all of my long-sleeve shirts together and colour coordinating them as well... surely every man on this planet does that? I'm sure the ladies will agree that a closet has to be organized. I don't have the tendency to check things multiple times but I do exhibit other traits.

Crisp clear thoughts? No, can't say that I've experienced that sensation especially when I'm deep in my research because I'll have 6 – 8 books open along with multiple websites and be darting back and forth to find something or to gather information. So, nope, no hypomania here, you're barking up the wrong tree.

4. Do you feel more talkative?

YES!

I've been informed and sometime reminded that I'm also repetitive or people tend to walk away because they can't get a word in edgewise. Or they just can't follow the conversation and have nothing to contribute,

so I may as well be talking to myself, which also happens on many occasions. Psst, don't talk to Wayne today, he's a babbling idiot but I'm not aware of it and they tell me later. But because people have made me aware of this, as difficult as it is, I will often gather with folks now and have little to say.

During a manic episode, a bipolar patient might also talk very quickly and jump from one idea to another—symptoms that are frequently found in those with anxiety as well. **I'm not known for talking fast, no.** So, to figure out if this "pressured speech," in Cohen's words, is truly related to bipolar disorder, therapists might ask themselves similar questions such as, "Is it hard to follow what they're saying?" **often, yes** or "Does it feel like they're talking a mile a minute?" **no** Cohen explains. Another key sign of bipolar disorder is a lack of insight, meaning when in a manic episode the patient doesn't usually realize that they're acting, speaking, or thinking differently. For example, anxious patients might say something like "Wow I'm really all over the place," while those with bipolar disorder likely won't have this moment of insight and will continue talking quickly as if it's the norm. **But then again; they never asked this question either.**

How am I doing so far? 4/4 = 100%? Cool! I always knew that I was an 'A+' student under the right conditions.

5. Have you taken on more projects than usual, such as at work?

You mean I've always had the option of just saying NO? In whose universe?

More often than not I become a workaholic, leaving co-workers in the dust and wonder why it is that they can't produce as much as myself with the same minimal margin of error factored in and I'll be in trouble for making them look bad... Yes, I'm serious. I've even had my office keys taken away for awhile because I was coming in too early and staying too late as far as the supervisor was concerned.

When having a manic episode, patients with bipolar disorder tend to have an "increase in goal-directed activity," Baldassano says. That's why therapists will ask patients about their recent workload. The clinician then has to parse out details such as negative feedback the patient says they're receiving from their boss or a comment that indicates they're being unproductive to figure out if their increased workload is, in fact, a symptom of bipolar disorder, Blumberg explains. If a patient's answer indicates that they're taking on more projects, and suffering from it without recognising they're having problems, these could be signs that they're bipolar.

I have also experienced the flip side of the coin… hey boss, here's that project you wanted… what do you mean I've missed the deadline… you said it was due Thursday, it's only Tuesday… oh, you meant last Thursday, My bad! They missed the boat on asking this one as well. Here's your sign! How many does that make now?

6. Have you done things that you would consider risky?

I wouldn't consider them risky, but others might think they are/ were even out right crazy and/or dangerous. Like starting an on-line business and spending $28,000.00 without batting an eye because the man said that I had to invest in myself in order to make money so I maxed out three credit cards.

You mean to tell me that four guys, four gals, who have rented a couple of hotel rooms for the weekend isn't normal? How about later on, we end up walking our dates out to a taxi because one of the ladies drank too much, threw up, so now all four of them have to go home? What the hell? Oh, did I tell you I have a very fast eye for detail? Then the same four guys meet one girl in an elevator. But, the game's afoot dear Watson because more than one thing is out of place here… upon further viewing, I realize that she is bare foot, not wearing a bra and by all appearances no panties either, hmm? Suddenly, in the midst of our conversation she reaches into her clutch, pulls out a reefer and asks for a light while suggesting she has more where that one came from should we care to share. I obviously oblige with the light of course, we share, continue with more than a conversation right there in the elevator and I end up escorting her to my room. I've just hit a home run!

What about picking up a fellow sleeping on the side of the 400 Highway, just outside of Toronto at 2330hrs and I drive him all the way to North Bay to his sister's house [address written on the back of an envelope] only to find out that he's walked away from a Mental Hospital in Hamilton and they've been looking for him for the past three days. Well, they didn't look very hard now, did they? Nothing to it… just helping out right? More to this story later. Hey let me drive you back, they may want to speak with me awhile, even keep me for a month or two while I'm at it.

Because bipolar patients in a manic episode are more impulsive, [**I don't have an impulsive bone in my body, I plan everything out… to the finest detail "Sure Roy" (inside joke)**)] therapists ask about previous irresponsible behaviours to try to figure out if they're just acting out or if these rash actions are different from their normal behaviours. For example, manic patients—more so than hypomanic patients—might tend to drive recklessly, **230 kmph on a dark deserted highway such as the 403 in Ontario at O' dark stupid isn't reckless. What about shutting my lights off in the middle of a pine forest road just to see how dark it really is on that Yukon highway** make poor business decisions, [**never**] and even get involved in dangerous sexual encounters, Baldassano says. Cohen also notes these risky behaviours <u>can</u> [**I like this word**] include "any sort of excessive behaviour that can't be controlled," such as even shopping too much. [**I like that… "Can't" be controlled! So, there… it isn't my fault that both of wives have told me that I spend too much $$ on a regular basis, but I just can't see it**]

6/6

7. Have you felt smarter, more attractive, or more accomplished?

YES, yes and yes! Who hasn't?

Looking back though, I'd have to say; No, not at all, I'd never be so arrogant. Psst, I've told more than one boss that I could do their job better than him/her and have proven it. I've worked my way up from the bottom or the middle of the company to the top on more than one occasion for no other reason, than… "just because I could!" But, then

I would either sabotage myself or get bored altogether and I'd walk out again... Felt more attractive? What guy hasn't? Especially near closing time and I don't want to go home alone and I still think that I have a shot with that red-head over yonder who's been continuously looking at me. Perhaps it's time to ask her to dance and if she'll buy me a drink. One time it was proven and I didn't have to do anything.... I like it when that happens... a buddy of mine and I were eating dinner in this sports bar when he decides to hit on a pretty lady. Couldn't blame him, she was really cute... but, ha... ha, she blew him off and came over to me to rescue her from him, hmm? A gentleman doesn't kiss and tell, but needless to say we went out for about 6 months after that and if only wallpaper could talk... what stories would they tell?

More accomplished? I know, repeat... but it was Proven! I'm the only one out of 5 kids who quit high school only to go back a few years later, graduated [98%], then went onto College [95% average], then to Bible College/Seminary never mind earning a PhD [4.0 average] with aspirations of earning another doctorate for no other reason then... wait for it... BECAUSE I CAN! And, there you have it boys and girls. I do just about everything and anything for no other reason then, because I can! Who's the stupid Ass now? However, I must add that there is a tad more to this one, then 'just because I can'. Nothing to it, any 'stupid-ass' [explanation later] can accomplish that, right? Right! And I'd set out to prove it once more. As their mood becomes elevated, so does a patient's confidence, self-esteem, and optimism. For example, a manic patient might walk into their clinician's office and brag that things are working out at their job, they're feeling great, and—in an extreme case—they're ready to quit the job without any concrete plan in place, [now, why would I do that?] Baldassano says. Many clinicians, however, don't ask this question directly to the patient. Instead, they'll discern if the patient's feeling "grandiose" as a symptom of bipolar disorder through observation [I suppose they weren't very observant then, were they?]—especially since manic patients don't have the insight to realise, "Oh yeah, I'm feeling way more successful than I did last week" nope, don't recognize that, no, really, I don't but it had been pointed out to me on a couple of occasions. So, if they could recognize it, why hadn't they explored that avenue a little further?

8. What's your family history like?

I don't know my biological father so I can't tell you anything about that side of my family. Mom was a hypochondriac, so I have no idea what she was really diagnosed with and I can't ask her because she's no longer with us. My siblings don't really know either because I've asked. I don't know anything about my maternal grandparents except that my grandmother had dementia, and granddad drank himself to death, so that's a tough question for me to answer... I guess we'll have to rule this one out.

While currently there isn't a way to determine bipolar disorder through a test, family history can be very helpful, Blumberg says. In fact, bipolar disorder tends to run in families and children with a parent or sibling with the illness are more likely to develop it, according to the NIMH. Both Baldassano and Cohen emphasise the importance of involving family beyond just medical records to help diagnose a patient. Because bipolar patients experience such dramatic moods swings, during which they might not have great insight as to their experiences and feelings, family members can be better reporters of a patient's symptom.

I have concluded that by determining which mood I'm in by how I am 'feeling today' and by charting these feelings will indicate when my overall mood is about to change or is in the process of changing or remaining the same. Mood swings can come and go at the flick of the switch though and I don't know why. I can be fine one moment than extremely irritated or agitated the next, but there is generally a trigger of some sort... I don't just go off of the deep end for no apparent reason. Looking back over the past little while, I had recognized when I was coming down off of that maniac phase... I suppose that's where the journaling comes in. But I hate journaling, it's boring and I never keep up.

I happened to mention something to my wife, to which she'd reply "don't go getting depressed" by that time it may have already been too late and I am looking for something to reverse the situation but nothing is forth coming except the continuing downward spiral. Her telling me to 'not to get depressed' was of no value whatsoever, but thanks sweetheart. It's only a matter of how low I will go at that point and how long will I stay down.

Sometimes someone will look at me strangely or say something [perhaps not out of the ordinary to them] and I'm flying off the handle or storming out of the room [or the house] not wanting to deal with that crap or engage them any further because I've already said too much as it is. More often than not, my mouth doesn't have an off switch either. Does calling it as I see it mean anything?

So, now that we've asked and given a short response to the 8 questions, how did you score?

87.5% actually! [Couldn't answer the family history question].

BINGO! Oh, sorry, wrong game.

Rats! I go to the head of the class. I win! Hey, Eeyore, imagination that! No dunce cap for me this time.

What's my prize?

A trip down 'who gives a 'rat's ass lane' because no one is paying attention to me anyways!

Oh, rats, I was hoping it was something fun and exciting… like going home with that red-head because I don't have enough excitement in my life as it is…

"Rat's ass in ancient times", it says: "In ancient Greek times people would sacrifice rat's ass to the gods. If someone didn't sacrifice any rat's ass, then it was said they didn't care about the gods. So, when someone says 'I don't give a rat's ass' (I don't care), that's where it comes from."

Ha, ha, I'm sorry. Not really… That's just a joke answer, but if people are actually going to read this, I'll explain more seriously:

To not give a 'rat's ass' is a rude slang for not caring for/about (something or someone). Therefore; they don't attach any importance to someone/thing. According to 'The Free Dictionary'

https://idioms.thefreedictionary.com/not+give+a+rat%27s+ass

Rats! Not particularly scholarly, but the use of "Rats" as an exclamation came into popular use in the Fifties, with a good deal of help from Scultz's Charlie Brown cartoons… it was politer to say "rats!" than to use a curse word.

Is it time to face an untold truth?

Past due, I'd say. Now, if only I can get the right people to hear me out… does anyone know how to make that happen? I'm all ears, really, I am.

If you aren't sure, ask a family member to answer these questions for you. You may be surprised at their answers.

Ha, ha, ho, ho, he, he, he… that's rich

No, I wouldn't be, really, I wouldn't be surprised at their answers at all.

There really is No need, Okay, but only if you insist… here goes…

Alrighty then, that was fun… no, not really.

There was a mixture of acknowledgment, realization of truth mixed with laughter and a few 'I told you so' tossed in for good measure. Thank you, thank you very much!

Come back later and we'll play another game… which chamber is the bullet in?

Go ahead, pull the trigger, I just might get lucky this time.

What Is Bipolar Disorder and What Causes It?

[this aught to be intellectually stimulating because I don't have enough to stimulate me now as it is]

Bipolar disorder, sometimes called manic depression or manic-depressive illness, is a <u>brain disorder</u> **[a brain disorder? So, I am crazy after all, I knew it and kept trying to tell them. But they weren't listening]** that causes extreme shifts in mood, energy level and behavior. Everyone has ups and downs, but people with bipolar disorder have higher "highs" and lower "lows." **[you don't say? Like living life on a rollercoaster?]**

They may repeatedly go from feeling very energetic or extremely irritable to feeling crushing sadness and hopelessness **[and more often than not, for no apparent reason, I switch right back again].**

Bipolar disorder is a lifelong illness with <u>no cure,</u> **[that... that right there... is enough to put me into a depressive phase]** but it can be successfully treated. **[there is hope? Sure, Roy! Next, you'll be telling me that my wall does have a window]**

There are several types of bipolar disorder, **you don't say? On that the experts can agree** each defined by the severity and pattern of manic and depressive episodes. Recognition of bipolar disorder is critical since, left untreated, it can have significant negative impact on a person's life **like every aspect of my life for my entire life?** In addition, the treatment of bipolar disorder is different from that for the more common "unipolar" depression.

Sorry, you've got the wrong #, there's no 'uni' here.

Though the cause or causes of bipolar disorder have yet to be uncovered, scientists are working on identifying a genetic connection. New research is looking at genes that are thought to be linked to the development of bipolar disorder as well as schizophrenia.

Here's a <u>serious</u> question for <u>anyone</u> in the mental/medical health fields;

Can Bipolar Disorder eventually lead to schizophrenia or dementia?

Are they linked in anyway that you are aware of?

No, seriously, can it?

I'd really like to know if I'm in for more of a world of real hurt than I'm already in?

How Do I Know If I Have Bipolar Disorder?

I don't, because if I had it, I wouldn't know it. It's like being crazy... if I know that I'm crazy, but they [the experts] don't know that I am, therefore I am not because if I were, then I wouldn't know that I was, therefore I am not.

Got it? Good, because I have no idea what I just said.

I only know it now because I've looked up a bunch of my feelings, behaviours, attitudes, symptoms, and actions over the years. I then put them all together with my past diagnoses which led me to explore the possibility of being bipolar.

Which way do I go now George?

Then I discovered and answered the eight questions as per above and, wouldn't you know it, I won a cookie. Make mine a Gingersnap, please.

Therefore; by reasonable calculations, I have concluded that I do suffer from bipolar disorder... I have suffered from this disorder all of my life but no one has caught it. Hey, if it's catchy, stay away from me...

I don't have a PhD for nothing you know.

Yes, I've put the pieces of the puzzle together for my self and found that by adding 2+2, I've managed to come up with five because I discovered other things that I was experiencing but hadn't realized what they were until I conducted my own investigation. So, now I know what they don't know and if they don't know what it is that I know, how do I make them come to know?

That again, is the $1,000,000.00 question, isn't it?

An equal number of men and women develops bipolar disorder. Men tend to begin with a manic episode while women more often start with an episode of depression. [**what about children?**] The alternating episodes of mania and depression that define bipolar disorder can differ greatly from person to person.

They can last from a few hours to a few months and may occur several times a year or only rarely. The defining characteristic of bipolar disorder is the occurrence of mania or hypomania. Hypomania is similar to mania but the symptoms are less severe and less disabling. Some people have symptoms of mania and depression at the same time. **How can that be?** Doctors call this a mixed state **make mine a double, <u>shaken and not stirred</u> with two olives please, because I like olives better than a lemon peel.** In between manic and depressive episodes, people with bipolar disorder often feel well **you mean like I'm feeling now?** and have no symptoms of the illness **other than the fact that the Eeyore Complex has a hold of me** Often people do not recognize their bipolar disorder as an illness, and some go undiagnosed and without treatment for years. **And years, and years, and years, Gee, I wonder why? Some days are Diamonds, some days are Stone...** John Denver 1981.

"<u>Shaken, not stirred</u>." The very phrase conjures up images of Sean Connery, natty in his tuxedo, about to break the bank at baccarat before bedding the beautiful double agent, doesn't it? James Bond has probably created more martini drinkers than all the gin joints in the world. The reason the debonair Bond wants his martini shaken is that he is an iconoclast. He's not drinking a martini at all! He's drinking a vodka martini. There's a difference, as we shall see. Let's start by looking at Bond's drink. He takes vodka and gin in them. Ian Fleming gives a recipe for his Bond's preferred libation in the first Bond book, Casino Royale (1953), chapter 7:

"A dry martini," he said. "One. In a deep champagne goblet." "Oui, monsieur."

"Just a moment. Three measures of Gordon's, one of vodka, half a measure of Kina Lillet. Shake it very well until it's ice-cold, then add a large thin slice of lemon-peel. Got it?"

https://www.straightdope.com/columns/read/1859/why-did-james-bond-want-his-martinis-shaken-not-stirred/

How Is Bipolar Disorder Diagnosed?

Help! [The Beatles 1965] I need somebody Help! Not just ANYBODY!

As with other mental illnesses, there are no lab tests or other physical procedures to help doctors diagnose bipolar disorder. To make a diagnosis, doctors consider a person's symptoms, how those symptoms have progressed, and his or her family history of bipolar or other mood disorders such as depression. Bipolar disorder can be difficult to diagnose for several reasons:

+ Signs and symptoms of bipolar disorder can vary widely in different people.

You don't say? Perhaps that is why it is so hard to diagnose. That and the fact that the quacks have never taken the time to listen long enough to hear my entire history. Or, in my case, they haven't listened to me at all! They hear one symptom and Bam! They know what it is... mention another experience and "Oh? okay, perhaps you're suffering from that, as well". Tell them how I'm feeling today... well yes, that's because it is apart of that... "no problem" he says. "I know just the medication that will help me with all of my problems and get me back to feeling as good as new in no time... it's called: Fuck-it-all, it's easy to digest and it's absolutely free!" The best part of it all is that I can take it as often as I like during the day or night, with/out food and I may even mix it with my favorite alcoholic beverage while I'm at it. Even

before I knew what manic-depressive disorder [or as it is now known today as 'bipolar disorder'] was I had been telling them that something just wasn't right with me. I was up, I was down, I was feeling fine, but then I'd be all over the map again. Well the quickest route between 2 points is a straight line, right? But of course, I never walked a straight line a day in my life, which led me to ask myself [I told you that I talk to myself]. What's wrong with me?

+ Symptoms of bipolar disorder are close to the symptoms of other mental illnesses. **So, they've told me. But they failed to do their homework.**

+ Depressed people may not recognize, report (or even be asked about) symptoms of mania or hypomania and may therefore be misdiagnosed as having unipolar depression. **They never asked me. Well they didn't.**

+ People with bipolar disorder may have other mental health problems at the same time, such as substance abuse, obsessive-compulsive, or panic disorders.

Although I've never knocked on or checked anything multiple times to make sure they were latched, closed or opened. I can however relate to Sheldon in some respects…"you're in my spot!" I have certain places where I like to sit or sleep, doesn't everyone? I do like things to be neat, organized and tidy… I've gotten better at being like that with 'just my things'. It used to drive me nuts if I walked into an office or someone's house and it was in a state of upheaval or the place would be tidy but something would be out of place that it would driver me batshit if I didn't/couldn't fix it. I swear that this one therapist would do this on purpose… she had a bouquet of artificial white carnations but in the middle of these eleven 'white' flowers, she would have one single red rose. It made a dozen but the red was so out of place. Every time I saw it I could hear the song from Sesame Street… "one of these things just doesn't belong here?" and I would pull it out every time and place it on the table by the vase. When the session was over, I'd

put it back. Sometimes I would say "have a nice unorganized day" but more often than not, I wouldn't say anything. I've never been anxious over anything to have a sudden panic attack either... and if you believe that... here's your sign as well.

+ Bipolar disorder may look like something other than a mental illness. Alcohol or drug abuse, poor performance at work or school, or problems with relationships may in some cases be signs of underlying bipolar disorder. **Does drinking from an early age count? Or starting the day with a double bourbon to go with my coffee because it's 5 o'clock somewhere. How about straight C's and D's year after year no matter what grade I was in? Until later in life that is. Friends were always over-rated. My childhood friend left me broken hearted in the early 1980's and the other two have died many years ago, neither have been replaced. So, no matter how I slice this pie, I am alone even though I am not by myself.**

What Are the Signs of Mania or Hypomania?

Oh, do tell, is this about to get even more exciting? Because if it is, I'm all ears!

Hey, stop hogging the popcorn!

In a manic episode, for at least a week a person must feel either so euphoric or so irritable that there is significant impairment of social or occupational function. In addition, if the mood is euphoric, he or she must have at least three of the following symptoms. If the mood is irritable, at least four of the symptoms must be present:

For at least a week? ONLY 3 or 4 symptoms? Can I design that T-shirt now? I've got that beat. This should be fun... He's Up, He's Down, He's All Around! Which way did I go George, which way did I go? I'm usually irritable more so than euphoric [I'm thinking of a T-shirt that has a tornado funnel cloud on it, and at the bottom of the whirlwind is the international symbol for bipolar disorder, that is if I'll be able to use the symbol. Yes, I think I'll design it and paten it, so you heard it here folks. If anyone else comes up with it, they've stolen

it from me] which would account for being easily upset and walking off a job so many times or walking out on people who piss me off so they don't get hurt or I'll say something that I might regret.

+ Increased energy, activity and restlessness **having multiple projects on the go count or is that just a state of being unorganized? I might still manage to get all projects completed or I'll begin too many of them at the same time that I won't complete most of them and I won't care. I've gone to the extreme of not caring to the point of telling the boss to do it himself to where I find myself being fired or I'll just walk off the job... but, I wouldn't care about that either. I'd often find myself getting bored rather quickly. What about staying up all night with a project of some sorts? It's all or nothing until completion and not even feeling tired. Can one have feelings of euphoria and be irritable at the same time? I'd venture to say yes, to that question. I would be 'happy' but then someone would do something stupid and I'd want to bite their head off. The other thing that used to really bug me was when some smart shit tells me that he knows what he's doing because he's too arrogant to ask questions for clarification. Later when I check up on him, I find that he's so deep in left field that he may as well be playing the ball game by himself. As far as I'm concerned there are only two types of stupid questions; the one that hasn't been asked yet and the one that had been asked, answered, only to have the same question be asked again.**

+ Racing thoughts, talking very fast and jumping from one idea to another

I've discussed that above... there just doesn't seem to be a braking system or a shut off valve anywhere. Check the blue prints again George, the architect had to have put one in here somewhere.

+ Inability to concentrate, very easily distracted

Like being on my way to do something and someone chats me up in the hallway that when I get to where it was that I was going, I don't recall why I was going there in the first place? "Now why did I come

in here?" Only to return to my desk in hopes that I'll remember. Nope, that doesn't happen either. Lately, the new one has been leaving my coffee cup on the Keurig, going to the bathroom and returning to my office without my coffee. Generally, I'm not a multi-tasker. Writing this book has been another challenge… inability to concentrate that my thoughts are all over the map. Does anyone have a GPS or a Compass that I could borrow?

+ Little need for sleep [**I told you there were repeats**]

How about staying up for 36hrs then getting 4 hours of sleep and I can still out do the <u>**Energizer Bunny**</u> **and go for another 36 or more.**

The <u>Energizer Bunny</u> is the marketing icon and mascot of the Energizer batteries in North America. It is a pink toy rabbit wearing sunglasses and blue and black striped sandals that beats a bass drum bearing the Energizer logo. https://en.wikipedia.org/wiki/ Energizer_Bunny

+ Having an inflated feeling of power or importance, or an unrealistic belief in one's abilities and powers

He's only 50lbs heavier and 6" taller, I can still teach him driving etiquette if I can manage to pull him out through his window that is. Oh, never mind, he's opening his car door for me, how thoughtful of him. Importance? No, I'm a nobody but then I'm everybody. Does informing a boss, he should be looking for work elsewhere because his attitude and performance suck count for anything?

+ Showing poor judgment, such as going on spending sprees or taking part in inappropriate sexual activity **Is trying to take a short-cut the wrong way up a one-way street count as showing poor judgement? How about doing it right in front of a squad car? Oops, I didn't see him there on the corner. What about going into a men's clothing store with the intentions of only purchasing a shirt and tie, but coming out with a new suit, dress slacks and a jacket to go with that new shirt and tie?**

- Abusing drugs, particularly cocaine, alcohol and sleep medications

Never did like the after effects of sleeping pills and alcohol is over rated as a sleep aide as well, but for some reason a bottle of wine generally helped me to sleep for a few uninterrupted hours. Never had the desire for other drugs, but I was addicted to pain killers for a time but they never made me sleepy, just happier than I already was. I was feeling very little to no pain which usually helped me to sleep.

- Exhibiting aggressive behavior

Oh, oh, Mr. Kotter, Mr. Kotter! I know the answer to that one… hitting a wine glass with my palm so hard that it shatters on contact, a large piece of glass is embedded in my hand while the remaining shards fly in all directions with such force that some even stick into the cupboard door. I then pulled out the shard of glass, covered it with a dish towel and drove myself to the hospital. Needless to say, it was Christmas time and I was in my slippers, had no coat, gloves or hat. Then the Mrs. called the cops on me, said she was concerned for my safety. Okay, and getting hit with an impaired driving charge would have just fixed everything now wouldn't it?

- Denying that anything is wrong

I'm not impulsive, argumentative, angry, or demonstrate poor judgement in anyway shape or form, everything is under control, you're the only one who sees anything wrong with all of this. Go on about your own business folks, nothing more to see here today.

The symptoms of hypomania are similar to those of mania, but they are less severe and often of shorter duration. Hypomania causes little or no functional impairment and does not result in hospitalization.

Go big or stay home I always say. Hospitalization? I've never been hospitalized a single day for anything in my life… I'm as healthy as a dead horse.

What Are the Signs of Depression?

Oh, this aught to be fascinating, I can't wait. Turn up the volume, will you?

In a depressive episode, for at least two weeks [**only two weeks? Nah, that has never happened, well okay, maybe a time or two**] a person <u>must</u> [**now there's positivity for you…'MUST'**] feel so sad, empty or hopeless that his/her life is significantly impaired [**or having a sense that doing anything is a waste of time. Or, perhaps wanting life to be over altogether comes to mind**].

<u>Must</u>: denoting things that are <u>essential</u> [**I like this word**] or highly recommended.

In addition, s/he must have four or more of these symptoms:

Only four? This should be easy. Hey, what's my prize if I win this time?

+ Feelings of worthlessness or guilt **buyers' remorse, drinker's remorse, shame for having slept with someone else again… why can't I control any of this? None of this is making sense to me and I don't know why. Not to mention the negative self-talk after sabotaging yet another job. The fact that I'll never amount to anything and am continuously proving it, rings a bell.**

+ Loss of interest or pleasure in activities once enjoyed, including sex **I can't say much about not being interested in or not being able to enjoy sex, but the other activities, definitely. Just going through the motions or not wanting to even try to do anything also rings a bell thanks to my buddy Eeyore. Remind me again why I'm writing this book? People tell me that I should get a hobby… what on earth for?**

+ Decreased energy **When I do manage to get some sleep [but never as per its definition] … from pure exhaustion only. What do you mean I have to get out of bed? I just got here… 10 hours ago, but whose looking at the clock?**

- Increased fatigue **How far did you say we're walking?**

- Difficulty concentrating, remembering and making decisions **Ya, whatever. What was the question?**

- Restlessness or irritability **Nope, can't say that has ever happened to me Here's a better question: When am I not irritable when depressed? Or is it just the fact that people have a knack of asking stupid questions or making insulting comments or committing stupid actions around me have anything to do with it? Would restlessness be wanting to just up and leave for no apparent reason other than the highway is calling my name and I have to go so bad that I'm vibrating inside because I can't answer the call have anything to do with being restless? Or, are you talking about the fidgety kind where I just can't seem to stay still or sit in my chair for more than a minute. Does pacing the living room at 2am have anything to do with it? Not being able to sleep comes to mind.**

- Sleeping too much or cannot sleep **Usually the cannot sleep. I'd be tired, go to bed [like last night] but be unable to fall asleep and find myself up several times a night [and it's not just to go to the bathroom] or I'd be up all night. More often than not, it's; why do I bother going to bed?**

  Interjection: 1414:10-07-2018; I didn't take a sleeping pill last night and went to bed at 22:10hrs and I do believe that I managed to lay there all night long without sleeping. I don't know how many times I tossed, turned and huffed because I just couldn't fall asleep. So, yes, why do I bother going to bed sometimes? I really don't know.

  Play it again Sam: 0600-19-07-2018; I didn't take the sleeping pill again last night. Wanted to see if I could fall asleep without it... Ya, right, who was I kidding? What a joke. I laid down at 2314hrs still awake at 0130 so I got up and I'm still up and will likely be up the rest of the day and the way I feel right now, I'll probably be up all night as well.

- Change in appetite or unintended weight loss or gain

Food is like sleep, it's highly overrated… as was discussed above. I believe the excess weight gain was due to the alcohol consumption, but I'm losing weight now because I've decided not to drink for a while. I'm down 20lbs in two months so I can't say that I've never experienced the unintended weight loss past the age of forty years. I do often wonder why it is that I'm gaining though.

Interjection: 2029-09-08-2018… I have a bad case of fuck it all lately so I dropped by the liquor store and purchased a 26er of Wild Turkey Bourbon and a 6 pack of beer and I don't give a shit what anyone has to say about it. Cheers!

+ Chronic pain or other persistent bodily symptoms that are not caused by physical illness or injury **some days it just hurts to open my eyes. Let me go back to checking my eyelids for pinholes, will Ya? My legs ache and I don't know why. I've had some knee pain as of late as well and this damn headache just won't go away no matter how many Tylenol tablets I consume, so I don't bother with them.**

+ Thoughts of death or suicide, or suicide attempts **who me? Never!**

How Is Bipolar Depression Distinguished from Unipolar Depression?

Patients with bipolar disorder are frequently misdiagnosed as having unipolar depression because mania or hypomania symptoms may not be recognized. They may have occurred in the past, the symptoms may have been mild (as in hypomania), or the symptoms of depression may be so striking that bipolar is just not considered. It is critical that patients with depression, including those without obvious mania, be questioned about the possibility of prior manic or hypomanic episodes. A family history of bipolar disorder may also point to the correct diagnosis. **I thought I told you that there's no UNI here, so, please, stop calling!**

What Kind of Doctor Do I See If I Think I Have Bipolar Disorder?

I do hope you find one that doesn't past the duck test.

A general practice physician may be able to diagnose bipolar disorder by eliminating other conditions but a mental health specialist, such as a psychiatrist or psychologist, is better trained to detect the signs and symptoms of bipolar disorder and would likely be more knowledgeable about the latest treatments **Really? I call Bullshit on that one! Then where have they been all of these years when I needed them?**

Does any of this sound remotely familiar to you? I think my record is scratched.

If any of this does sound remotely familiar, and you may be experiencing something similar as to what my experiences have been, then you may want to see your doctor sooner rather than later, trust me... it may tell you a lot about yourself that you may not have already known or why you weren't able to put 2 and 2 together.

If any of this confirms your suspicions that you've had the feeling that something is/was wrong, then there is a high probability that you may be suffering from bipolar disorder and the good news is: You Aren't as Crazy as I thought I was.

There is help... Well, that's what they've said. You may save yourself from a life of living through a hellish nightmare.

Maybe? Perhaps? Not now, Eeyore... Oh, okay let's stay positive, shall we?

Please seek help, <u>NOW</u>! Don't put it off any longer!

Put this book down and take care of yourself, I'll be right here when you return.

Email me, I'd truly like to know how you made out.

SECTION TWO

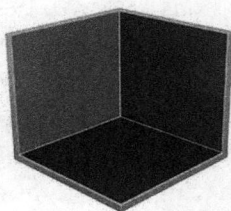

NATURE OR NURTURE?

I have been living with Bipolar Disorder which has not been diagnosed and therefore has gone untreated for all of my life. I'm approaching my 60th year on this earth and most of it has definitely been a '**living hell**'. More often than not, I asked myself: "what's wrong with me?" and thought that I was either crazy or going crazy. Looking back, I often wondered if my behaviour was normal or have I been crazy from the get-go? There have also been many attempts to take my own life as well as multiple thoughts of taking someone else out with me.

Someone please wake me up when it's all over so that I can have a proper life, if that's even remotely possible… thank you!

Saying that life has been a living hellish nightmare is an understatement and some what of an exaggeration to say the least because it has actually been worse than that in many respects. But, I really don't know of any other words or expressions to use to describe it for you. Not only have I been tortured and tormented, but I've carried my skeletons into adulthood and I've harmed my family in one way or another as my skeletons have managed to break forth from their closet. I'm sure I've put my loved ones through hell leaving them wondering; why they have ever stayed with me? It's having me ask myself that very question and more. Perhaps that might answer my question as to why my children don't stay in contact with me as often as I think they could or should? I know I'm loved in some respects, but why does my wife love me, why has she stayed with me, why hasn't she shown me the door years ago? Why? Why? Oh Why? Ah, I can't think of a single reason right now. It might come to me later, but I highly doubt it.

For some reason, the song entitled 'Woman' by John Lennon; released January 1981, has just popped into my head.

So, to has "Easy like Sunday Morning" by The Commodores; released march 18, 1977.

I want to take life as "Easy like a Sunday Morning" but I am internally being chained to do no harm only to break free once again to rape and pillage, so to speak. However; with each cycle I find that I am tormented no matter which way I turn.

Why this book and why now? I don't know how many times over the years that various people have suggested that I write a book. Not only about my upbringing but also of places I've been and things that I have seen and done. However; inhibitions to sit down and actually go for it, have prevented me from doing so. Until now, that is. It's not that I'm a procrastinator or anything, far from it. I've had many thoughts about this subject running in circles around in my head over the past couple of years but I figured I may as well stop chasing my tail and 'just do it' and share 'some' of my life with you. Besides, everyone who has ever earned a PhD has at least one book in them, right? Well, that's what they've told me. There's no time like the present so, let's get to it then, shall we?

One time [no, not at band camp, although I had gone to band camp one year] I had written my autobiography for a psychiatrist who didn't even bother to unseal the envelope and read it. "It was an exercise for me" he said… How was he suppose to help me if he wasn't going to even glance at the homework he had assigned? What was its purpose? I knew my life history… I was so pissed that I walked out of his office never to return. I went home and destroyed the copy that was on a stick because I didn't want people to know how terrible my life had been. I'm wishing now that I hadn't. The memoirs would have come in handy right about now if for no other reason than for cutting and pasting. But no worries, I have everything locked away in my steel vault of a mind [well, that's what my wife calls it]. They say that elephants never forget either… ha, I'm pretty sure I have them beat. Now, what was that combination? Just kidding. Somebody, get me a flashlight… it's awfully dark in here. Have I ever told you that I hate spiders? I'm not afraid of them, I'm just not a fan. Will someone also bring me a broom to sweep out these cobwebs? Oh, thank you.

Most of my thoughts concerning my writing a book were more in the form of questions for myself really: Why bother? Was the number one question. Who's going to want to read what I have to say? What do I have to say that hasn't already been said? [Lots apparently] What do I have to say that would interest other people, never mind paying for the ramblings of this maniac and the babblings of an idiot? My thoughts go all the way to the opposite spectrum to suggest that I just might be able to assist one suffering soul, it would have been worth it. It might also be worth it if other people could see their loved one here and seek help for them. Or, perhaps someone though they had a bad upbringing and when they read about mine, they may figure that theirs wasn't so bad after all. Or, parents may have a child who suffers from ODD and they may have recognized it here and seek help. Who know?

Then there were other jumbled ideas of: will people really believe me or am I making all of this crap up? I've never fancied myself as a fictional novelist, but one never knows? I know there are a lot of good horror, suspense, and fictional stories out there, but believe me, you can't make this shit up, honestly, you can't... well, I can't. What you are about to read is a combination of horror, non-fiction, drama, suspense with perhaps a hint of terror as well as humour and education all rolled up into one... so, look at the bang you're getting for your buck on this one. If you don't believe me... well that too is your prerogative and it's your loss.

Some might say that I'm writing this book just for the attention? After all, I have been known to cry Wolf! Have I not? That too is their prerogative. Then, I had the thoughts of how long will it take before the ridicule and the scoffing will come followed by a ruined reputation. Well, in certain circles my name is already 'mud' here in Canada anyway so I may as well go down swinging and alienate myself in the United States and in other countries as well. No matter, because right now I'm experiencing that in between phase and I don't care anymore what the people who are in so-called 'spiritual authority' think, I can still assist my fellow man because God has asked me too and I do not require man's approval nor authority to do so. Many Denominations desire that a man/woman have an alphabet behind their name before they will hire him/her as a Pastor or Counselor or what have you. Well, I went out and accomplished just that... I not only have a few letters behind my name, I also have acquired a couple of titles prior to my name as well. So, in essence I have given them what they wanted but I have still been rejected by these 'spiritual authorities' for one reason or another... Live by God's law first, not man's laws or desires. No matter what Church you desire to attend, a mainline 'Denomination' a 'Non-Denominational' or an 'Interfaith', make sure they are 'Bible' based teaching and not full of man-made rules.

Then I had my worst thought of them all… the fear of my secrets coming out, as I bare my soul for all who read my book to see. I had thoughts of being arrested for past crimes, and the fact that you now know that I was capable of hurting someone or being mean to others while in a maniac state just because 'I have to be heard' and the truth must be told. Well, steps 4 and 5 of a 12-Step program has one taking inventory then sharing with God and another human being of those wrongs. Confession in the Catholic Church would amount to the same… Confessing before God, and man while asking for forgiveness, direction and strength not to do it again. Which of course led me to thoughts of shame, embarrassment and about hurting my family and others… well, it is for them that I have decided to leave names out completely.

I wanted to protect the innocent whomever, they may be… siblings, wives, children, step-children, grandchildren, past girlfriends, ex-lovers, long lost friends [I did have them once upon a time], acquaintances, class-mates, the bullies, teachers, social workers, medical professionals, mental health professionals, addiction counselors, psychiatrists, police officers, rescuers, EMT's, MP's, Padre's, friends who have been laid to rest, dear old mom and even step monster. Have I missed anyone? If so, I do apologize.

However, after reading this book, should you decide you want to acknowledge the fact that we are related, or acquainted, Cool! Should you read this book and you decide to disown me? That too is your prerogative and it's been a slice! Perhaps we'll meet again on the other side of life. Presently, thanks to the disorder and to my Eeyore Complex, I don't really give a shit either way. But, I may have different feelings later during a maniac episode. But, you'll never know, now will you?

However; whoever you are don't bother writing me to say Bullshit! You weren't there 24/7/365, I was! We all have our own stories to tell and our own perceptions of those stories and the truth. Ask ten people who witnessed the same traffic accident and you'll get ten perceptions of what actually happened and it's all… the… truth… according to them. Well, the same goes for my life. There is only the account from one eyewitness here that really matters and that eyewitness is Yours Truly… Me… Myself… and I, and we have you out numbered.

Besides, who out there is perfect? As far as I know, there was only one man who was perfect and they crucified him over 2.000 years ago so what does that tell you? Show me ONE, Just ONE family on God's green earth that isn't <u>dysfunctional</u> by its very definition. Just in case you don't know: dysfunctional as an adjective, is something that is not operating <u>normal</u>ly or properly. Synonyms are: troubled, distressed, unsettled, upset and/or distraught. So, if you think that you have a '<u>perfect</u>' little family, well good for you and may God Bless!

Now, define '<u>Normal</u>': as a noun: it is the usual, average, or typical state or condition. As an adjective: conforming to a <u>standard</u>; usual, typical, or expected. Synonyms: standard, usual, typical, average, the rule, etc.

The major problem with this definition is that everyone's 'normal' is different. It means various things to you and me and everyone else on the planet. So, go ahead and lead a 'normal' life, if you can, I dare you! God Be with You, because Luck, has nothing to do with it!

<u>Perfect</u>: adjective; having all the required or desirable elements, qualities, or characteristics; as good as it is possible can be.

Ha, Ya, right, I got you there… and that describes any family today? There aren't such things as 'usual' or 'standard's' nor is there anything 'typical' or 'normal' about families or any one person in any society on the globe and there has never been since the fall of man nor will there ever be until the Lord returns. Speaking of '<u>standards</u>,' what are you using to measure this so-called 'standard' of yours? Religious writings such as the Bible, the Quran, the Torah, Vedas, the Egyptian Book of the Dead, Tao Te Chin, Upanishads, Bhagavad Gita, Buddhist Sutras, Non-Religious Ancient Books, the writings/sayings of the Dali Lama, Confucius, the Satanic Bible, the laws of the land, your horror scope, going to a psychic, a palm reader… come see me and I'll paint your palm red for you… Lol, or something else that you've dreamed up? I heard that there was a new religion on the horizon; Pastafarianism or some stupid shit like that. Apparently the 'Flying Spaghetti Monster' is their deity and there are 13 steps required to join the church… check it out, it's on Google and Wikipedia. Sounds like something someone dreamed up while smoking bad week if you ask me. Right… so, by who's or what 'STANDARDS' are any of us living by? More than not today it comes down "to each their own" [hopefully within the confines of the law] but what is wrong and what is right? Again, a definition that cannot really be defined nor explained.

Isn't having difficulty staying on track one of the symptoms of bipolar disorder? I do believe it is. I've derailed again, oh well. It happens a lot in this book so you may as well get use to it.

Back to my thoughts: How can anyone go through all the crap that you are about to read and live to tell about it, you may ask... Well I'm glad you have, asked, that is. Sad to say, but perhaps there was a will and determination somewhere with in me... or, as mom use to say... "God isn't finished with him yet" and the last time I checked, I do believe He is more powerful than I. So perhaps "God isn't finished with me yet." Others would say that I am really making my guardian angels working overtime, or that one day my luck will run out. Oh, well, won't 'luck' run out for all of us one day anyway? So, with that in mind, yes, one can and I have, lived through it because I'm here to tell you about my living hell.

There are many times that I had wished and even prayed that the old man would have killed me so that he'd have gone to jail and it would have saved the others from living a life of hell under his roof. I even prayed that he'd be in a car accident or get some disease that they couldn't cure and he'd be gone and we'd live a peaceful life or that he'd be arrested for brutalizing us, but that never happened either. Needless to say, my childhood prayers were never answered and the torture continued. My experiences are similar yet different from my siblings, but I'm not here to tell their stories, I'm here to relay mine to you. So, please, do take this seriously, even though there are some funny antics here for your amusement if for no other reason, but these things really did happen to me.

I also do realize that going back over my life while writing this book will open old wounds for myself and others but, that's life and I make no apologizes to them except to submit that you work your way through your skeletons and let me deal with mine as we see fit and get over it already. To steal and rephrase the words of Winston Churchill... this is my FINEST HOUR! So, I'm going to take it whether 'they' [my siblings] let me have it or not. I feel that it is finally time for my skeletons to come out of my closet, if for no other reason than having that 'Last Waltz' with them and finally burying them once and for all and I'm not giving up the location of their bodies.

Should you desire to contact me and learn more, or whatever, I have submitted my email address on the very last page, please feel free to use it and I will attempt to answer your questions and/or concerns with gratitude. Hell, I'll even accept and answer your hate mail… at lest I'll know you've read my book. So, let me thank you in advance. Sorry, no refunds or credit vouchers will be mailed to you, and this book is not something that you may exchange either, so don't ask. If you don't like what you've read then perhaps you may know someone who maybe a fellow sufferer and might have the desire to read it, if for no other reason than for them to know they aren't the only one who really isn't crazy. Maybe, just maybe, mind you, they'll see themselves here and will be able to laugh or, if they haven't been diagnosed, I hope that they've been encouraged enough to seek help. So, please, feel free to pass it on, sell it, use it as a paper weight or burn it. It is your book after all, to do with as you please. 'Just Do It!'

Just like your life… it is/was yours and yours alone, no one else's. My truths are just that… MINE! And mine alone! I may be delusional but the events which I shall unfold for you have occurred according to the team of ME, as I had experienced or have recall of them. So, I'm here to tell you MY story, not someone else's and I'll leave it at that. Are we clear? Crystal! Good! I know, I know, I've repeated myself, but I had wanted to make a point!

The darkest has overshadowed my world once again, just when I thought that I couldn't sink any lower than a snake's belly, I may have sunk to the lowest I have ever been and I find that eating dirt doesn't taste very good. Neither does eating crow in case you were wondering. I've been hospitalized before but I don't remember my previous experiences to be anything like my most recent stay at Club Mental Health [CMH]. Just a short week ago I was released from a Mental Health Unit about an hour away from my home where they kept me longer than I had anticipated and against my will too I might add. Damn the mental health act!

If you're wondering what that's all about, you can check it out:

For Alberta: www.albertahealthservices.ca/info/mha.aspx

For B.C.: http://www.bclaws.ca/civix/document/id/complete/ statreg/96288_01

For Canada: www.mentalhealthcommission.ca/English/what-we-do/ mental-health-and-law

For everyone else... just Google the mental health act for your Province or State and I'm sure you'll find your health department info on the subject.

I Googled "mental health act, Texas" for example and this came up: https://www.dshs.texas.gov/mhrules/

I've read through most of the information provided in these websites and they are rather a fascinating read. Especially if you're looking for something to help you fall asleep at night.

To eat crow implies, at its mildest, an unpleasant action since the flesh of the crow is believed to be unpalatable. As an expression, it denotes the anguish of humiliation at having to admit to wrongdoing or fallibility, usually in the wake of hubristic actions or words.

This is my personal opinion: Unless you're in absolute dire straights, never ever and I do mean NEVER EVER [I know, never say never but I did twice, so get over it] go the ER with suicidal tendencies or else you'll end up in a mental health ward where in my opinion, you'll receive very little to no psychological help whatsoever but they will retain you against your will if for no other reason than because they can! In the guise of the interest of 'your personal safety' that is. Of course, I have no knowledge of what the facilities are like in your general area, but here St. Paul, Alberta, Canada the food is atrocious and unfit for human consumption. Yes, I have submitted complaints to the appropriate authorities expressing both my professional and personal opinions of their facility. The lady on the other end of the phone said that she would get back to me after they have conducted their investigation, but I highly doubt that they will conduct and investigation or get back to me. I submitted my complaints in May and it's now the middle of September… see, I told you no one would get back to me. The showers are cold and so is the washing/shaving water. I don't mind shaving in cold water but I prefer a warm shower thank you. The beds are comfortable and the nursing staff are [mostly] nice people but you won't receive the mental assistance you require to move forward. Partially due to the fact that they're just aren't enough Psychiatrists for the number of patients in the area [so they say] and they can't do justice for everyone so, everyone suffers because of it. Thanks to Rachel Notley and her NDP government, I'm sure, but that is speculation on my part. Sign of the times I suppose? The other problem [in my opinion] is that the shrinks are too busy with their 'out-patients' and they neglect their 'in-house' patients in the process. Oh, and the so-called 'optional' therapy classes… yes, they are optional, but sorry guys, I'm sure you have a curriculum that you are required to follow and not everyone is on the same playing field, but p-l-e-a-s-e… [eyes rolling] those sessions were very immature and mediocre at best. I've produced Bible studies for preteens that had more meat to them, but nice try fellas. I will give you an 'A' for effort. If nothing else, you let me stir the pot which got everyone riled up and participating… so, in essence, I did you a favour. To say the least, that was fun, it made for some lively discussions which everyone participated in which made for a most memorable moment while in your company. So, Thank You for that and I hope I never have the privilege of meeting you on the inside again because I like being on the outside looking in.

But… should you find you have nowhere else to turn, Please, use the 1-800#'s on page 4 or dial 911 anywhere in North America, or make your way to the ER rather than taking your own life. Every life, is worth living.

A grievous darkness has overshadowed my existence taking control of my every thought and my life, as I knew it… was/is all over… once again… at least, in my mind it may as well have been. Severe depression [Severe as an adjective is described as being something bad or undesirable which is very great or intense] mixed with alcohol, stupid impulsive actions, not giving a damn along with jumbled thoughts of killing myself have plagued my every waking moment [and we all know that I don't sleep much, so that's a lot of waking moments]. Running away had occurred to me as well, but then, where would I go? How would I survive? Do I even want to survive? Statements such as; What good am I? You 'stupid-ass' you've done it again, when will I ever learn? No one cares about me or whether I live or die, or if I ever existed in the first place... flooded my brain every second of the days that preceded my being hospitalized to the point where the voices were inexhaustible and demanded to be obeyed. But I can't this time, I've tried that unsuccessfully so many times before, what makes me think I'll succeed this time? I can't do anything right, remember, I am a "stupid-ass" who can't even kill himself properly. "I'll never be able to do anything right, but yet I'll never amount to anything either, so why bother remaining alive?" The Eeyore Complex continues to haunt me, torment me, forever bringing doubts to myself about my shitty existence. But this is deeper than the Eeyore complex. This time was different, the pit of despair was so deep and dark that it was difficult to even see my hand before my eyes. Death at that point would have been received as a warm welcome invitation extended from the other side by a friend who has gone on before me. "Come join us" he calls out from the abyss. Anything at that point would be better than the hell I was going through once again and everyone would be better off without me.

"Goodbye Cruel World" no, not yet! Damn, foiled again.

If only I had a gun, I'm sure it would have been all over and you wouldn't be holding this book in your hands. I couldn't obtain one so I stepped out in front of a big truck once again... damn brakes and/or slower speeds, shitty timing on my part, I don't know? Maybe it was God intervening because He isn't finished with me yet, but the scene wasn't a good one let me tell you. I'm surprised someone didn't call the cops. Or had they? I don't know because I hadn't stuck around long enough for them to show up after I was pulled out from under the vehicle, shoved off of the road and back onto the grass. As of yet, I'm not sure if I'm thankful for that truck stopping or not. Should I survive another 15 or 20 years, perhaps

I'll write a short sequel so you'll know how things have turned out for me, or perhaps not??? Keep a copy of this book, just in case I do write a sequel... anyone producing this book [dust and all] at time of purchase will receive a 25% discount as my thanks for your continued support.

By now, I'm sure you've noticed as I have, that I like to use the word 'hell' a fair bit... okay, a lot but the thing is... many people don't see it as a swear word while others just think it isn't a nice word to be saying, but I heard it all the time growing up so it often comes automatically. The other thing is, that I know what its biblical definition is [do you?] but just for shits and giggles I thought I would include it here at this point for your amusement and/or education just in case you aren't familiar with its definition or haven't experienced it personally for yourself or you don't really care. Either way, here it is... whether you've asked for it or not...

Hell: a place regarded in various religions as a spiritual realm of evil and suffering [sounds about right where I grew up] Often traditionally depicted as a place of perpetual fire beneath the earth where the wicked are punished [continuously] after death.

Here is the Wikipedia explanation of Hell: https://en.wikipedia.org/wiki/Hell

Hell is a place of unquenchable fire, of memory and remorse, of misery and pain, a place of frustration and anger, of separation of eternal torments, and punished with an everlasting destruction [now there's something I don't know anything about. And if you believe that, I have some swamp land in the Yukon to sell you]

It sounds like a perfect description of what living with the monstrous step-dad was like all of those years in combination with living with an undiagnosed bipolar disorder. Oh gee, I get it from both sides so it didn't matter which side of the fence I found myself to be on, I was hooped. Which way do I go George? Which game do I play first? Tag, you're it! So, Yes, going through the never-ending phases of this disorder has been and truly is a living Hell in and of itself, never mind the torment I was subjected to on a regular basis by a mean son-of-a-bitch I was suppose to call 'dad'. I dare any fellow sufferer to deny it or come up with a better description to describe bipolar disorder for me because I'm out of options and I'm all ears. Please; use my email on the very last page and let me know your thoughts and share your experiences as I would love to hear from and to converse with you.

Once again, the darkness engulfs me and I'm face to face with my nemeses... staring into the blackness I am unable to see my reflection as it too is sucked into the nothingness. It has the soul of a hardened black wall of despair, which may or may not have a window [despair is another inadequate word in our English language to describe the true hell I'm enduring]. I never know how long it's going to last or what rabbit hole it will lead me down next, or how dark it will be before the dawn [and they do say "it is always darkest before the dawn"]. How long will I be tormented this time? Will it be days, a week, a month, several weeks or several months? I really don't know for sure because each is cycle is different from the last that there is no point in writing a program because the theme and the entertainers of this production will change each day. Sometimes my environment has a lot to do with it. Sometimes it's the company I keep or am forced to be amongst.

Despair: as a noun; loss of hope, hopelessness; As a verb; to lose, to give up or to be without hope. Sounds about right!

Each time I cycle through, it varies depending on life's situation at that particular moment in time, what's ahead and/or without explanation a maniac/depressive phase will come to an end and I find myself adrift. Reprieve! No, not really, I'll only cycle through again, and again, and again... now my record is scratched. To be tormented for as long as I walk this earth. But, can I hang on this time?

How do I hold on? Do I even want to hold on? It's not like only going "7 seconds on a bull named Fu Man Chu" [Live Like You Were Dying, by Tim McGraw]

Because the '7' seconds are never up, the horn never blows and I'm hanging on for the ride of my life. When my current divider has finally been breeched I find myself to be in the foggy state of indecision and a mood that tells me that: 'I don't give a <u>shit</u>' ['<u>shit</u>'; an exclamation of disgust, anger, or annoyance]. I may find myself in this state for days, weeks, or even months… as it's been 3 months this time around. Again, I never know who or what will pull me out of it… I may even spiral back down into the depths of despair once again before the uprising will come. At least riding on a roller-coaster I know what's coming because I like to ride up front for full vantage and effect of the ride. The never-ending question is: how long will it be before I find myself winding up once again? The other problem is; none of it makes sense to me. Flip a coin, now count the number of times it flips before you catch it again, only you don't catch it and the flipping is perpetual [currently, I find myself to be stuck in the Eeyore Complex while I'm writing this book. Hell, I don't even know why I'm writing this book in the first place. I suppose someone thought it was a good idea so as usual… when I find myself to be in an Eeyore Complex, I just go along for the ride because I don't know if I should turn left or right but either way I can not remain on the straight and narrow path even if you were to put a gun to my head. Go ahead, pull the trigger, you'd be doing me a favour] and I don't feel like doing anything or going anywhere or seeing anyone and I end up just going along with the flow like a boat which has it's sails out but there is no breeze to fill them to carry me to who knows or who cares where and I find myself to be without a paddle to assist with the forward or reverse motion. So, I am adrift on the current not knowing or caring where I'll be taken to this time. But then, hopefully, I'll start the upswing and God only knows what trouble I'll find myself in, but what a ride it will be! No, seat belts are not required, they wouldn't do me any good anyway. You can call this in-between phase what you will, but I refer to it as 'coasting.' I'm neither reversing or slowing down, nor am I powering up getting ready to be propelled full throttle in a forward motion. Coasting is just moving along without using power to get me to where it is that I'm supposed to be or to wherever it is I'm suppose to end up this time. And, just where that is? I have no idea, so don't ask. Oh, you already have… well, [can be a very deep subject] I don't know because I can't find it anywhere on my map of life which is forever changing!

I welcome sleep but I am unable to find it without alcohol or chemical assistance and even chemical assistance can be highly over rated as well. For years I'd use alcohol and other things to assist my slumber but found out I'd never really acquire more than a few hours anyways and what little sleep I could manage to find was never really all that restful, nor peaceful, nor deep enough to remember dreaming. REM sleep continues to elude me. I haven't remembered a dream in years. I don't even know if I dream anymore and would venture to guess, that I do not. I was going on another three days with perhaps three hours of sleep in total when I decided to self medicate once again. Then, and only then, was I able to rest for a full eight hours or more with not wanting to get out of bed the next morning. I always hate that dopy, groggy feeling the next morning after taking a sleeping pill, it's worse than a hangover. My biggest problem at that point was that the morning always arrives way too soon and I have to face another day. Or do I? I'm unemployed once again so who cares if I get out of bed or not? I sure as hell don't. Sometimes I don't and I lie there half awake/half asleep. Sometimes I doze off, sometime I do not, but either way, several hours [or has it only been several minutes?] will pass before I venture forth and begin another cycle of restlessness, irritation and an all-around sense of fuck-it-all. Okay, since discovering this one, it has become my new best saying. But in all reality and to be polite, I suppose I should stick to using my Eeyore Complex. So, I shall endeavor to do the best that I can with this. I've gotten so use to functioning on three or four hours of sleep a night that I'm seriously beginning to believe that sleep is highly over-rated as well. Another problem is though, that I can't really function unless I'm in my maniac phase. Then and only then am I like the Energizer Bunny that just keeps on going and going, kind of like that song that never ends, it just goes on and on my friends.

Insomnia for me is caused by not having an off switch in my head. Whether I'm maniac or depressed, my mind won't stop thinking, pondering, wondering, about anything/everything and then nothing at all for hours on end which in the middle of the night can seem like an eternity, or has it only been a few minutes?

The minute hand quietly clicks down another hour… kind of like, hickory-dickory-dock, three mice ran up the clock. The clock struck one and the other two escaped with minor injuries. Yes, I'm grievously injured and I have another headache from laying here for so long trying to go to sleep when I know better. It's now 2:00am, I had been lying there since 2300hrs unable to sleep; so, why do I even bother lying down? [so, I get out of bed and make my way back to my computer] How many "O dark stupid" mornings have I seen while attempting to sleep? What is this now, the third or fourth night in a row? I can't recall because my days blur into my nights and my nights meld into my days. If the sun didn't rise each morning, I wouldn't know if it were night or day… heck, today I had to look at the calendar three times before the day of the week sank into my noggin. I often lie there on my back motionless, starring blankly towards the ceiling, into the darkness without a thought running through my head. Hey, have you ever tried counting those little black dots before your eyes while starring into nothingness? It's practically impossible, they keep moving or disappearing only to reappear in a different location and the counting starts all over again. It's better than counting sheep. If you haven't tried it, you really should. It's pretty wild!

Then [in the summer time] there is the fact that the room is never dark enough in the land of the midnight sun and the birds start chirping again at 03:30, ugh! I can only imagine what it's like further up north. Then there is the never-ending blasted ringing in my ears, [which of course has nothing to do with bipolar disorder or does it?] it's enough to drive me batshit all by its self. [Batshit; adjective, completely mad or crazy] See, I don't make this stuff up ladies and gentlemen. You should try the Urban Dictionary, it's a blast. I've looked up many things just for the heck of it and almost fell on the floor laughing… but really, it's about time someone put all of our modern slangs and ethaniums into a book so people would use them correctly. I don't think there is anything worse than someone trying to appear to be smart by making up their own words or using existing words out of context. But, that is just one smart ass's opinion.

More often than not with this one, most people will say "batshit crazy" but you don't have too because batshit means "crazy" so in essence, you are calling someone 'crazy, crazy'. There, you've been educated on the proper use of that phrase. Oh, you're welcome, it was and always is, my pleasure. I paid for my education but I may as well educate you for free... oh wait, it wasn't entirely free was it? You did have to pay for this book after all, so I thank you!

Or, the music, that sometimes is a never-ending serenade of piano, violins, [more often than not, its violins, I just love the sound of a violin and a tenor sax] often mingled with horns and percussion, that won't stop playing yet there isn't an electronic source [I know, because I've scoured the entire house on numerous occasions looking for a source] for the sounds which now I know, only I can hear.

Another problem [gees, how many problems do I have? I just did a word search count, apparently there are 78 of them in total, isn't that just funtastic?] is that I haven't listened to Mozart, Kenny G or any other type of classical or jazz music in a few days so, why am I hearing it now when I'm trying to go to sleep? But if I tell anyone, they'd think I'm weird or just plain crazy. To be honest with you, I'm not sure which I am either, but no one listens to me anyway, so I've just stopped trying to tell them. Hey, you better stay away from Wayne, he hears music in the night. Oh, and for your information, it isn't just during the night. Today I was on my way home from the grocery store and I didn't like the song on the radio so I turned it off and immediately I heard a mariachi band. Why in the world would I be hearing a mariachi band when I was just listening to Country Music? Not only that, but I've not been to Mexico in months. Huh? Sometimes I'll be driving down the road and the radio will be off but tunes are playing out inside my head which are very audible but only to myself. It's like having a front row seat at a concert for one. Cool! The best part is, the seat is free and who doesn't like free shit? Eh?

What about seeing things? I've already discussed that previously, but it happens to me more often then I care to admit. Why, when I was waiting to be admitted into the hospital, I thought I saw an elderly woman lying in a bed in the emergency department. The doc said that I could go into 'that room'... pointing in the general direction where I saw the woman.

"No, there's a lady lying in the bed" I said… he looks, "no, it's available," he said and so it was. When I took a second look that is… but where did she go? I could have sworn she was real. Holy shit WAyneman, have you been eating those magic mushrooms again? She was so real in appearance, I swear I thought for sure that I could have reached out and touched her. However, upon closer investigation, the bed was completely empty. It's a real riot, I do hope that you get to experience it sometime. But again, Sshh! You can't tell anyone or they'll lock me up and throw away the key. I'm always seeing shadows passing by but when I blink or do a double take… there's nothing/no one there. But, they keep telling me, what? What are they telling me? Oh, I know… they aren't telling me anything, because NO ONE IS LISTENING! So, I guess there's nothing to worry about because there isn't anything wrong with me… or is there? I'll let you be the judge… All rise! hear ye, hear ye, this looney tunes court is now in session. Our honourable Judge whac-a-mole presiding.

Looney Tunes is an American animated series of comedy short films produced by Warner Bros. from 1930 to 1969 during the golden age of American animation, alongside its sister series Merrie Melodies.

https://en.wikipedia.org/wiki/Looney_Tunes

Whac-A-Mole is a popular arcade redemption game invented in 1976 by Aaron Fechter of Creative Engineering, Inc. A typical Whac-A-Mole machine consists of a large, waist-level cabinet with five holes in its top and a large, soft, black mallet. Each hole contains a single plastic mole and the machinery necessary to move it up and down. Once the game starts, the moles will begin to pop up from their holes at random. The object of the game is to force the individual moles back into their holes by hitting them directly on the head with the mallet, thereby adding to the player's score. The more quickly this is done the higher the final score will be. Just in case you weren't sure what it was… it can be fun.

What about voices?

What about them? Who said that? Am I on Candid Camera? Don't tell me you can hear them too… Are they my own thoughts, or can I hear yours? Are they something subliminal? Is it someone else's words in my voice or do I actually hear other people's voices? Wouldn't you like to know? Have you ever seen a movie where someone is reading a letter from home, but we have a narration of the other person's voice who wrote said letter? Well, it's kind of like that. I've already alluded to hearing voices or what some might refer to as 'self-talk'. However, these words are often in the voice of my step-monster, who is informing me that I'm good for nothing, that my family would be better off without me, that I can't do anything right, calling me a 'stupid-ass' once again and shit like that. Yes, sometimes he even tells me to go kill myself because no one loves me anyway. Awe, but is it the devil trying to get the better of me? Some have even gone as far as to inform me that I'm possessed… and have prayed over me to rid me of the evil spirits who reside within. Or, are the sounds really my voice echoing his words in my head from my childhood because that's all I ever heard and now that I'm proving him to be right once more, that he continues to haunt me? I don't know, you tell me… More often than not, it's the old man's voice I hear… and not my own voice repeating his words. Like I said, he's still in my head especially when I royally screw up, and when don't I? Royally screw up that is. And, I've royally screwed up once again. The problem with this is that I haven't lived with the man in 42 years. Oh my, it's terrible how the actions and words of others during our informative years are buried so deep within our subconscious that they haunt us for the rest of our lives. But I can't afford to let bitterness overtake me or I'll go out the same way my mother had… she lived with him for about 20 years, she was separated and divorced from him for approximately 36 years and she died a lonely bitter old lady because she just wouldn't/couldn't let go of the past or the anguish that man caused her that she brought that crap into every relationship there after. So, he won out in the end, hadn't he? I would venture to say, YES! Sad to say, he had.

Have you ever had an argument with someone and then replayed it in your head while hearing and listening to both sides of the argument but in various voices as if you were a spectator in all of this? Why am I going over this? Political correctness does have a baring upon me and I know that it isn't 'who' is right or 'who' is wrong, but 'what' is right and 'what' is wrong that really counts. I've often heard that it's okay to talk to myself but when I start answering back or carry on a conversation with myself it's cause for concern. Well, we're w-a-y past the point where it's a cause for concern! I will continue to play out countless scenarios only to not use a single one of them when confrontation time finally arrives. I eventually give up trying to go to sleep because the voices won't let me and I'll arise because for some reason the sleeping pill isn't working that night either. Does that happen to any of you, or is it just me? But how is it that the sleeping pill won't knock me out? I just don't get it. I guess my mind is more powerful than a chemical substance... cool!

Oh, and they've tried to hypnotise me in the past and that didn't work on me either. The mind can be a powerful thing, when one knows how and chooses to use it. When I can't sleep I would often go on the computer and do research or write sermons [I can identify with Father McKenzie in Eleanor Rigby by The Beatles 1966, who writes words to a sermon that no one will hear] or play games until I'm bored and try going back to bed a couple of hours later and maybe this time [just maybe, mind you] I'll get some sleep. Ya, right... who am I kidding? In this case it's... here's my sign, cause that ain't happening.

Oh, and warm milk doesn't work for me either. Warm brandy, perhaps, but not the moo-juice.

Just to prove how much of an insomniac I can be, and how much I have accomplished during a maniac phase of insomnia... I actually have five years worth of Sermons put together that might require minor adjustments just prior to presentation. I have six years worth of Bible Studies and over one-hundred sessions for discipleship and leadership classes that I could conduct. I'll let you do the math. Oh, and since I'm bragging a little here... I was conducting my research for my Doctoral Thesis while studying for my Master's Degree, but then every good student does that, do they not?

So why doesn't anyone listen to me? Why hadn't they asked all of the right questions?

WILL SOMEBODY, ANYBODY, FINALLY PLEASE HELP ME?
HELLO? IS THERE ANYBODY OUT THERE? ANYONE?

There, I've screamed once again for help, but will anyone hear my cries this time?

I just had a funny thought… maybe I should write to Dr. Phil? So, I did.

https://en.wikipedia.org/wiki/Phil_McGraw

Interjection: 1032-08-09-2018: I still haven't heard from Dr. Phil's staff, so I don't suppose I will.

Answer me this:

"If there is no one in the forest and a tree falls crashing to the ground, does it still make a noise?"

"Yes, most definitely!"

"How do you know if you aren't there to hear it?"

Do you ever feel like that? I feel like that all the time. I feel like that tree in the forest who is making a thunderous clamour but no one is out there to hear me, so what's all the commotion about? Well, if you feel like that tree, just keep on clamouring until someone finally listens to you. They may think and feel as though you're crying 'wolf' but get a 2ND 3RD or even a 4th opinion if you must until finally someone listens. That's what I've finally decided to do this go-round. I'm sick and tired of this crap. I swear I'm going to keep kicking-in those doors until someone finally pays attention to me, Once and For All! Why? Because, I'm sick and tired [how sick and tired am I?] I'm so sick and tired of being sick and tired! I don't know how much more of this bullshit I can take. Really, I don't!

Does the phrase: "Dead Man Walking" mean anything to you?

Dead Man Walking is a phrase traditionally used in U.S. prisons to announce a condemned prisoner being walked to the place of execution. Its use has expanded as a euphemism for anyone facing an impending and unavoidable loss. Sounds about right! And that's how I constantly feel like.

It's no wonder people go <u>postal</u> in our society today, or so many gunmen are shooting up our schools, or that we're finding out so many homeless people have mental instabilities. But, perhaps that is why they are homeless in the first place. They can't work, they're unable to pay the rent and in most cases... they are unable to manage their finances to be able to have proper shelter never mind affording their medications. Hey there's another Google search for you... Homeless, Mentally Ill, and the Neglected! It makes for an interesting read, trust me... Especially our American friends, you guys are really fucked up, let me tell you. But hey, our Canadian statistics aren't all that better I suppose, given our smaller population.

Here is a small sample: The Mental Health Commission of Canada reported between 25-50% of the homeless population in Canada suffer from a mental illness(es). More critically, the National Learning Community on Youth Homelessness found that well over 50% of the 1,054-youth experiencing homelessness in their 2014 National Needs Assessment reported a mental health issue of some kind. Now, we all know that there are more than 1,054 young people on the streets today... so, what would be the actual number... staggering thought, isn't it?

http://homelesshub.ca/blog/mental-health-and-homelessness-canada

<u>Postal</u>: Gone crazy or insane; irrational. It came into use after a number of workplace shootings by disgruntled U.S. Post Office Workers.

Well, according to Dr. Margorie L. Baldwin PhD, who wrote an article for 'Psychology Today' says that "It's easier to get homeless people with mental illness into jail than into care" [I told you, they'll lock me up and throw away the key if they get their hands on me]. Dr. Baldwin was addressing a Rotary Club, her topic was how society has failed to assist people with serious mental illness and how we have abandoned and left them on the streets of our fair cities across the nation (USA). To prove her point she stated "My brother-in-law is a real estate developer in the city. Before my talk, he took me on a tour of the homeless encampments in town—one of which is on property he owns. Every six months or so he receives a notice of violation from the city, informing him that the encampments are in violation of city codes and that he must remove the people from his property [I thought that was the job of law enforcement. I guess not]. He does so, which costs his firm thousands of dollars. Where do the homeless go? They rebuild their encampments in another part of town until they are removed from there, at which time they move back to my brother-in-law's property [wouldn't it be cheaper to erect a fence?] Clearly, the notice of violation is no solution to the underlying problem."

There are of course many underlying issues but the biggest factor is that many people with mental illnesses don't even realize that they are sick. It's an interesting article which makes me wonder how the mentally ill and homeless are being treated here in Canada. You may read the entire article for yourself at: www.psychologytoday.com/us/blog/beyond-schizophrenia/201608/homeless-mentally-ill-and-neglected

I've been to Toronto, Montreal, Vancouver, Detroit, Los Angeles, Seattle, Atlanta, San Diego, and various other large cities in both Canada and the United States and have seen these 'encampments' for myself… not a pretty site and can be a scary place to be walking past at night time. And, what are we doing about it? Very little to NOTHING except making them move about the city or to migrate to warmer cities come winter time.

Well, enough of the chit-chat, lets get down to some of the Hellish things I've gone through in my life time which are the reasons for this book in the first place… I think? But which may have also contributed to my bipolar disorder to begin with. Remember, this section is called Nature or Nurture… you be the judge.

Perhaps I should change the title to 'A Living Hell!' What do you think? In case you haven't noticed I like Google, man, you can find just about anything through a Google Search… Fire Fox search engine is alright, I've come across Two Cows and others but I like and prefer Google. So, I Googled 'a living hell' [by the way, 30,200,000 results came up] [just for shits and giggles, I went to Microsoft Edge, which I believe is 'Bing' search and only 16,500,000 results popped up. So, have fun with that] and these are just a few samples of what I have found...

"A 'living hell' can be defined as an extremely unpleasant place or experience. That's a start! Hey, that's what the 'Free online Dictionary' called it as well.

It may not be a single experience; but, it will be a continuous cycle of such experiences [again, sounds like living in my step-dad's house and living with bipolar disorder at the same time if you ask me] so that the person having such an experience will feel life as a "living hell." [told Ya]

"The person is highly depressed with so much of unhappiness, nothing works out favorably, everyday he/she feels sicker and sicker of living his/her life and does not understand the purpose of life at all" uh, huh... sounds accurate.

+ feels that no one cares about him/her, feels empty and useless. Go on with you, I guess I'll go eat those worms again.

+ feels that they had not committed any mistakes, but, is being punished without any reason or by just life itself. You don't say? I told you it wasn't my fault but the beatings continued until the moral improved and so had the bullying in the hood and at school.

+ there is a feeling that he/she is unnecessarily tortured by everyone for no reason and people are making fun of them not just feeling... they still are and they were making fun of me and they use to beat me up on a regular basis too. I'm really surprised that I was able to have children when I grew up because I took so many shoots to the nuts.

+ feels that s/he should not continue to exist to bear such a useless life any longer. Hence the constant desire to end my life. But, I can't even do that right. Go figure.

Sound familiar? Well it should for those of us who suffer from bipolar disorder or, if you are someone living with a fellow sufferer, it can be a 'Living Hell' for you as well!

Or, you just might be living with an abuser… someone who tortures you mentally and/or beats you physically… you don't have to put up with that crap. How/why can you love someone who treats you like shit? You don't deserve to be treated like that. You're better than that and my advice to You would be to <u>GET THE HELL OUT, NOW!</u> Don't wait, take your kids and leave. You can always return with a Sherriff, a Marshall, a Police officer for protection to collect what belonging you need. There are <u>50 ways to leave your lover</u>… listen to the song, it just might be inspirational and give you some ideas. [You just slip out the back, Jack. Make a new plan, Stan. You don't need to be coy, Roy. Hop on the bus, Gus. Just drop off the key, Lee and get yourself free!] You owe it to yourself and your children to have a safer, better, happier, healthy, loving life… if you're single, you owe it to yourself to get out of Dodge and do it NOW! While you still can. And Seriously, <u>RUN Forest RUN!</u>

<u>50 Ways to Leave Your Lover</u> by Paul Simon 1975 https://www. youtube.com/watch?v=ABXtWqmArUU

<u>Run Forest Run</u> is of course a famous line from Forrest Gump; a 1994 American romantic comedy-drama film based on the 1986 novel of the same name by Winston Groom. It was directed by Robert Zemeckis and written by Eric Roth, and stars Tom Hanks, Robin Wright, Gary Sinise, Mykelti Williamson, and Sally Field. The story depicts several decades in the life of Forrest Gump (Hanks), a slow-witted but kind-hearted man from Alabama who witnesses several defining historical events in the 20th century in the United States.

Now let me be perfectly clear here… as a Minister of the Gospel and as Counsellor, I do not endorse separation and divorce, especially among Christians. However; there are Biblical circumstances where Christ says that it's okay and the Apostle Paul announces conditions for remarrying. Many Denominations are now just looking at Mental and Physical abuse as "breaking of the marriage covenant" and are accepting these reasons for a divorce and permitting remarriage… it's about bloody well time if you ask me. Also, I don't advocate sin, but if you are without Christ, divorce and remarriage are forgiven when you come to Christ. Write me via email and I'll send you my research on the subject of divorce and remarriage. It is quite a fascinating journey. Psychology today has an article on 15 ways to leave your love with love... by Dr. Lissa Rankin, 2011. I've read through it and it is rather interesting from a 'worldly' perspective.

https://www.psychologytoday.com/us/blog/owning-pink/201104/15-ways-leave-your-lover-love

For the Christian Couple who are struggling to 'hang-on' and can't let go, there are a lot of Christian 'Self-Help' books if you will, but which author do you trust? Dr. Chuck Swindoll has an excellent book called "Strike the Original Match" [which I own a copy of, of course] it may be purchased through Amazon and it may be helpful. Of course, you could always go for counselling with your Pastor, or a Christian Psychologist or, you might think about **Joe Beam** who founded **Marriage Helper,** an organization that provides marriage help to hurting couples. He has written an excellent article "What to Do When Your Spouse Wants Out"

https://www.crosswalk.com/family/marriage/divorce-and-remarriage/what-to-do-when-your-spouse-wants-out.html

Here is a link to his seminars: http://www.joebeam.com/seminars.html

But as we all know, there are a dozen of so 'Biblical Scholars' out there who share their opinions on this touchy subject... you just have to find one whom you are familiar with and trust the most.

Okay enough talking about marriage and separation and such, and back to my book. See, I can't stay on course...

Perhaps we should start out slowly and go from there; shall we? I happen to like the question [from the point of a second party] and answer format for this type of thing... so, I'll use that approach from this point forward. Hopefully it will make it easier for me to follow the progression of my living hellish nightmares or my 'living hell' as I shall continue to call it as I face my... **<u>Wall without a Window</u>**

How did you come up with the title for your book?

"Does my Wall have a Window?"

My wife and I sarcastically tossed around a few ideas while sitting in front of the campfire one evening while I scribbled them down on a piece of paper. I even wrote down "My Living Hell" as one of my choices but it just didn't 'zing' for me... it was catchy but it didn't jump up off of the page, you know? But when I started to read my list out loud to her, and even making fun of a few of them along the way, we found that we had liked this one the best... so, here we have it. Isn't that usually how the best things in life come about sometimes? All too often and sarcastically out of nowhere, so it would seem. A wall and a window can mean various things to each individual but in our lives, we come face to face with so many challenges right from the moment we are born to that very last second when we take our last breath and give up the ghost. Some things come naturally of course, such as seeing, hearing, eating, eliminating, breathing, thinking, some moving about and things of that nature, but that's about it.

We have to learn everything else such as; social interaction, right from wrong, good from bad, we learn to crawl, then walk and before we know it, we're running all over the place and falling down. The question is... will there be anyone there for me when I fall down to help me get back up on my feet again? Many of these challenges or hurdles, if you will, in life can either aide or hinder me along my journey and I am either assisted or left to figure things out on my own.

Or not! Isn't that the <u>Law of the Jungle</u>; survival of the fittest? I do believe it is... I wasn't very fit, but yet some how I have managed to survive... perhaps because I outwitted them all and continue to do so to this very day. After all and the trophy doesn't always go to the swift nor to the sure and 'fit' doesn't necessarily always mean physically.

"The law of the jungle" is an expression that means "every man for himself", "anything goes", "survival of the strongest", "survival of the fittest", "kill or be killed", "dog eat dog" or "eat or be eaten".

https://en.wikipedia.org/wiki/Law_of_the_jungle

I have encountered more 'walls' in the way of hinderances and hurdles than assistants in my life and more often than not, I was left to figure things out for myself as I progressed on through my years. Then of course, there was being beaten into submission by the king of the jungle I was forced to dwell with. Fear based obedience came into play at a very early age because I was afraid of the consequences should I disobey… however; I was beaten anyway because there was never pleasing the monster, so what was the point in even trying to be submissive? Either way it was always a crap shoot and I always, yes… always lost. Perhaps that is why I don't gamble today.

For example; everyone should learn about their physical anatomy, their reproductive system, why the sexes are different, where babies come from and how they got in there in the first place, right? Think again… so, when it came time for me to enter puberty or when step-dad thought I should have some knowledge of what was about to change in my body and how girls undergo their transformation as well, etc. He brought home a book from the doctor's office. Throwing [yes, throwing] the book at me he says; "here, read this, if you have any questions, don't ask." "Oh, okay, thanks, I think?"

The only other thing he said on that subject was a couple of years later; "if you're going to have sex, at least have the forethought of wearing protection so that you're not making any babies." "Okay, what's protection?" But I didn't dare ask him. Besides, I already knew. I don't think sex is a small hurdle in a young preteen's life… it's major stuff we're talking about here and all I get is a book thrown at me and told not to ask any questions. Oh, and it wasn't a very good book either. I learned more from commercials, magazines, my mom, some girls and other women on that subject than I ever learned form him and that stupid book. In fact, I hadn't learned anything from him about any of life's important matters except maybe… how NOT to be a dad to my children and how

NOT to parent them. Thanks for the education, asshole! I thought men were suppose to talk to their sons about things of this nature? You know, the birds and the bees, how to make friends and how to be one, how to be a good husband and father, how to help out other people and other interesting life skills of that nature, how to be nice to the ladies, etc., but how was he able to teach me that sort of stuff when he was constantly knocking my mom and me about the house every chance he got? In his case, I thought wrong, and he proved it on every occasion and more often than not, it felt as if the occasion came daily. I could not rely upon him for anything, except to be beaten into submission of course. I viewed this never-ending type of shit as a wall in my life. "Don't do drugs, they're bad for you." "Okay" But, what are drugs and why are they bad? "Just because your friend has one, doesn't mean I have to get you one as well" but I never asked you too. It felt as though he was never home either, and why? "Because I work for a living!" 24/7? "I work for a living so you can get out and earn your way as well" Sure, but at 10 yrs old? I was selling poppies, delivering catalogues for Sears, advertisements, delivering flyers/papers, cutting grass, shoveling walks, driveways, etc., whatever I could do to earn some extra money during the summer vacations, winter weekends, holidays, or what have you.

Old Man: "Have you shoveled anyone's driveway today?"

Me: "No"

Old Man: "It's snowing, get the hell out there!"

That man was so cheap: How cheap was he? He was so cheap, I'm surprised that he didn't charge me rent on the use of his shovel.

A <u>wall</u> has many uses. A wall may be a support, it may be used to divide, to enclose, to contain, it may also be a barrier which must be understood in order to be conquered and overcome. It may be viewed as an obstacle, a hinderance or an aide in life. There are multiple variables left to my mood and to my imagination as to what type of wall I would be facing on any given day.

Wall; as a noun is a continuous vertical brick, stone, or wooden structure that encloses or divides an area of land or is an upright support for a building or structure, [it may also be an invisible barrier of one's imagination].

Of course, there are numerous types of ramparts, but metaphorically speaking, it is an extremely dark clouded barrier found within the caverns of my mind which must some how be dominated before I am able to find relief for a short spell, only to find myself confronting yet another obstacle which became a never-ending cycle for me.

While in the military they taught me to adapt and overcome, but when shit hits the fan, in life, it's difficult to overcome anything to say the least especially when operating on sleep deprivation. Relief for me are the phases in between my maniac and depressive states. No Man's Land if you will, where nothing has control over me and I can almost, yes almost… feel like myself… whomever it is that I think I am. Who is Wayne? That is a question that has often been asked but an answer is not forth coming. But it is I'm sure, something in the nature that I am feeling now… and I'm feeling okay actually. For now, I can laugh, the idiots in traffic don't bother me, I'm polite to people, I hold open doors, I joke around… wow… who is this guy and where did he come from all of a sudden? Hey, I'm perfectly fine when being treated as nicely as I give out, but when people use or abuse me, then I'm not so nice… why is that, and I often ask; why should I be?

Because Christ compels us to treat people regardless of how they treat us, that's why.

No Man's Land is land that is unoccupied or is under dispute between parties who leave it unoccupied due to fear or uncertainty. The term was originally used to define a contested territory or a dumping ground for refuse between fiefdoms. In modern times, it is commonly associated with World War I to describe the area of land between two enemy trench systems, which neither side wished to cross or seize due to fear of being attacked by the enemy in the process.

https://en.wikipedia.org/wiki/No_man%27s_land

For me, tackling this barrier is like a Knight in shinning armour taking on the dragon who is terrorizing the villagers, burning down their crops, their houses and eating people as they run from the sheer terror of it all. It's 'kill,' or be 'killed', there is no third option because dragons are not known for taking prisoners, nor are they tameable. There are no Puff the Magic Dragons in my life or in my dreams.

Puff, the Magic Dragon is a song written by Leonard Lipton and Peter Yarrow, and made popular by Yarrow's group Peter, Paul and Mary in a 1963 recording.

A wall therefore, is no minor hurdle, it's more like a formidable hinderance which hampers every forward progression and I haven't the materials or the knowhow to construct a catapult to blast that puppy into oblivion. More often than not, when I come face to face with this blackened, dense, dank, fog, I encounter what I may perceive to be an impenetrable force and just merely turning up the collar to my favorite winter coat isn't going to keep me warm or safe through this one. Somehow, I know it isn't real but it is an invisible roadblock with such power that it appears to be impregnable just the same, or is it? Keeping in mind that I do hallucinate so it is as real as I am sitting here typing away on this key board.

I therefore, [I like that word, 'therefore', it sounds so 'as a matter of fact'] therefore, I have two choices: the first being that I somehow conquer this obscure veil to continue my life's journey on my own. The 2nd obvious choice is to simply give up and wither away while death overtakes me, I like tiger lilies, thank you.

The question that I and everyone else must ask [whether you suffer with a mental ailment or not] [and these days who doesn't?] and answer is: Am I a fighter or a quitter? Do I have what it takes or do I not? Am I a lion or a mouse? [Pass the cheese, please. Make mine an old cheddar].

While investigating my new-found troubles, I'd query that I have a third option… and that third option for me is that I'm neither, but yet I'm both simultaneously. I am a fighter and will lead the charge because I'm not a quitter but I appear to be, why else would I attempt suicide? Therefore, I must be a quitter! Fight or Flight? I win either way, don't

I? Or, do I? Ah-ha, hence the 'bi' in **bi**polar… being that of having two opposite poles which do not attract but are so different from the other that [for me] they appear to fight their opponent for dominance while repelling one another. The third option I spoke of is the Eeyore Complex and I wouldn't care about a wall in the first place and just stand there doing/accomplishing nothing while hoping this wall will eventually go away all on its own.

Why is life so complicated? Does anyone care? **CARE**, Care, care, care…

Do you Hear that? Hear what? Exactly! No response. No one cares anyway, so, why should I? And fuck it all takes dominance once again. Somewhere in my head I hear a voice which tells me to use my toolbox! "Use your tool box!" "Eh, what's that?" Am I hearing things again? But how do I scale this partition without a rope or a ladder? How do I penetrate a solid barrier without a hammer and chisel of some kind? How do I dig under without a shovel, or go around something that appears to go on and on for all eternity? How do I accomplish anything without the right tools? "Use your tool box!" A whisper that is barely audible echoes again within the canyons of my mind. How do I utilize the tools I've been equipped with if I don't know how or when to use them, or even know that I have need of them in the first place? But I do know that I have them and I should know how to use them because I've been screaming for years for help and have been put on many courses to learn how. Somebody, just shoot me already. Please, anybody, end this misery for me, will you?

For the longest time I, like many others didn't even realize that I was ill and during a maniac episode, who cared? I didn't! Full steam ahead and steady as she goes, or not, only to find myself beached once again.

You couldn't convince me that anything was wrong. I was on cloud nine and I'd make up things as I went, let's just get going already! But where are we going? What does it matter? Who cares? Lets just get there already. What's your problem? I'm going this way whether you're coming along or not because, I'm gone already.

What does a window represent for you?

A window is a-hole-in-the-wall, or perhaps an opening through any type of barrier. Like a skylight in the roof, that if transparent, permits the sunshine to burst through and if opened, allows the flow of fresh air. Sunshine might represent a ray of hope for the future or it could be just a reminder that it is day time and I really should get my butt out of bed. The fresh air is a representation that the worse is over and I can breathe new life again unless it's damp with the smell of rain which would indicate that a storm is brewing on the horizon. A window might also represent an escape route from my dilemma thereby being an aide in life which may perhaps be another blessed hope, of something good that is yet to come. There just might be a chance and a slim one at that mind you, that there will be something better should I only dare to venture up and through finally breaking forth to <u>freedom</u>.

<u>Freedom</u>! As a noun it is the power or right to act, speak, or think as one wants without hindrance or restraint.

I'd say that bipolar disorder would classify as a hindrance, a restraint to the brain and therefore, I have never, nor will I ever, experience true freedom [as defined here] while going through this personal 'living hell'. A window might present an opportunity worth attempting to climb up to and quickly escaping through. God forbid I should fall back down in my attempt to be free only to face the menacing obstacle once again while the cycles continue their never ceasing anguish. But then, I must at least try but people who don't want to listen to my entire dilemma seem to be the hindrance, but why are they holding me back? What's their problem? Then the vision of numerous rats in a cage comes to mind. I'm the one who has found a way out and am trying to escape but the others fear that escape is impossible and they're continuously pulling me back, down, to remain with them in misery. Well, they do say that misery loves company, don't they? Then I come to believe that perhaps that window is just an illusion, why else would they not want me to make a break for it? Perhaps there is some looming danger out there that I am not privy too? This window, if it is real, may also be so far out of reach that I don't bother to climb up for fear of raising my hopes too high only to be dashed as I collapse in utter failure while resolving to kill myself once again. The window may even be so far down the wall the more I walk towards it the further away it appears to be, just like a mirage in my hallucinating, dilutional state of reality. I can't decide if it is really there, or if it is not. To be or not to be, that is the question! [William Shakespeare: Hamlet Act 3 scene 1]

https://www.poets.org/poetsorg/poem/hamlet-act-iii-scene-i-be-or-not-be

Answer your own question for us then: Does my [your] Wall have a Window?

To answer that question honestly; I can not simply offer you a Yes, or No answer, so I won't [not right away, I'm being tormented so I thought I'd pass that a long].

I would have to say that it would depend upon which cycle I'm in, or what phase I'm going through in any particular cycle. Just like that wall, is it really there or am I hallucinating? I have no positive or negative evidence to the fact nor to the contrary, so why do I doubt myself? Conditioning perhaps? When we were kids and someone complained about something that no one could do anything about... we'd give the fella a quarter and tell him to call "1-800-who gives a shit", [the quarter was for the imaginary phone booth] or... we'd ask the fella "would you like me to call you a wambulance?" because you're not getting any sympathy from me, so suck it up princess and get over it already.

So, I had given up any hope of relief and went along with the prognoses [that is if there ever were any while growing up] of the so-called 'experts.' But yet I knew deep in my heart [and in my head] that wasn't the entire deal here. I wanted the full-meal deal whatever that might be... give it to me straight, just the way I enjoy my whisky... without ice, no watering down the good stuff and let's sort this shit out once and for all. I'm not severely depressed right now but I'm not in the 'maniac' phase either.

Most of the time I would say that I can't see a window and would ask you to point it out for me. Even if you were to tell me it's there, "look, it's right there" as you point your outstretched boney finger towards it's general direction, I probably wouldn't believe you because you'd be making fun of me just like the old man, my brothers, the bullies from my childhood, or my co-workers wanting to keep me back by telling me it's an impossible task while they steal all of the glory.

It's often like looking at an island out in the lake and thinking, "I can swim to that." Only to get about half way and suddenly realizing that it's a lot further than it looked and I don't think I'm going to make it and drowning isn't an option either but if I do make it to the island, I still have to swim back. So, I turn around and give it everything I have to make it to shore from whence I first ventured out only to collapse with exhaustion in the shallows. That would be the case of a healthy functioning mind. But we all know that I'm neither healthy nor functioning to full capacity.

In a maniac state… "are you kidding? That's not far, I'll race you to it." And I'd splash into the water before you even got up off of your beach towel.

In a depressive state, I may have only attempted it on a dare. Once I discovered I wasn't going to make it [just as I told you I wouldn't] it would take a lot of encouragement for me to make it back and I wouldn't care if I'd make it or not and give up and drown, [I'm going down for the third time, is anyone going to save me? I suppose not, just like I knew they wouldn't "Good-bye cruel world"!] Blub, blub, blub, and I'd vanish beneath the surface never to be seen or heard from again. Then, from the great beyond, you'd hear me say, "I told you I couldn't make it". My words would haunt you for the rest of your life, and you'd deserve it too.

During my Eeyore Complex, I would look at you, look out towards the general direction of the island and say; "eh, who cares, knock yourself out while I sit here and watch." Then I'd be called all sorts of names… baby, scardie cat, chicken, mama's boy, etc., etc., etc. Why should anything ever change?

Then out of nowhere Maniac Man appears and asks: "Window? What Window? Who needs a window when there's no freaking wall?" Everything is wide open, we're good to go, and its full speed ahead and I'll take no prisoners along the way. Resistance at that point is futile because you're either with me or you're against me. You either come along with the herd or you'll be trampled by it, the choice is yours. But not really, I generally won't give people a choice because the slightest sign of hesitation on your part will be met with... "suite yourself" and I'll leave you in my wake because that ship has sailed and you've missed the boat.

So, does my Wall have a Window?

NO!

Not at this particular moment in time, I'm afraid that it does not! Come back perhaps in a month or so and I might have a completely different answer for you. Oh, but wait... it's been a couple of months already since I've started this book. Hold on, let me check... Nope, I don't see a window, not now nor in my immediate future. I know, that was a long explanation to a question which you might have thought would have been a simple answer. Well think again buster... there isn't anything simple about my life or any of this for that matter. Not from my vantage point anyway. I just had to get that out. Thanks.

It's probably a good thing that there aren't any train tracks around here. I'd more than likely find myself sitting on them playing solitaire while waiting for the noon express from Edmonton. Oh, sure I was often depressed, I resented authority, I quit more jobs than eighty people might have had in a life time and moved around a lot, okay too much, but by who's standards? Okay, so much so to last a normal person 100 life times, there, happy? But I grew up moving around and thought that was my 'normal.' Then leaving home, joining the Navy the moving just naturally continued, so I didn't know anything was out of place, because I hadn't known anything different. I can't imagine people growing up, living in their parent's house and eventually dying there, that too is just not <u>logical</u> and is absurd, and creepy... but moving was my idea of normal.

<u>Logical</u>: adjective; of or according to the rules of logic or formal argument.

I once knew these two farmers in Southern Alberta. Two brothers who owned and operated a grain farm. Both were married but had to buy homes in town for their wives because neither of the women would live on the farm. I don't know why, it was a decent house and there wasn't much in town for them to be active in anyway. Their family farm was about eight miles or so from town and they never ventured beyond a couple of hours drive from there. They'd go into Calgary or Lethbridge regularly but never any further. Huh? I'm serous. I can't even imagine that because I've been in about 30 countries by now and a few of them several times. I've been in every state of the Union some of them many times and have lived in just about every province here in Canada. No, you haven't… Yes, really, I have. What do you mean you've never been more than 2 hours away from home? To me, that's crazy! But that was their 'normal' not mine. To each their own. Right? See what I mean by normalcy… it's different strokes for different folks… hey, wasn't that a sit-com in the 60's or early 70's, why, yes, I do believe it was. See, I can't even stay on topic…

Seriously though, I'm hoping a move is forth coming because I don't like it here and by my estimation, we've been here too long already. Speaking of moves, I found a piece of paper with most of my addresses on it and I filled in the blanks as best I could. So here goes…

5915 Primrose, Cold Lake, AB since 2014
270 Vernon Road, Winnipeg, MB – 2009-2014
347 Chippendale Cres, London, ON – 2006 – 2009
1744 89th Street? Edmonton, AB. 2004 – 2006
245 Mons Ave, Lancaster Park, AB. 2002 – 2004
3766 Greenlane Rd., Beamsville, ON 2001 – 2002
4294 John St. Beamsville, ON 2000 – 2001
10 Saturn Rd. Port Colborne, ON 01/2000 – 08/2000
Pine Crest Motel, Hwy 3. R.R. 1 Dunville, ON 11/1999 – 01/2000
1940 Regional Road 12 – R.R. 1 Smithville, ON 09/1999 – 10/1999
Kings' Court Dr. Waterloo, ON 06/1999 – 09/1999
7 Amherst Dr. Kitchener, ON 05/1999 – 06/1999
#7 – 350 Wellington Road, Port Colborne, ON 1996 – 1999
7 Apollo Drive, Port Colborne, ON 06/1999 – 09/1999
12163, Braun Rd. Wainfleet, ON 1995 – 1996
Dune Village Rd. Kitchener, ON 1994 – 1995
R.R. 2 Bamberg, ON 04/1994 – 07/1994
#7 Morgan Road, Richibucto, NB 02/1994 – 06/1994

Hwy 126 Lot 34, Adamsville, NB 10/1993 – 02/1994
1054-C Churchill Avenue, Kitchener, ON 04/1992 – 10/1993
2 addresses in Regina Beach, Sk.
1 Address in Lumsden, Sk.
RR1 Lumsden, Sk. Poultry Farm
Keeler Sk.
Alliance, AB.
Vauxhall, AB – Sheep Ranch
Wetaskiwin, AB – Poultry Farm
Longview, AB – Poultry Farm and Ranch
2 Address in Calgary, AB
King Edward Ave, London, ON
Putnam, ON - Turkey Farm
Thamesford, ON - Turkey Farm
Emery St. London, ON. – went back to High School
King Edward Ave, (1st residence)
Wonderland Road, London ON
Norton Cres. London, ON
PMQ's in Shelburne NS
Residence Shelburne NS
Barracks @ CFS Shelburne
2 Apartments in Dartmouth, NS
Barracks @ CFS Stadacona, Halifax, NS
HMCS Protector, Halifax, NS
CFB Borden, ON – Trade course
CFB Cornwallis, NS Boot Camp
Elgin St. Waterloo, ON (grade 10)
York St. Kitchener, ON (grades 6 – 9)
High St. Waterloo, ON (grades 3 – 6))
7 State Court, Waterloo, ON (grades K – 3)
Apartment downtown, Waterloo, ON (age 3 – grade K)
Avondale Rd. Kitchener, ON
Collingwood, ON
2 Residences in St. Catherine's, ON
Victoria. BC (born here)
OMG! That's what? 55 residences? Crazy or what, eh?

I don't know about you, but I count 8 provinces… and a few several times, so, go ahead, count them for yourself… And that ladies and gentlemen is the best I can do for now. I could spout off quite a few of my employment situations but I really don't think that there is a need for that. I think you have enough to give you an indication of what a living hell I've been through. I don't even remember how we got on to this topic in the first place but once I started I suppose I had to show off a bit… oh well, shall we carry on?

Two questions some psychologists have asked over the years [but never really followed up on] were:

Did you have a happy childhood and if I ever felt loved growing up?

I can hear the roar of the Sunday crowd, ah, you're killing me with laughter! LOL can not begin to express the tears rolling down my cheeks from those hysterical questions. Does rolling on the floor laughing my ass off mean anything to you? Well, it should and would if you knew anything about my happy, loving childhood.

No, seriously…those were two legitimate questions and this really isn't supposed to be a comedy show…

Sorry! Let me compose myself. Okay, I'll be alright. Maybe.

Are You sure you're quite finished?

No, but let's continue… snicker… chuckle, ah, you're killing me.

Sorry, that was just me laughing out loud again, "Woooooooo I'm dyyyyyyyyin'!?"

Happiness and love were only words in a dictionary for which I hadn't the foggiest idea of what they meant… what an ignoramus… I know, eh? Not only had I not known the meaning of those words, I neither had the occasion to be bothered looking them up when I was a child and there wasn't a remote chance of them echoing through the corridors of any of my residences for that matter because I lived with an Ogre who aren't known for their niceties you know. You can look up Ogres for yourself to, or do I have to do everything for you?

Not to be a smart-ass or anything, well, okay, I am, so I'll answer the question with a question;

What is happiness?

What does it mean to be happy? [okay, 2 questions]

Psychologically, **happiness** [oh, this aught to be rich] is a mental or emotional state of well-being [lol] which can be defined by **positive** or **pleasant** emotions ranging from <u>**contentment**</u> [that too may be my problem, I have not yet learned to be content] to intense joy. Joy was a girl I knew once in grade school, but I don't think she's involved here in anyway... That's about the closest I ever came to being 'happy' while growing up in a monster's lair. There were no 'positive', pleasant emotions floating in the air to cause happiness in my house.

<u>Contentment</u>: noun; a state of happiness [there's that word again] and satisfaction. Oh. Okay. Ya, right, satis-what? The Stones song "can't get no satisfaction" come to mind right about now.

I can definitely understand what the Apostle Paul is saying here in Philippians 4:11-13: "[11] I am not saying this because I am in need, for I have learned to be content whatever the circumstances. [12] I know what it is to be in need, and I know what it is to have plenty. I have learned the secret of being content in any and every situation, whether well fed or hungry, whether living in plenty or in want. [13] I can do all this through him who gives me strength." I know what it is to have plenty, I understand want and need, because I've lived through them both but that 'contentment' part... I have no idea what that would even look like in my life. I agree that I can do all this through him who gives me strength, when there is that connection... and I know Christ promised to be with me always. However; more often than not, I 'feel' so all alone in that sense... I can understand what Mother Tereasa meant when she wrote in one of her letters about "Understanding the Dark Soul". You know that famous 'Foot Prints' picture... where we see two sets of foot prints in the sand and then we only see one set of prints. At that point we're supposed to be encouraged because it represents the time in our lives where Christ carries us... well, for me, it represents the times in my life when I've been abandoned once again and I am truly alone facing my demons while traversing my living hell in an attempt to remain alive. Why is it that I wish to live? For whom and/or what am I living for?

Oh, I'm familiar with the word and I understand its definition but I've rarely, if ever have experienced 'happiness' or what some might refer to as 'true-happiness'. I would say that there is no such critter [okay, perhaps I am delusional]. I have found temporary 'happiness' when I was left alone to play by myself or when step-dad was out of the house or when I was out of the house at Cubs, Scouts, Cadets or Work but those moments were fleeting and far and few in between. Perhaps I'd find a glimmer of 'happiness' with friends, but not to any great extent mind you because I really did not know what happiness or contentment was/is. Plus, I also had a hard time trusting people and I never knew when these so-called friends would turn on me for whatever reason or for no reason at all. That is why I didn't have any friends in the hood or at school because most of the kids were bullies and only pretended to be my friend should I have something they wanted. If I didn't share with them, they'd just take it away so I generally made sure I didn't have anything in my possession that they would want to have. But they still picked on me anyway. So, just like at home, I couldn't win either way. There were people I hung out with while at Cubs, Scouts and Cadets but they were not my 'friends' by any stretch of the imagination. What were they? Mere acquaintances with the similar interests. Most of them I wouldn't see outside of these activities. I can tell you somethings that made me 'happy' for that particular moment in time, but as a euphoric all-around general state of 'being'? It's nothing more than an illusion that everyone is in pursuit of... ["Hey have you found happiness today?" "No, but he's around here somewhere, I can feel him close by"]. Ya, right, whatever. Whose dilutional now?

"The American Dream" is a happy way of living that is thought of by many Americans as something that can be achieved by anyone in the U.S. especially by working hard and becoming successful

♦ With good jobs, a nice house, two children, and plenty of money, they believed they were living the American dream.

As described by Merriam-Webster Dictionary:

https://www.merriam-webster.com/dictionary/the%20American%20dream

Old Man... "Because of You" by Reba... [Recorded with Kelly Clarkson and released August 16, 2005]

Because of you, I never stray too far from the sidewalk, Because of you I learned to play on the safe side so I don't get hurt. Because of you, I find it hard to <u>trust</u> not only me, but everyone around me... Because of you, I am afraid. Or better yet, I am untrusting because I lived in fear every waking moment of every day and slept quite lightly for the same reasons. I never feared anyone after I broke free from his clutches though and it often got me into trouble. More often than not, I really don't care what other people think of me either. Or, had I? I would venture to say not, for the most part that is.

As a child, being out and away from 'his' house caused other anxieties because I always had to return while never knowing what frame of mind the brute would be in. Would he be hungry for skin and bones or had his appetite been quenched with beer? Or has the alcohol made him meaner and hungrier for my flesh and blood? If quenched with malt, how was his overall demeanour? Would I be able to sneak in and make it to my room before the devil realizes I'm stalking about? <u>Anxiety</u> disorder? Who says I was anxious? If he wasn't home when I arrived, I always worried about his disposition when he too would have no choice and finally be forced to return to his hidey-hole [I've always been a light sleeper and still am to this very day, thanks again to you know who]. Would I be left alone in my slumber or would I be woken up by their fighting downstairs, or would they skip round 4 only to sneak upon me and I'd find myself being ripped from my cozy cot to be beat upon once again for some imaginary atrocity that I may or may not have committed during his absence. I generally slept on the top bunk so, being torn from my bed also meant falling to the floor, which could cause some minor damages in the process, depending upon how I landed. More often than not, when I'd walk by the prick and he'd reach out and SMACK… me while laughing "that's for what you're thinking, just wait until you really do something." You don't even want to know my thoughts at that point… I'll leave that up to your imagination, but if you're thinking they began with 'f' and ended in 'u', you win a cookie. But I didn't dare say anything because I'd get another smack, or worse.

He dragged me out of my bed in the middle of the night to deliver a beating on me more instances than I care to remember. One night I thought I was safe. I put the television in front of the door so he was unable to enter at his whim. Well, you can all imagine how well that went over and what happened to me the next day… I got it worse because he hadn't been able to get a hold of me when he had wanted too which gave him time to stew and brew about it just like a witches' cauldron [Double, double toil and trouble; Fire burn, and cauldron bubble]. He was fuming when he caught up with me the next day lecturing me about how it may be 'my bedroom' but it was 'his house' and he'd go wherever or do whatever he damned well pleased and if I didn't like it I could leave any time… while he's pounding on my shoulder with his fist naturally. You try going back to sleep when your ass is burning, or your shoulders are aching, or with lumps on your head, or a bleeding nose, or a sore eye, or a fat lip… and I was supposed to get up for school the next morning… R-i-g-h-t, and exactly how do I do that?

Needless to say, that I learned to sleep lightly or to barely sleep at all. Many times, I'd hide under my bed or in the closet so he couldn't find me. But, you know he always had. Except that one time I heard them fighting and I hid in the crawl space of the house. He didn't think of looking in there. I figured if he couldn't see me in my bed, he wouldn't bother looking for me. But that only worked when I was in my mid teens and had a part-time job which sometimes kept me out until 2 a.m. on a Friday or Saturday night…. he'd just figured I hadn't arrived home from work yet so, that maneuver had out smarted him a few times.

This one time, we were at his father's place at the beach… step-dad and I were playing horseshoes… problem with that was, I was constantly looking over my shoulder because I never knew how close he'd stand behind me because he had a habit of grabbing the shoe just as I'm winding up to swing with all my might so the shoe makes it to the opposite peg… that sudden stop almost ripped the shoulder out of my socket… "that hurts" I call out… "don't be such a baby and play the damn game" he'd say. This one time I blurted out "Fuck-off" but luckily it wasn't loud enough for him to quite hear what I said… "what did you say?" quickly thinking… I answered "back-off, that hurts" he laughed called me a "baby" [again] so I dropped the horseshoes and walked away form him. "Where are you going"? "Anywhere, where you're not" I replied and kept on going. I'm surprised he didn't come after me… he just called out "Big Baby!" And of course, I said aloud for no one to hear but myself… fuck you, and I really wanted to give him the finger but knew better than that… needless to say I never played horseshoes or any other game with that man again.

Anxiety: People with anxiety disorders frequently have intense, excessive and persistent worry and fear about everyday situations. Often, anxiety disorders involve repeated episodes of sudden feelings of intense anxiety and fear or terror that reach a peak within minutes (panic attacks).

Shakespeare Quote of Double, Double Toil and Trouble…

https://www.shmoop.com/shakespeare-quotes/double-double-toil-and-trouble/

Terror: noun, meaning extreme fear.

I'm surprised I didn't have stomach ulcers by the young age of 10.

You asked: **Did I have a happy childhood?**

If you call happiness walking on Lego Bricks in my bare feet constantly being in fear of EVERYTHING including my own shadow… while never knowing what kind of mood 'Cousin It' would be in, not knowing if/when he'd reach out and smack me just because he could, or in fear of making too much noise on a Sunday morning and waking the brute who is forever looking for the slightest excuse to break forth and devour little ole me, or being afraid of breaking something, or ducking when he quickly raises a hand to scratch his head and I think I'm about to get clobbered while the son-of-a-bitch laughs, etc., – then yes, I suppose I had a happy childhood. Thinking about it now, I'm surprised I don't have some sort of underlined paranoia disorder as well. Who's there? What was that? Am I being followed? We've done it now, here he comes… run and hide! It's everyone for themselves! Or, do I?

Paranoia: a mental condition characterized by delusions of persecution, [huh? no delusions here] unwarranted jealousy, or exaggerated self-importance, typically elaborated into an organized system. It may be an aspect of chronic personality disorder, of drug abuse, or of a serious condition such as schizophrenia in which the person loses touch with reality. Loses touch with reality? That wasn't reality to begin with… that was a never-ending hellish nightmare. Come to think of it, I'm really surprised that I'm not schizoid as well. Well, I'll be darned.

Schizophrenia: noun; a long-term mental disorder of a type involving a breakdown in the relation between thought, emotion, and behavior, leading to faulty perception, inappropriate actions and feelings, withdrawal from reality and personal relationships into fantasy and delusion, and a sense of mental fragmentation… or am I? But that's what I'm trying to tell you, it was my reality, there was no 'losing touch' about it.

Didn't you know that children were to be seen but underlined never heard? Try tip-toeing through those tulips Tiny Tim!

Never: adverb; at no time in the past or future; on no occasion; not ever.

Tiny Tim: musician; https://en.wikipedia.org/wiki/Tiny_Tim_(musician)

Moving on with the 2nd question, then shall we?

What about Love?

Seriously, What about it?
Oh, I'm suppose to answer that question as well?
Again, almost rolling on the floor laughing my ass off… excuse me, I think I have to pee…. answering the question with yet more questions;

What is <u>love</u>?

I've heard that love is a many splendid thing, I've heard that it can also be fickle and it is better to have loved and lost, than never to have loved at all.

But seriously, is that a person, place or thing, can I eat it, smoke it, shovel it, or is it another one of those 'state of being' you keep wanting to talk about?

'Love is in the air' [John Paul Young, released in 1977] sounds like a wonderful concept.

I asked Google how many songs there were which contained the word 'Love', it was unable to answer the question. That many huh? Love is just another word that meant absolutely nothing to me while growing up. Read my lips... okay, you can't see my lips, but read the word: N-O-T-H-I-N-G!

This is what Wikipedia says about love in it's first paragraph alone:

<u>Love</u> encompasses a variety of different emotional and mental states, [how do they do that? Put emotional and mental states in the same sentence?] typically strongly and positively experienced, [he, he, he, that's rich, positive experience, what a maroon, what a nincompoop] ranging from the most sublime virtue or good habit, the deepest interpersonal affection [deep what?] and to the simplest pleasure [nothing pleasurable there]. An example of this range of meanings is that the love of a mother differs from the love of a spouse differs from the love of food. Most commonly, love refers to a feeling of strong attraction and emotional attachment. Love can also be a virtue representing human kindness, compassion, and affection, as "<u>the unselfish loyal and benevolent concern for the good of another</u>" [you're kidding, right?] It may also describe <u>compassionate</u> and <u>affectionate</u> <u>actions towards other humans</u>, one's self or animals [the only affection I ever felt from the behemoth was from his belt, the back of his hand or from his fists]. What do you say in a moment like this when you can't find the words to tell it like it is? Reba... "What do you Say?"

https://en.wikipedia.org/wiki/Love [oh, that was rich, I needed a good laugh, thank you].

Pass a Kleenex please, my eyes are tearing up from this hysterical moment that I can't even read the words on the page. I need to pee again, excuse me... oh, that was good. It always helps to have a good old-fashioned belly laugh.

There wasn't an air of unselfish, virtue representing human kindness, compassion and/or affection anywhere in that man's body let alone displayed towards myself. I often think the only thing he was compassionate about was his time away from 'his house', his drinking time with his buddies and I have to include his time with the various ladies who were stupid enough to have him in their beds. I believe he only worked because it was a means to his ends. He went out for: Darts on Monday evenings at the Legion; Cribbage on Wednesday evenings at the Legion; Bowling on Friday evenings [just conveniently a block away from the Legion]. When I was old enough to leave the house by myself I went to: Cubs on Tuesdays; Scouts Wednesday. As of the age of 13: Cadets on Tuesday, Band practice on Thursdays and Sunday afternoons... see the connection? Then he almost always visited to the Legion on Saturday afternoons while I was left in the car in the parking lot or at home during the winter months... yes, alone, and from an early age [try that today and a parent would be slapped with child abandonment charges]. Then he went back out to the Legion on Saturday nights.

So, where was this Children's Aide Society back then and just exactly what was their mandate if it wasn't to protect little kids like myself who were constantly being tortured, neglected, rarely had proper meals to eat or clean clothes to wear? Sometimes the parents would come home with groceries and sometimes they would not. Saturday nights, if he wasn't working the bar, [driving taxi for extra cash], during the dances he was trying to pick up every woman present. Married or not, it didn't matter to that hound dog. How do I know? What do you think he and mom fought about more often than not? Like she was one to talk... apparently, he couldn't have children [so the story went] so, she went out and had 5 children with 5 different men, so give me a fucking break already. We all know a woman doesn't usually get pregnant on the first go-round, so what does that tell you? I know because she'd bring some of these tom-cats' home from time to time and I'd hear the two of them in her bedroom or on the couch making funny noises. Sometimes I snuck down the stairs to find out what all the funny noise and quiet laughter was all about… [well, more often than not, they weren't very quiet] and before I was old enough to realize what that was all about, I saw her naked with a fella who wasn't step-dad doing funny things to her on many occasions throughout my younger years.

I remember the cartoon strip called "Love Is" that came out in 1975 by Kim Casali. I think the artist portrait something like 800 or so, various things that 'love is', but I had not experienced any one of them, no NOT a single ONE of them growing up in the freak's house. Nor had I ever heard those three 'magical' words either.

"I love you." I'd probably have shit my pants for sure if I ever was to hear them.

I only heard the other four words of praise once in my life when I was 17. Those words were: "I'm proud of you." Which of course were quickly negated when he asked which Navy trade I had chosen and he called me a 'stupid-ass' upon hearing my answer. So, what's the point? Garbage in, garbage out they always say and I always thought of him as garbage that I wished I could have taken out to the curb to forget about, never to be seen or heard from again. Good riddens, I say!

My mother never ever uttered those three words that I can remember either, not even while lying on her death bed in the hospital. Nor would she tell me who my biological father is/was… I honestly can't help but wonder if she even knew herself because she'd been with so many guys in her younger years.

I am aware of the world's definition of this mysterious word 'LOVE' for which we utter all too often without meaning or thinking about what it was that we have just said. To me, it was nothing more than just another word found between 'lovat' and 'loveable' on page 588 of my Webster's Dictionary, without expression of life or meaning. When I became a teenager, I quickly learned though that 'love' was a word I said to a girl when I wanted to have sex with her, but I never really knew what it meant or recognized its true sentimental value or the deep impact that it would have upon another human being until I was married… but aren't Love and Happiness the very two things that the majority of us are looking for in life but lacking the most?

Oh, I intellectually understood the concept and had been the recipient of people's 'love' as they expressed it in many ways, especially my wives and their commitment to stand beside me through whatever hell I was facing or dragging them through at the time. I even remember the first girl who uttered those words to me… she wanted to get married at a young age, but I didn't, couldn't… how was I suppose to move out and support us? We were still in high school for Pete's sake. I went off to the Navy and she went off and got married to someone else as soon as she was 16. I saw her later in life, just as beautiful as I remembered her. She had three lovely daughters but a lousy choice of men and she blamed it all on me because I wouldn't marry her. I never heard those words from my siblings either while growing up. My siblings and I utter that word now from time to time, but not then. The word was just not in our vocabulary. Love was a mystery to say the least. Another elusive beast that I am forever on the hunt for.

I have long since then, come to learn and understand the Greek philosopher's four definitions of the word 'love' as well as the biblical meaning of what 'love' is to God because "God is Love" 1 John 4:8, and John 3:16 is but one Huge monumental demonstration of God's love towards mankind while we are yet sinners. Other than being the recipient of my wives' love, I had never truly experienced it in life while growing up. The toughest thing about this concept was that I couldn't understand how it was possible for a Heavenly Father whom I could not see, was capable of loving me, when an earthly Father, whom I could see and interact with on a regular basis does not? I'm sure many people face this same dilemma, so they understand my position and it is for that reason alone, that many people do not believe that there is a God in Heaven who is capable of loving them. Not to mention, not being able to understand how a 'loving' God could allow such atrocities to happen to an innocent child over and over and over and over again. Because of the fall of man there will always be sin in the world and God is not to blame but people don't make the connection and God, always gets the bum wrap. I think now would be a good time to search your heart and speak to God. Whisper a prayer and let Him speak you your heart right here and right now:

1. We must acknowledge God as the Creator of everything, accepting our humble position in God's created order and purpose. Romans 1:20-21

"For since the creation of the world His invisible attributes are clearly seen, being understood by the things that are made, even His eternal power and Godhead, so that they are without excuse, because, although they knew God, they did not glorify Him as God, nor were thankful, but became futile in their thoughts, and their foolish hearts were darkened."

2. We must realize that we are sinners and that we need forgiveness. None of us are worthy under God's standards. Romans 3:23

"For all have sinned, and fall short of the glory of God."

3. God gave us the way to be forgiven of our sins. He showed us His love by giving us the potential for life through the death of His Son, Jesus Christ. Romans 5:8

"But God demonstrates His love toward us, in that, while we were still sinners, Christ died for us."

4. If we remain sinners, we will die. However, if we repent of our sins, and accept Jesus Christ as our Lord and Savior, we will have eternal life. Romans 6:23

"For the wages of sin is death, but the gift of God is eternal life in Christ Jesus our Lord."

5. Confess that Jesus Christ is Lord and believe in your heart that God raised Him from the dead and you are saved. Romans 10:9-10

"That if you confess with your mouth the Lord Jesus and believe in your heart that God has raised Him from the dead, you will be saved.

For with the heart one believes unto righteousness, and with the mouth confession is made unto salvation."

6. There are no other religious formulas or rituals. Just call upon the name of the Lord and you will be saved! Romans 10:13

"For whoever calls on the name of the LORD shall be saved."

7. Determine in your heart to make Jesus Christ the Lord of your life today. Romans 11:36

"For of Him and through Him and to Him are all things, to whom be glory forever. Amen.""Repent, and let every one of you be baptized in the name of Jesus Christ for the remission of sins; and you shall receive the gift of the Holy Spirit." (Acts 2:38)

If you decided to receive Jesus today, welcome to God's family. Now, as a way to grow closer to Him read the Book of John, then Matthew, The Book of Acts, the rest of the Gospels and then go from there. Follow up in your commitment by finding a Bible believing Church… Get baptized as commanded by Christ, tell someone else about your new faith in Christ. Spend time with God each day in prayer and in His Word. It does not have to be a long period of time. Just develop the daily habit of praying to Him and reading His Word. Ask God to increase your faith and your understanding of the Bible. Seek fellowship with other followers of Jesus. Develop a group of believing friends to answer your questions and support you.

Okay, I squirreled again but that was a good one. Email me and inform me as to where you are in all of this. wayne_driver@outlook.com because I really want to know and to help you in your new walk of faith in anyway that I am able too. God Bless.

Personally, I always thought that my step-dad had always been and always will be, incapable of loving anyone but himself and his booze never mind possessing the ability to express it to anyone, especially to yours truly. Oh, okay, so the truth be told; he had to stop drinking years ago because the doctors took out half of his stomach because he developed bleeding ulcers because he drank too much. But he was nothing more than a <u>dry drunk</u> who was forced to stop drinking. It is my personal opinion, but I feel that he became meaner than he already was [as if that were possible] after he was forced to stop drinking. How that man has managed to have had 4 wives let alone 1, with a few lady friends along the way, I'll never know. Come to think of it, three of the four have all died of various cancers while he yet lives… funny thing is, this 4th one has cancer of some sort as well.

The term <u>dry drunk</u> is believed to originate from 12 Step recovery groups. It is used to describe those who no longer drink alcohol but, in many ways, behave like they were still in the midst of their addiction. The dry drunk may be full of resentment and anger. Instead of finding joy in their life away from alcohol, they can act as if they were serving a prison sentence. The only change this person has made is to stop drinking, but in other respects their life remains the same. Friends and family can complain that the dry drunk is almost as hard to be around as they were when drinking. In AA, they describe it as a person that hasn't touched alcohol in years but have not yet managed to get sober.

So, <u>No</u>, I had NEVER experienced 'LOVE' growing up while living in that 'persons' house!

But you know what really made me sick to my stomach over the years? Was that I **had** to kiss that bastard 'goodnight' before going off to bed, yes… even after he had just beat on my ass. A kiss on the cheek, and off to bed I'd go. Shortly there after, they would go out drinking. I was elated when the day came when that loathsome ritual had ceased forever. Oh, and the praying and the saying of grace as well… if we can't talk about this 'shit' as he put it, in his house… what was all that about? One day I just finally decided that I wasn't going to pray [because God never answered my prayers anyway] nor say Grace at the table any longer. Perhaps they had learned from the Corn Flakes War and hadn't given me a hard time about all of this. And, the kiss good-night before going to bed? What was that all about? Why should I show affection to some prick that just beat me half senseless? I remember me standing there at 10yrs old with my arms crossed…

Him: "It's time for bed, come give me a kiss good-night"

Me: "No, I'm not giving you a kiss goodnight anymore"

Him: "Why not?"

Me: "Because you're always mean to me and beat me and I don't know why."

Him: SMACK

Me: "There, you just did it again."

Him: SMACK again… "Get the hell out of my sight"

Me: to myself… gladly, and off to bed I went and have not kissed him over the past 50 years and he has no one to blame but himself.

"Good-night" indeed. "Ya, right… I hope you get drunk and drown in your own vomit you bastard" were many a night's thoughts for me, praying to God [if there was one] that He would make it happen. [I never really believed in God as a child because he never answered any of my prayers, nor had he ever saved me from any of the beatings and I don't know why]. If that had have happened, then and only then would I truly have a 'goodnight' not to mention a peaceful rest of my life. And maybe, just maybe mind you, I might have come to believe in this mystical heavenly Father who was so foreign to me.

Did you know that if you haven't got an answer, then you haven't got a question? And if you haven't got a question, then you'd never had a problem, but if you've never had a problem then everyone would be 'happy' and if everyone was happy there'd never be a love song… Harry Nilsson, "Joy" [10 July 1972]

I suppose I should have written a lot of love songs, shouldn't I? I do have a couple of poems that have been published out there, somewhere, once upon a time.

Tell us about your humble beginnings then.

"How much time do we have?"

"Take all the time you need, it's a book remember."

"Oh Ya, it's a book, so I'll take all the time I need, and as many pages as I require as well too. Thank you,"

"You're very welcome."

I'm the second oldest of 5 children (3 boys, 2 girls) born 6 minutes after midnight on **Friday January 23, 1959** [just in case a fan wants to send me a birthday greeting] to a pair of retched, miserable, always fighting alcoholic parents. Some of the war movies I've seen over the years made it look like an adventure compared to my upbringing. More often than not, it was like witnessing a war movie unfolding right before my very eyes within the confines of my house and then just for the hell of it, flack would come my way. Perhaps you thought cats and dogs didn't get along. Huh, those four-legged fur balls couldn't hold a candle to these two. Especially on Sundays for some reason [Oh! Oh! Mr., Kotter, Mr. Kotter... I know why, because they were 'forced' to be in the same house together for general living purposes other than lying down to sleep] it was... more often than not... like watching a middle-weight vs a fly-weight... and in this Corner, weighing in at 182lbs, standing 5'8"... 'The Monster' and in this Corner... weighing in at a mere 105lbs [soaking wet] standing 4'11" "the Cape Breton Contender"! and believe me... there were no holds barred and anything went and usually did... everything from hair pulling to kicks to the groin to being thrown down the stairs... or being violently raped. But, the fly-weight got in her slaps, punches, kicks, bites, chunks of hair pulled out and kicks to the gonads on many occasions that I personally witnessed. One time I had to run away to laugh because she grabbed him by his kahunas, brought him to his knees, shoved him backwards and then ran like a scared rabbit out the back door not to be seen or heard from for several days. Needless to say, that she was knocked about when she returned. I asked her many times, "why don't we just leave?" "I have nowhere to go with 5 kids" she'd say and leave it at that. On one occasion, I believe I was about 10 when I heard them fighting in the bedroom. All I kept hearing was her yelling, "stop!" "don't" "you're hurting me" I don't know what the hell I was thinking, maybe I thought that I could save her or something? I'm invincible, remember? I ran into their room and the first sight I saw was both of them naked from the waste down. He had her pinned face down on the bed and he was standing behind her. Of course, I had no idea what he was doing and yelled out "you leave my mom alone!" I was yelled back at to "get the hell out" and he kicked at me as I scrambled away to which I then heard the slamming of the door and the tumbling of the locking mechanism and her yelling at him some more. Of course, I received a beating afterwards for barging in on them and was told that I was never to go into their room again. As far as I can remember, I never had after that frightful incident.

"Monday's Child" (1967) is one of many fortune-telling songs, popular as nursery rhymes for children. It is supposed to tell a child's character or future based on the day of birth and to help young children remember the seven days of the week. As with all nursery rhymes, there are many versions.

Monday's child is fair of face, Tuesday's child is full of grace, Wednesday's child is full of woe, Thursday's child has far to go, <u>Friday's child is loving and giving</u>, Saturday's child works hard for a living, And the child that is born on the Sabbath day Is bonny and blithe, and good and gay.

According to this… I'm suppose to be a 'loving and giving' person… how can I be loving when I had no idea what love was? I could be 'giving' though and very helpful while growing up… but back then as in today… it would all depend upon what phase I am in at any given moment I'm sure. I'm a Dr. Jekyll and Mr. Hyde [is a gothic novel by the Scottish author Robert Louis Stevenson first published in 1886, which became a film in 1931] or Bruce Banner and the Hulk, [we all know who they are] kind of guy… it's complicated, but then, that's what this book is all about, isn't it? The complications of living with an undiagnosed bipolar disorder. I can be the most loving person you'll ever meet, until you do me wrong… I know, it isn't right and I'm just figuring that out as I obviously have a disconnect but what goes around comes around I suppose. But we'll get into this a little later.

Over the years though, I've been known to do great and wonderful things for people. I'd give away a fair amount of money, buy meals for folks on the street, purchase groceries for the single mom, give rides to strangers, loan out tools, my vehicle, cut grass and shovel snow for neighbours, bring strangers into my home for a hot meal, a bath, a bed and give them my clothes if they fit, or I'd wash theirs for them… but looking back, I have discovered that I wouldn't necessarily have to be in a maniac cyclone to help someone… that was just my nature. What? Are we talking about me? Yes, we are. I've even ran into a burning building on not one, but two separate occasions in an attempt to save souls. Now truly, tell me, who does that other than trained fire fighters?

Oh, yes, we were talking about my humble beginnings, sorry… can't seem to stay focused I guess. See… and what were one of the symptoms? Oh yes, being easily distracted.

In my opinion, humble or not as it may be, step-brute was a mean-spirited, ungenerous, harsh, nasty, heartless, malicious, hateful, spiteful, vindictive, deplorable, detestable, insufferable, revolting, repulsive, disgusting, vile, dreadful, abominable, abusive, horrid, vindictive, malicious, malevolent, hurtful, hateful, violent, cruel, inhumane, obnoxious, offensive, insulting, unmannerly, sadistic, evil, retched [have I used enough adjectives for you to get the picture?] drunk of a man. The more he drank the meaner he became when around me anyway. As if everything was my fault or something… okay, perhaps some things were, but not everything. When I was in my early teens, sometimes I'd be up late with friends and playing Monopoly or something and he'd want to join in after a night of drinking at the Legion. Sometimes he would 'goof' around but he always 'played' rough and I'd get hurt… for some reason he always liked twisting the arm that got broken. Again, the name calling would start and I'd walk away. Who needs that crap? So, more often than not, I would spare myself the agony and just walk away when 'he' wanted to 'play'. There were many times though I told him that he couldn't play Monopoly with us because I deemed him to be too intoxicated. To which of course he responded with a slap to the face and he shut our game down. So, yes, there's a loving dad who nurtured me in a happy environment.

Hold up… weren't there 5 children?

Yes, but I'm not here to tell their stories, only my own. So, I'll use the singular as if I were an only child, it's my book and right now, I'm the only one who matters. It's the team of me, Remember? Me, myself and I are the only ones who count at this point... Go Team Wayne!

Oh right... Sorry, I forgot...

That's okay, just don't let it happen again, now on with the show!

Monsters' idea of discipling was by [rarely, just] spanking but [usually] beating on me while calling me names, or by telling me 'not' to do whatever it was I had done, again. There were a few times I remembered just being 'spanked' but those moments were extremely rare and far and few in between, so much so that it's hard to recall those rare moments. As more often than not, he started with a 'spanking' to get the truth out of me and then when the truth [according him] was made known, he then took it up a few notches and I was beaten senseless. More often than not, I had to tell him what he wanted to hear [truth or not] because he hardly ever believed what I had to tell him. Mom was a bit more fun loving but a hypochondriac at the same time who appeared to be allergic to everything on the planet or had every [unseen] sickness known to man who gobble down whatever pills the doctor would prescribe her. But, she seemed to be constantly busy nursing an ailment of some kind or another and never had time to spend with me. She appeared to be hungover or have some kind of headache or sinus troubles until the evening rolled around that is, when she would go out drinking again. I've heard her call-in sick on many occasions just so that she wouldn't have to report in for the evening shift, but that hadn't stopped her from going out drinking until the cows came home [who do you think I learned to tell lies to my supervisor from to get me out of work?] Many of their fights were also about how one of them would disappear for awhile and the other would want to know where the other was... I can only guess... can you? Let's just say, the cars were bigger back then and had larger back seats. If she was working the evening shift, she generally joined him at the Legion before for last call or she'd bring someone home for 'last call' while knowing that her husband wouldn't be home for sometime yet to come. Come to think of it, I don't believe the old man ever walked in on her with someone else. I do recall a few fellows giving her a few bucks after their little play time. But again, I was too young to know what that was all about. She wasn't so mean-spirited as the beaster was, but she wasn't without her moments either and was definitely the farthest thing from a saint… quite the opposite really. There were many times when she'd blame me for her troubles and told something or other to the old man and I'd get a beating when he got home while she'd stand idly by watching the show with that stupid smug smile of satisfaction on her face. "Mess with me, will you, you little bugger?" "Just wait till your father gets home!" "Oh shit!" I'm in for it now… oh well, what else is new? When mom said: "Just wait until you father gets home!" I may as well continue whatever action it was that I was engaged in and make it worth my while because she always followed through on that threat. So, I'd ignore her and continue doing whatever it was I was just told not to do. Why not? I'm already in trouble anyway, so what did it matter? It was already game over for me. Her idea of disciplining though was yelling, grounding, smacking me with the wooden spoon or threatening to tell the old man on me. Misbehaving in her mind was anything that a kid could do that would annoy her… and that was just about everything from running through the house to laughing too loud at the cartoons. Kids fighting I'm sure was never pleasant but it seemed as though no matter what I did, it bothered her.

Next to 'telling the old man" her other favourite was threatening to call the "Children's Aide Society" [whoever they were] on me. They apparently were people who would come and take me away and I'd never see them or my siblings ever again and I'd have to grow up with strangers, blah, blah, blah… I heard that speech so many times I knew it by heart. Hey, Make My Day! Never mind, let me dial the number for you… I didn't want to live there anyway. Hell, if that was suppose to be a threat… oh, try me… I dare you! And, of course, I'd misbehave on purpose after that… like I just said, "I didn't want to live there anyway!" I wanted her to make the call, she'd be doing me a favour, in my opinion. Mom was also a yeller, and I can't stand people yelling at me today, or any yelling at all for that matter. To be honest, when she started her noise, I'd tune her out but more often than not… [just to be a brat] I'd put my fingers in my ears as I walked [more like a stomp in hopes of drowning her out] out of the room and I'd just go play in my bedroom so I wouldn't have to

SECTION TWO: NATURE OR NURTURE?

listen to her screeching. You know how when you run your finger nails down a chalkboard and people don't like that sound… well, that's exactly how her voice sounded to me when she'd yell at me. A couple of times I remember yelling back at her and getting a slap across the face "Don't you raise your voice to me, you little bugger"

Double Standards or what, eh?

"Well, if you don't like it, what makes you think that I enjoy it any more than you do?" And I'd get another smack for talking back and be sent to my room.

In many respects, I think the gaffer may have been resentful of me because I wasn't even his kid. I was born a sickly child [how sickly were you?] [keep reading, you'll soon find out] who took up most of mom's attention [but I don't remember being the recipient of her attention] for so many years and of course their money went for medication which meant he had less money for beer. In retrospect, had I been diagnosed with bipolar disorder, I doubt the bugger would have even filled my prescriptions. I'm sure he'd be in denial "it's all in his head" I can hear him say to this very day. Just like when I needed glasses… two of my siblings were wearing them but when it came time for me to get glasses…

Step-dad: "it's all in your head"

Me: "yup, my eyes are in my head"

Smack! For mouthing back. Well, they are, aren't they? He was informed that I should have had an eye test and been wearing glasses when I was probably in the sixth grade. I finally got my first pair of glasses when I was in grade nine. Another example of his love and tender care which aided to my overall happiness and well being. But that didn't stop mom from having more children after me. Nor did that appear to slow them down from their drinking because I remember plenty of times when there was more beer in the fridge and liquor in the cabinet than food in the cupboards.

Again, this is MY opinion... but neither of them should have been permitted to raise children. They didn't know how to care for/or nurture me and it's only by the Grace of God that I survived that hell to even be able to tell you about it today.

The grand-sire was so mean... "How mean was he?" He was so mean, that when I broke my arm at 16, an elderly couple picked me up off of the road and took me home. He wouldn't even take me to the hospital because...

Me: "I fell off my bike and I'm pretty sure my arm is broken"

Step-dad: "You 'stupid-ass' you got what you deserved for being so stupid as to ride your bike in the rain... you could have walked your bike you know and you wouldn't have fallen off in the first place"

Me: Just standing there looking like a deer caught in the headlights...

Step-dad: "You do have two feet and a heart beat, don't you?"

Me: "Yes, I do"

Step-dad: "then you can walk your 'stupid-ass' over to the hospital all by yourself."

There you have it, yet another perfect demonstration of his 'love', 'caring', and compassion, need I say more? Oh yes, and this was only a small example of my living in his 'happiness' while he expressed his love and concern towards little ole me. They shoot horses, don't they?

I knew as soon as I hit that sign post that I had broken my arm. That was interesting. It burned more than it hurt. So, after putting my arm in a make-shift sling [of course I knew first-aid, I had been in Cubs, Scouts and Cadets remember], I walked myself the few blocks to the ER. Mom worked at the hospital at that time and when I reported in, they called her down.

Mom: "Where's your father?"

Me: "At home, drinking, or he went out to continue drinking, I don't know, I don't care, what does it matter?"

Mom: "Is he not here because he did this to you?"

She knew him all too well, didn't she?

Me: "No, I fell off of my bike but he couldn't be bothered with me so, I walked over in the rain by myself."

Needless to say, that by this time it was pouring down pretty hard and I was soaking wet.

You mentioned that you were a "sickly child". What was wrong with you?

I was so sickly; "how sickly were you?" now you're getting it! I was so sickly that I had almost died right after child birth and a few more times before the age of 10 if I remember mom's stories correctly. I was really sick up to about the age of 12 though and I suppose it fizzled out from there or something, I don't know. I remember many stays in the hospital it felt as though it were my second home because I was so sick. Truth be told, I don't like hospital stays today. I will visit someone who is forced to be a resident, but I don't like being a resident myself. I also remember taking this medication that tasted like black licorice. I love and crave black licorice to this very day. As a matter of fact, I generally have a bag of it in the glove box of my truck, and a few bags about the house some where. It's hard to keep black licorice in my presence because I can eat the entire bag in one sitting even though I know I shouldn't, sort of like I'm doing right now while I'm writing. The Dr's were surprised though that I even made it out alive actually.

I was born premature, under 5lbs. I don't know how common it is today **AIHA** is a relatively rare condition, affecting one to three people per 100,000 per year but apparently it was rare in 1959. I remember mom telling me that the doctor's informed her that my white blood cells were 'eating' my red blood cells which was the simplest explanation they could come up with. They flew in a specialist from Seattle Washington to attend to little ole me, ain't I special? "Yes, very!"

Apparently, I had several blood transfusions and a bone marrow transplant somewhere throughout my early years. After I was born though, Mom was told that I wouldn't live out the day so they brought a priest in to administer the last rites. She told him to leave me alone, that "God isn't finished with him yet".

Every time the Grim-reaper came a calling, a priest would be brought in because I was not expected to make it through the night and each time, mom would say "God isn't finished with him yet!" A priest came a calling so often it's a wonder that I can't recite the words in Latin myself.

It's quite the interesting disease really. Yes, I Googled it!

Autoimmune Hemolytic Anemia or AIHA which is a blood disease in which a person produces substances that cause their own body to destroy red blood cells, resulting in anemia.

Here is one website I found to be helpful... should you be interested in learning more.

https://www.ihtc.org/payors/conditions-we-treat/other-hematological-disorders/autoimmune-hemolytic-anemia/

Last rites: in Catholicism, are the last prayers and ministrations given to many Catholics when possible shortly before death. The last rites go by various names and include various practices in different Catholic traditions. They may be administered to those awaiting execution, mortally injured, or terminally ill. But 'last rites' are also known in other religions. Mom was raised a Catholic, He was Anglican, if that matters?

https://en.wikipedia.org/wiki/Last_rites

Needless to say, I had missed a fair bit of school as well. I don't remember much of Kindergarten, 1, 2, part of 3 or grade 4 for that matter. Thinking back, I only remember bits and pieces of grade 5, but I do remember grades 6-12. Growing up, mom was supposed to watch me like a hawk, but how could she with 3 other children right behind me? She had 5 children in 7 years. So, I suppose she was a busy lady. An older brother 14-months ahead of me. A younger brother 11-months and 3 weeks, sister 2 ½ yrs, sister 5 ½ yrs younger. She had her hands full and I was often ignored so I'd find myself in some form of trouble or another. I probably spent more time in a play pen, in my room, or confined to the backyard by myself more than any other kid in history… unless he lived in a bubble or something. Ha, ha… Ya, right? You can't be serious. Or, Can I?

Funny I should mention that: it's another interesting read… bubble boy;

https://en.wikipedia.org/wiki/Bubble_Boy

I keep telling you, I don't just make these things up for your entertainment or enlightenment people… are you just crawling out from under a rock or something? Come-on, live a little, get out on the web and explore, it's a 'wonderful world' after-all. [Classic 1939 movie staring Claudette Colbert, James Stewart, and Guy Kibbee].

Should I cut or scrap myself, I would swell up like a balloon quite quickly too I must add. Mom called it <u>blood poisoning</u>.

<u>Blood poisoning</u> is not a medical term. But as the term is often used, it refers to the presence of bacteria in the blood (bacteremia) or an infection in the blood — and not a poisonous substance in the blood. However, bacteremia and infection can <u>potentially progress to sepsis and septic shock,</u> <u>serious illnesses that require prompt medical attention</u>. Did you catch that? **PROMPT MEDICAL ATTENTION!**

Which of course is not something the fiend adhered to on more than one occasion during my childhood.

Keep reading this gets interesting to say the least. More popcorn anyone?

Here I always thought she was making that up when I was a kid. Cool, I have blood poisoning, aren't I special? [okay, I've already established the fact that I am, so I'll move along] Where/whenever an injury opened my skin, the area would get all red, pussy, and extremely swollen. Then it would spread rather quickly around the opened wound. I couldn't walk on my foot for days or use my hand and the time I ripped my knee on barbed-wire, I couldn't bend it for about a week or so without suffering from some sort of pain. Then the fever would come and another trip to the emergency room... they must have loved to see me coming.

"Right this way Wayne, we have your room ready and waiting for you, Sir."

Why, thank you very much... [hold my calls please, I'll be busy for awhile] how thoughtful of you, what's on the menu for supper tonight? Not to mention the geezer having to spend more of his precious beer money on my medication.

Hmmm, looking back at it now, perhaps I got even on more than one occasion, LOL, I kill me... I know, don't give up my day job, oh, wait, I already have, oh well.

You know how other little boys come home with toads or frogs in their pockets or grasshoppers and crickets in their hands all covered over so the critter won't escape... well, they're pansy's in comparison to myself. I always, okay, almost always came home after having put a nail through my foot, a cut knee form barbed wire, a tear in my leg from a screw nail, or broken glass, a scrapped-up knee, elbow, leg, head or some other wound of some sort from fighting with the bullies or haven fallen off of my bike or something or other and back to the hospital I'd go. Hey, maybe step-dad should have had stock options there as well. I was injected with so many <u>tetanus</u> shots that they should have taken stock out on that too and perhaps they'd at least recoup some of their losses.

<u>Tetanus</u>: because established tetanus is often fatal, even with expert treatment, prevention is of paramount importance. Prevention, like it was my middle name or something... Ya, Right! The farthest thing from it, I'd say.

Prevention.... Ha, ha, that's a good one. In my maniac phases, I doubt that even Superman could have kept me pinned down long enough to keep me out of trouble. My oldest kid followed after me too there for a while as we called her bumps and bruises because she was always getting banged up.

<u>Tetanus</u> continued: The immunization is highly effective up to 10 years...

What? Wait a minute, did he say 10 years? Why did they give me shot after shot then after every little owwie? Damn them again! Oh Ya, I had AIHA, I suppose they couldn't take any chances. Oh, how I love needles! Not! I'm sure I had enough of those to last 100 kids over a life time.

https://www.webmd.com/children/vaccines/understanding-tetanus-prevention

Here is another example the monstrosities caring love which contributed to my overwhelming sense of happiness, and wellbeing. When I was in grade 6 while living in our first house on York Street in Kitchener [only a few blocks from the hospital] I do recall going into the garage one time after step-dad ordered [he never asked anything of me, he was barked a demand or an order, how rude] me to fetch a tool for him. The old codger had left a few pieces of wood on the floor, for some reason or other, [who's the stupid-ass now?] and for no other stranger reason then, because I could... I stepped on the boards instead of stepping over them. Well of course, I saw the boards on the floor, but I hadn't seen the rusty nail that was sticking up out of one of them and it went deep into my foot. Oh shit! Shit... shit... shit, here we go again. After pulling the nail out of my foot [which hurt just as bad as it had going in], I returned with the tool in hand, but I was limping.

Old man: "What the hell's the matter with you?"
Me: "I stepped on a nail"
Him: "how the hell did you do that?"

Now you know why I subconsciously use the word 'hell' quite a bit. Because that and a few other choice words were constantly echoing in my head while growing up. I don't think that man could put an entire sentence together without using at least one bad word in it.

Me: "I stepped on the boards that were on the floor in the garage"
Him: "why didn't you step over them, stupid-ass?"
Me: "I don't know"
Him: "You stupid-ass, let me see"

Yes, he used that phrase quite often… every chance he could I'm sure. So, I took my shoe and sock off. It bled a fair bit and my sock was soaked with blood but it was only a pin prick according to him.

Him: "you'll be alright, go clean it up and put a band aid on it"
[famous last words… he, he, he. Just wait until mother gets home]

Well, if you were paying any attention to the previous pages, you know that I wasn't going to be… 'all right', that is. I don't remember where mom was, probably at work, but she arrived home, only to discover me watching television in the living room with my foot up on a stool and a cloth wrapped around my foot with an ice inside of it to help reduce the swelling [like that ever worked for me].

Mom: "What happened to you?"
Me: "I stepped on a board which had a nail sticking out of it and the nail went deep into my foot"
Mom: "Did your father take you to the hospital?"
Me: "No, he said it was only a pin prick, told me to wash it up and put a band aid on it"

But I hadn't put the band aid on it as of yet because I knew that wouldn't do any good.

Mom: "Let me see"

By this time, the wound was oozing a neat colourful greenish/yellow puss, [colourful, ain't it?] and my entire foot was red and swelling fast… the swelling was begging to encroach upon my ankle.

Mom: "Damn that man" she muttered, as if I wasn't supposed to hear what she had just said.

I already knew he was in for it, but she confirmed my suspicions... I love this part, go get him mom!

Mom: "It looks painful" she said.
Me: "It is"

Well of course it was... what part of my breathing through my teeth and pulling back when you touched it don't you understand?

I thought it looked awesome though and I knew I'd be home from school for yet another week. Missing school was always my favorite pass time and it was always absolutely fine by me. Although, there wasn't much on day-time television. Come to think of it, there still isn't. But I did watch a lot of news and learned more about the Vietnam War than did most adults had I'm sure.

Mom, yelling out, calling him by name...!
Mom: "how can you be so stupid? This kid needs to go to the hospital" laying into him when he finally emerged from outside.

Him: "Don't be so bloody stupid woman, it's a tiny hole, he's just being a big baby"
Bloody was one of many he used.

Mom: "baby my ass, look at it"
he grabs my foot, yanks it towards him...

Him: "you stupid-ass, can you walk?"
Me: "I think so"
Him: "then think your ass out to the car"

He, he, he.

Thankfully I didn't come home for a couple of days because I'm sure he paid all hell for that one [again] for not taking me to the hospital right away… you can mess around with mom most of the time when it came to all sorts of things but NOT when it came to her precious 'little man'.

Mom did always know best when it came to me and cuts, scrapes and/ or puncture wounds. Damn, I ate up his beer money with medications once more. Oh well! Sucked to be him now, didn't it? I don't know about you, but I'm busting a gut laughing, it's so fucking funny telling that story after all of these years. The things we remember eh?

What about the barbed-wire?

Oh, okay, long story short… I believe I was about 9 when several of us were taking a short-cut through a famer's field [which we were told to stay out of on account of the bull… [bull-scmull, I'm invincible? I'm sure I can outrun a lazy old bull]. While climbing over the wire fence, I got hung up somehow, [because I can never do anything right] and caught my knee on a barb… that little 'catch' ripped my pants, put me on my ass on the ground while tearing up my knee in the process.

Of course, the other kids were laughing. Ouch! Ya, that was more than an ouch. I didn't even bother going home and went right to Emerge. Had cell phones been invented back then, I would have had them on speed-dial I'm sure.

Operator: "K-W Hospital, Emergency department, how may I assist you today?"

Me: "Hi, it's Wayne Driver again; I'm on my way home."

Operator: "Thank you for the heads-up Sir, we'll get your bed ready and have a team on stand-by awaiting your arrival."

Me: "how thoughtful of you, thank you, see you soon!"

If only eh? I told my younger brother to tell mom what had happened and that I'd meet her at the hospital. He laughed,

Brother: "you know you're going to get it from the old man when you get home, don't you?"

Me: "Ya, I don't give a shit about that right now, I have to get going before I can't walk anymore"

'Shit' was another word I constantly heard. Never really thought of it as a cuss word really.

Brother: "See you later 'stupid-ass'" he said, laughing again as we parted ways.

For some reason, my getting into trouble with the beast always amused my brothers... always! I remember a few beatings they took that weren't so funny though. But those aren't my stories to tell. I walked to the bus stop, didn't have a dime for the ride but given the circumstance the driver let me on... "where are your parents?" "I don't know, probably drunk again." I told him. He didn't say another word. I traveled to the hospital, limped off and into the Emergency room... "Why hello, again Wayne, thanks for the phone call, everyone is waiting for you... right this way please?" And off we'd go again. I'm sure they'd have my mom on speed dial as well. I swear I could feel my knee getting larger with every step I took and with each minute that past I felt warmer and warmer. By the time I arrived at the hospital, I was hot and sweating and it wasn't just from the exertion of limping... and if you're a medical professional reading this, who thinks it could not happen that fast... just remember... I had AIHA so, yes... it can and did happen that fast, according to a little kid. Not to mention the fact that I was a scrawny little rat with a buggered up immune system. They called the parents but couldn't reach anyone on the telephone. My brother must have relayed the message, no doubt laughing the entire time [mom never drove] so step-beast always had no choice but to show up... except when he was drinking [which was practically all of the time, so it seemed. So, you know what that meant? He rarely showed up, that's what] she would call a friend or a cab, [which meant wasting even more money on my account]. I should add that mom never drove because asshole was too intimidating [and that's putting it mildly]. I remember her getting behind the wheel with him in the passenger seat only once while I was in the car. She didn't want to drive but he had one too many [as usual]. It was during Christmas season so the cops were out doing their annual checks and Thing 1 shouldn't be driving. But wait, isn't your teacher also suppose to be sober when someone only had a learner's permit? I think they were... anyway, this particular time he was very angry... with her second mistake he was darn right mean and had called her everything from a dumb whore to a useless bitch. Which of course are words a little kid shouldn't be hearing but I heard them all the time so they weren't anything new for me. I can't say that I blamed her, but you can't leave me alone with him either... "hey, where you going? Take me with you!" She didn't even bother pulling over... she stopped right there in the middle of the road, grabbed her purse and after slamming the door, she walked away. Come to think of it, she never ever drove with that man again and had never obtained a driver's licence. Who'd blame her? I never drove with him under any circumstance. Once I achieved my learners permit, I paid for my own driver's education at school.

Him: "Hey, I have to go get something at Canadian Tire, do you want to drive?"
Me: "Who? Me? Drive? With you?
Him: "Ya, of course"
Me: "Not bloody likely"
Him: "Why not?"
Me: "You don't remember that incident where mom left us in the middle of the road and walked away, do you?"
Him: "What the hell are you talking about?"
Me: "Exactly, never mind, ah, no thank you."
Him: "Suite yourself, suckie baby."

I did suite myself thank you very much and I never asked to borrow the car from him either.

Oh right, I was in the hospital again... this time mom had called a friend because the wormwood was out drinking [as usual on a Saturday afternoon]. I swear my knee was almost three times it's normal size by the time she had arrived. Okay, this might be a slight exaggeration, but I was a kid, give me a break. They only required her presence to sign the paperwork of course. If they were smart, they would have had a few blank forms on hand with her signature scribbled out upon them for unexpected future incidents such as this one, and trust me... there were many of such incidences yet to come. It's not like she could stay or anything with the other kids at home. Not that I required her presence anyway, it was always more fun with the other kids in the hospital when she wasn't around anyway. And, Yes, all from a little scratch from a little barb. The barbs on the wire back then were longer than I've seen some today. Well, okay it was more than a little scratch but I told you, 'I was a sickly kid' and it was a cut really and it was deep and all the same difference really because it tore open my skin. I still have the scar to prove it. Ah, scars upon our person are mementos of childhood antics gone by. Scars upon the heart and our emotions though are harder to heal and represent the battle scars of childhood trauma's that we aren't meant to carry. When the shit finally came to pick me up a couple of days later, the hospital staff offered up a pair of crutches, but the miserly fellow wouldn't pay for them. So, needless to say that I hobbled everywhere over the next week. I was surprised that we hadn't already had a pair somewhere in the basement. But, with every ripped-skin, torn elbow, skinned or scraped knee or whatever episode that involved opening me up in some fashion or another... it meant a trip to the hospital and with every trip to the hospital came an intravenous cleansing, intravenous antibiotics and a prescription for 7 – 10 days which meant the guardian was always pissed because every single incident meant that I gouged into his coveted drinking money! Not to mention another new pair of jeans, a new shirt or new shoes from time to time for that matter. I was even blamed once for getting hurt so that I would get a new pair of pants and you know what the bugger did? He gave me extra chores to help cover their cost. Now how cheap is that?

Oh, 'pissed' and 'pissed-off' were two more I heard almost on a daily basis… he seemed to be always 'pissed' about something and let me know about it verbally if not physically at every chance he got.

There were plenty of times when I wasn't even allowed to leave the yard though because he couldn't trust me not to fall and rip myself open somehow on something or another. That's okay, I could always find some source of mischief to entertain myself with, even within the confines of my own back yard. Climbing up an old oak tree to the very top which towered above the house wouldn't count as 'finding' trouble, now would it? I didn't think so either. I guess in some respects, I'm surprised I never fell from such a lofty height. The Chap caught me up in the tree one time...

Him: "what are you looking at?"
Younger brother: "Wayne, he's way up there and I can hardly see him."
Him: "Where? I don't see him." "hey, stupid-ass, are you up there?"
Me: "Yes"
Him: "well get the hell down before you fall and break your bloody neck."
"Bloody" yup, another one!

Just for fun, I'll tell you about another incident where I ripped open my leg... I don't remember what grade I was in, but, I was taking the garbage out to the dumpster which was located in the parking lot of the townhouse complex and I brushed the bag up against my leg [because I was playing around and swinging it back and forth]. How'd you guess? Oh, you're getting good at this... Yup, another Owwie! There was so much blood that it looked like a wound from a MASH hospital patient. A piece of broken glass was in the bag which cut right through my jeans [which of course it meant he had to buy a new pair] and it cut my leg open... another trip to the ER, six stiches later, another week of antibiotics... and a few smacks about the head for being a 'stupid-ass' [No, I'm not kidding, he was always hitting me for no apparent reason]. It wasn't my fault the broken glass was in the garbage, but it was my fault for swinging the bag in the first place. But you see why he was always pissed at me? Because, I was always swallowing his beer money with medicine instead of him enjoying his favorite libation... it's a good thing he didn't have to pay the hospital bill as well. Hey, shit happens.

[I'm tired, tired? I just woke up from a 2 hr nap a ½ an hour ago, I know but Iim tired No, keep writing, I'll eventually wake up. Oh, Okay, if you insist].

Even when I was an adult, things didn't always go according to plans with just a 'regular' washing of the wound. One time I was looking into hauling cattle... wouldn't you know it, my very first gig and a stubborn steer wouldn't come out to play. I was backed up to the stock yard chute but the lighting was poor and I couldn't quite see where the critter was. I had already zapped him once with my cattle prod, but they didn't tell me…"whatever you do, don't go into the trailer after them" well, I wished they had of passed on that little tidbit of information because it sure as hell would have saved me a great deal of hurt… needless to say I went in after him but almost didn't make it out alive. That bugger caught me with his horns, tossed me over his head, smacked me above an eye with a hoof, ripped me open and I flew into the opposite wall. I think it took about 14 stitches to close up my eye and a few more for the lower abdomen. He was pretty close to ripping my boys off and it's a good thing that hadn't have happened, I'm fairly attached to them. Well, I woke up in the hospital three days later and my eye was practically swollen shut because they hadn't cleansed it out properly and it was grievously infected… of course, not to mention a hoof in the head would tend to cause swelling and a concussion. It was oozing yellow-green cheesy stuff, Cool! It looked rather gross actually, so no, Not Cool! They had to reopen a part of the cut, clean out the wound, close me back up again and they gave me some awfully strong antibiotics that made me sick to my stomach. Needless to say, that was not fun!

Play it Again Sam!

Another time I had the same eye ripped open, and I never told anyone this, because it's embarrassing, that's why… but I was 'trying out' at a pig farm in Saskatchewan… I've never worked with pigs before and never have since that day either, thank you very much. I'll stick to eating pork, not raising it. I was in the wiener pen scraping it clean of manure when I slipped and fell bashing my head, just above my left eye on the shovel… I sprawled to the floor seeing blood and stars. The thing is, under no circumstances do you want to pass out in a pig pen because pigs will eat you. I quickly got to my feet before passing out, hopped over the rail and laid out on the walk-way between the pens. It took awhile to gather myself because I was seeing too many stars to walk straight. Once I recovered, I walked out to the supervisor, who took me to the showers and helped me clean up. They brought in the first-aide kit, patched up the wound and drove me to the hospital and called the girlfriend. Well, it was the same scenario all over again, not a thorough cleansing, severe infection, more strong meds and a whole lot of fun. My girlfriends five-year-old fellow and I were fooling around a few days later and he accidently kicked me in the head... Oh damn... that hurt... he may as well have been the bull because it hurt that much all over again. The thing that really annoyed me was that she laid into the little guy for hurting me. It was an accident, we were goofing around and it was just as much my fault as his. Any way, cheezie schtuff oozed out and it was back to the hospital to be cleaned out, more meds and the headache that I already had was worse now more than ever. Oh well, another job opportunity down the drain, but I didn't really mind on this one, trust me. So, I've always had problems with infections when my skin was opened at every age. Yes, even still today.

Yes, pigs do eat people... the news is full of stories

https://www.dailystar.co.uk/news/latest-news/433815/Farmer-eaten-alive-pigs-shocking-attack-Romania

This one time... at Band Camp? [no, not at band camp, stop asking will ya] in the turkey barn I wasn't quick enough and I grabbed at a rat from in between the straw bails. I made a grab for him because I forgot my pitch fork, okay. I meant to catch the body but I only managed his tail and the bugger turned around and bit right through my work glove... by the time I got to the hospital there was a greenish discharge. The wound was swelling, red and painful that I couldn't touch peter pointer to my thumb. I didn't think a little rat bite would hurt so much... needless to say, he wouldn't be biting me ever again and the cat had a gourmet meal.

Yup: 'Bugger' is another one!

Blood Poisoning Continued: <u>Without prompt treatment</u>, bacteremia or infection can spread to other areas such as heart valves or other tissues, or progress to severe sepsis and septic shock, <u>which may be life-threatening</u>. Cool!

See... 'without prompt medical treatment'... bacteremia or infection can, and does SPREAD!

As if I didn't spend enough time in the hospital with the anemia, I was in for blood poisoning more times then I care to count and I'd miss a few more days of school, or work. Cool! I always enjoyed missing both, or did I tell you that already?

https://www.mayoclinic.org/blood-poisoning/expert-answers/faq-20058534

A couple of times now, you've mentioned that there was little to no food in the house and that eating to you was like sleeping… which "was highly overrated" I believe you said.

Yes, I did say that.

What's that about?

Well, it's about mom and step-dad being so caught up in their drinking and buying cigarettes that sometimes they'd forget to buy groceries. Or, perhaps it had something to do with going through bankruptcy a couple of times that they couldn't afford to buy enough food because the "Needs of those Two, Outweighed the Needs of us few" [an adapted Star Trek quote, said by Mr. Spock. I'll let you look that one up for yourself] were more important than feeding their family and we'd have to survive off of whatever they could get from a food bank, or wherever they got it from. We ate a fair amount of pork and beans, mac-n-cheese, canned ham and my all time favorite; Corn Flakes! I never ever remember them going without their basic needs which were booze and cigarettes during the time I spent growing up. I do remember powered milk though. Oh God, can there be anything more disgusting? To make the milk stretch, they would make up a batch of that powdered shit and mix it with the 2% milk…. blah! Come to think of it, that could be another reason why I wouldn't eat the Corn Flakes.

Yes… Shit is another word I'm sure I heard it on a daily basis as well.

Probably another reason why I don't like 'powered' or processed eggs either. It's another nasty invention. Come to think of it, SPAM is better than some of the stuff I've eaten and that's saying a lot about SPAM. I also learned to go without food because I was either so finicky that I wouldn't eat and get sent to my room or to school on many occasions without anything in my stomach while my little brother ate my portion [before it went soggy]. No wonder he grew to be bigger than I... I wouldn't eat my Wheaties. Or, they would give me too much and of course I couldn't finish it all. But, one of the rules of the house was that I had to 'clean' my plate before I was allowed to leave the table. But, being the stubborn brat that I was, that was just about an impossible task on the best of days. I do remember a couple of times mom telling me to clean my plate, so being the 'stupid-ass' that I am, I licked the plate clean and got a smack from the has-been for my troubles... Many a time I remember being sent to my room because I would not consume whatever crap she decided to dish out and put in front of me that she dared to call 'food'. Did I mention that mom was not a very good cook? If she couldn't heat and serve whatever came out of a can or a box, we didn't get it. Mom just usually sent me to my room but not mom's partner... no, he had to make a major production out of it each and every time...

On the stage for you this evening we have a really big shoo, all the way from Victoria B.C., please welcome your host and our favorite maniac... ME!

More often than not, I was called back down after dinner and given a second chance to eat. Oh Joy! I'm sure if she was invited for supper, she wouldn't eat that slop either. If I wasn't going to eat it the first time, when it was hot... what makes you think I'm going to eat it now that it's cooled down to room-temperature? Does any of this make sense to any of you? It sure doesn't make sense to me. But hey, let's play this one out for the stupid people whom I lived with. Now, for no other reason than for your viewing pleasure; picture this in your mind... the overseer spoon in hand feeding a stubborn 6, 7, or 8-year-old kid who is more than capable of feeding himself but absolutely refuses to do so! What is a parent to do, right? Well I can tell you one thing you don't do... You don't beat him senseless for God's sake.

Old man: "Pick up your fork and eat"
Me: "No"
Smack across the mouth
Him: "I said, pick up your fork"
Me: shoveling shit... and spitting it back out.

SMACK!
Him: grabbing my fork…"Open up!"
Me:"No!"
SMACK!
Him:"I said, open up, damn you!"

Damn you… yup, another phrase often heard.

Opening up meant getting a spoon full of peas or something or other disgusting cold slop shoved in my mouth and I'd spit it right back out. SMACK! Again, I'd cry and open up and get that <u>same</u> mouthful [that I just spit out] shoved back in… me, half gagging, half choking on some imaginary glob of goo that won't go down my throat even if you used a tiny plunger and I'd get smacked again for my theatrics. Oh, and I wasn't permitted to wash it down with water either. Drama queen or what, eh?

Him:"Open up and don't you dare spit it out!"

More often than not I'd swallow without chewing if and when I could and for no other reason than not to be smacked again. If I actually complied in the first place, that is.

With another spoonful…

Him:"OPEN UP!"

Me:"NO"

Smack, another back from the monster… then he'd give up…

Him:"take off your clothes"

And he'd take off his belt and I'd be butt naked there in the kitchen getting it again and then being sent back up to my room with nothing to eat that evening. Which of course was fine by me. Sometimes, he'd hit me so hard with the belt that I would pee on the floor, then I'd receive a few more blows for making a mess and would have to clean it up before making my way up to my room.

The other classic is "The Corn Flakes Wars" Sounds funny doesn't it?

Well, after what you just read, you won't want to miss that, I'm sure it would be a block buster extravaganza. Well, to be honest with you, it wasn't really all that funny while it was being played out but I'm sure you'll enjoy this just as much as I am presenting it to you. It's a riot! Now that I'm looking back. You haven't read anything yet... and after it all, you'll be wondering... why was this kid so damn stubborn, or stupid? I'll never know either. Keep reading, this will bust a gut for you. Hey, I should send this into the people at Kellogg's, I wonder if they'd get a laugh from it as well?

"The Corn Flakes War" Proudly brought to you buy Wayne and the people who looked after him!

I don't know who or what mom thought she was feeding half of the time but she never learned either and she always, YES, ALWAYS! gave me too much or something I didn't like. Come to think of it, I didn't like much when it came to food she was serving. I was never a kid who went for those 'sugar' cereals either. Yuck!

Mom pours my bowl of Corn Flakes, but as I said; generally gave me too much so I could never finish them up and would leave the table with half a bowl of Corn Flakes left and off to school I'd go. Or, the Corn Flakes would get soggy too fast and who wants to eat soggy Corn Flakes? Another disgusting invention.

I'd come home for lunch and that same bowl of Corn Flakes [yes, the same bowl of mushy Corn Flakes] would be brought out of the refrigerator, the plastic cellophane would come off and the bowl would be placed before me for my lunch. Oh, joy! [who invited her for lunch?] I'm sure Joy wouldn't eat that crap either... soggy Corn Flakes, yummy, my favorite. I'd sit there the entire lunch time, not saying anything, or eating for that matter, just starring at that bowl of mush [wishing that it would evaporate or something] and pouting while the other kids would eat a sandwich or something.

Oh, I just thought of another disgusting so-called edible delectable... Chef Boyardee Anything! Who the hell came up with those perverted imitation foods? It's just my opinion, but I'd rather eat canned Spam than that crap! That stuff is worse than the slop they tried to pass off as food at the hospital in St. Paul... OMG! There was another product I absolutely refused to eat and we'd often have a war over those vial products as well. More often than not, I'd want to barf just smelling them. Mom would open a can of that crap and I'd be nowhere to be found, unless you looked for me in the general direction of the school because that's where I was headed without lunch.

Now... how easy would have been to just down that bowl of soggy Corn Flakes and move on? Eh?

Pretty easy I'd say, but no way man... there was no way in hell I was ever and I do mean NEVER going to give in... I know, let's get Mikey, he'll eat anything.

Little Mikey was a fictional boy played by John Gilchrist in an American television commercial promoting Quaker Oats' breakfast cereal Life. The ad was created by art director Bob Gage, who also directed the commercial. It first aired in 1972. The popular ad campaign featuring Mikey remained in regular rotation for more than 12 years and ended up as one of the longest continuously running commercial campaigns ever aired. https://en.wikipedia.org/wiki/Little_Mikey

The problem with that was that Mickey hadn't been invented yet so I was on my own. My younger brother came close but even he wouldn't eat my soggy Corn Flakes for me. I have no idea how many times she'd tell me to eat, but I wouldn't.

She'd even try the old guilt trip thing on me... nice try lady!

Mom: "You know there are kids starving in Africa who'd love to have a bowl of Corn Flakes right about now"

There was always kid starving in Africa... or India... wherever those places were. As far as I knew, they were fictitious far away places found on the television.

Me: "Good! Mail it to them, cause I ain't eating this shit"
Smack! A slap for swearing...
Me: "well I'm not!" and I'd push it away.
Mom: "Then I guess you'll go back to school without lunch"
Me: "I guess I will then" and with that, I was out of there faster than a fox being chased by a hound so she couldn't smack me again for talking back.

Damn! Here we go again... I suppose they wouldn't learn that this kid was more stubborn [ODD, perhaps?] than they were because that same bowl...

Yes! Damn it, that same bowl... how many times do I have to tell you? I introduced you to it at lunch time, well... play it again Sam, cause here we go again.

You're kidding?

I wish that I were. No, I'm not kidding!

That same bowl of soggy Corn Flakes would come right back out of the refrigerator and be set before me for my dinner. Yummy! But this gets more interesting, trust me.

"Play it again Sam!" "Alright Wayne, whatever you say, You're the Boss..."

I like Sam, he's a great guy!

And, we'd go through it all over again. Everyone would be eating their dinner except for yours truly. Of course, the thug had to have me sit next to him so he wouldn't have far to reach out and 'touch me'... if you know what I mean, during dinner time. I'd get a smack or two along the way, but I still refused to pick up that bloody spoon and put that shit into my mouth even after he had made my nose bleed. I would sit there with my arms crossed while blood dripped down onto my folded arms and onto my shirt just staring at that damn bowl of gross, soggy, disgusting Corn Flakes while a tear or two might roll down my cheek. OMG, shoot me now! After everyone had eaten, I'd be told to take my clothes off and I'd get the belt and be given another chance to eat, but I wouldn't. I was made to sit there in my chair butt naked until I ate every bite… oh, we didn't have a dog so I couldn't give it to him/her either. I would sit there just staring at that cursed bowl because there was no way in purgatory, they were going to make/force me to eat them. I'd die choking on those cursed things first. He could have put me on a rack and stretched my limbs until they ripped off of my little body and I still wouldn't eat. Sometimes I'd sit there stark naked until bed time without eating that bowl of mushy pig slop.

You mean you'd sit there at the table from about 5:30 until 8:00 not eating, not doing anything while life went on all around you?

Yes, that's exactly what I'm telling you.

Stubborn, eh?

Or, Stupid… take your pick.

Mom would clean up the table, do the dishes, sweep the floor, turn off the lights and away she'd go, without saying a word to me. If it were winter time, I'd be left there in the dark all of that time. Bully would return just prior to my bed time [or on his way out to out somewhere] and I'd still be sitting there [in the dark] with just as much of those Corn Flakes in the bowl as there was when he had first left me there. I wonder if any of the milk evaporated?

Him: "Are you going to eat?"
Me: "No, I'm not"
Him: "adopt the position"

I was already naked, so, all I had to do was lean over the chair.

Me: "fine by me"
Him: "We'll see just how fine it is when I'm finished with you."

and I'd get it again then be sent up to my room for bed, and yes, that was the second beating that same night. And, Yes, I still had to kiss him goodnight. Mom would come out and flush the Corn Flakes down the toilet.

I'd arrive to the breakfast table the next morning and everyone would get breakfast except for me.

Me: "Where's my breakfast?"
Mom: "I flushed it down the toilet last night"

I catch on rather quickly...

Me: "So, I don't get anything?"
Mom: "That's right, you don't. You get to go to school hungry today and maybe you'll appreciate what's put in front of you"
[not bloody likely]

Me: "Fine!"

and off to school I'd go without eating anything. So, here we are the next day and in 24 hrs, all I've had to eat is a half a bowl of Corn Flakes. Needless to say, that scene played out numerous times in our house over the years. Sometimes I would be the evening entertainment three or four nights in a row. Funny thing is, I eat Corn Flakes today but you can be darned sure I eat them fast so they don't have time to go soggy... Oh, and if they do... I flush them down the toilet for no other reason than... because I can... Ain't I a stinker?

Again, you can't be serious.

Yes, I'm dead serious! I'm not making this up just to entertain you.

I told you... I was/am stubborn. Is it just me or does anyone else see oppositional defiance disorder [ODD] in any of this? If you haven't already, look this one up as well. It wouldn't matter if I were depressed or maniac, I was stubborn... the only difference was... depending on how I was feeling at the moment would depend upon the amount to which I would mouth back. I told you [or are we not there yet?] that my mouth got me into just as much trouble as my brain did. I didn't care what they did to me, there was no way in perdition were they going to force me to eat those soggy Corn Flakes. Uh, uh… ain't happening in this life time, or the next, nor in ten life times. They even tried force feeding me on many occasions by pinching my nose so that I would have to open it to breath… which gave him the opportunity to shove that slop in my mouth… well of course I spit it right back out into the bowl, I'm not that stupid… or am I? Spitting it back out meant that I'd be butt naked over the chair again, and again, and again, and so forth. Well, I survived, hadn't I?

There were many of mornings when I'd come to the table for breakfast…

Me: "what's for breakfast?"
Mom: "For you, Corn Flakes"
Me: "Why just for me?"
Mom: "because, you're going to learn one way or another to appreciate what's put in front of you… that's why."

Ya… In your dreams bitch… because that ain't happening today either.

Me: "No, thanks"

and off I'd go without breakfast once again because that's the only two choices I was given… Corn Flakes, or Nothing, and when faced with that dilemma, nothing won out every time. Nothing got to be mighty tasty after awhile. I swear she use to feed me Corn Flakes just so my tormentor had a reason to beat on me. I eventually learned to live with being hungry that hunger no longer bothered or affected me and I chose to go that route than to eat the Corn Flakes. And that my friends… is my story about "The Corn Flakes War"

So, let the records show, that I did it my way… I paid a price, but what the hell.

That was an awesome war. Defeat nor retreat were in my battle plans no matter who my enemy was. I took my lumps for sure, each and every battle, but I won the War!

So, now maybe you'll believe me when I say today that "I'm not hungry" it truly is because I AM NOT hungry!

I can and have gone 3 or 4 days without eating and still not feel hungry. Nor do I have an appetite either... I just don't understand what it means to be hungry.

So again, appetite and hunger are only words in my dictionary because I have no physical concept of their conditions.

Hunger: noun; a feeling of discomfort or weakness caused by lack of food, coupled with the desire to eat.

Sorry, that doesn't make sense to me because I do not get a feeling of discomfort or weakness caused by the lack of food.

Oh, and that was another way I happened to get welts and bruises upon welts and bruises... or are we not at this point yet either? I can't remember... oh well.

I couldn't help notice that you've used the word 'beating' several times;

What is your definition of a 'Beating', verses a 'Spanking'?

A spanking would be where a child might receive one, two, or three but not more than a few wacks on the buttocks with an open hand or perhaps a wooden spoon, a belt, a paddle or a switch of some sorts and I'm sure most parents would permit a child to keep his/her clothes on. Or perhaps a child might receive a couple wacks across the palm of their hand depending upon the offense I suppose. I rarely received such 'special' treatment. If I did, I got off luck for some reason or other. But I was never fortunate enough to my recollection.

Have you ever watched these guys in 'cage fights'? Well, that's not a beating... they're pussies comparted to what I received as a child and as a teenager. Have you ever watched Rocky? Now, there was a guy who could take a beating. Him and I are soul pals for sure. Rocky is a 1976

American sports drama film directed by John G. Avildsen and both written by and starring Sylvester Stallone.

https://en.wikipedia.org/wiki/Rocky

A <u>beating</u> would be and was, a <u>flogging</u> [you're cold] <u>battering</u>, [warmer] a <u>pounding</u> [getting hot] and sometimes a <u>pummelling</u> [you're burning up] with so many strikes with the belt or blows from his fist that I ached for days and sometime for a week or so. There was no way I dared lift a hand to protect or to defend myself because I got it all the more and harder too. That is if he didn't break my arm first or rip it out of my shoulder socket for daring to raise a hand to him... [which I thought he would do on a couple of occasions when I dared to protect my face]. I remember trying to run away a couple of times when I was younger. He'd grab my arm, hold me up so that my tippy-toes were just barely touching the floor, or he'd lift me up completely off of the floor while beating me with his belt. When he was finished, with me, he'd drop me. I'd crumble to the floor and he'd kick me while yelling at me to get to my room. I think I grew up mostly in my room? Yes, by my lonesome, but I was never lonely. I liked playing with myself... I mean, by myself. The underlined words above define being brutalized by being stricken repeatedly with whacks, slaps and/or punches so many times we couldn't count. He didn't care where he connected; the face, legs, stomach, the head, the back, the scrotum, where ever the belt, or fists landed was okay by him.

"Come on seriously?" "Surely you're exaggerating!"

"Am I?" "Were you there?"

No, I wasn't... but,

"But nothing!" "No, you weren't there so stop interrupting and let me tell you how it was!" "Keep reading... for the rest of the story, you haven't been told the half of it yet!" And you thought the Corn Flakes War was traumatic...

<u>Beating</u>: a punishment or assault in which the victim is <u>hit repeatedly</u>;

Flogging: noun; a punishment in which the victim is <u>hit repeatedly</u> with a whip or stick. Verb; <u>beat</u> (someone) with a whip or stick as punishment or torture.

In this case the weapon of choice was his leather belt, until I got older, then he used his fists. But more often than not it all started with a few slaps about the head first just so he'd get warmed up.

Flogging: definition; https://en.wikipedia.org/wiki/Flagellation

<u>Flogging</u>: images; Google it for yourselves if you don't believe me... then keep reading. Go for it! You know you want to!

It gets more gruesome I promise you that.

<u>Battering</u>: the action of <u>striking repeatedly</u> with <u>hard blows</u>;

<u>Pounding</u>: <u>repeated</u> and <u>heavy striking</u> or hitting of someone or something;

<u>Pummelling</u>: <u>strike repeatedly</u> with the <u>fists</u>!

Have you noticed the 'repeated' words?

He would hit me so hard and so many times that he caused <u>welts</u> and black/blue <u>bruises</u> that wouldn't heal sometimes for weeks.

More often than not I had bruises upon welts and welts upon the bruises because the previous beating hadn't had sufficient time to heal and I'd be beaten again. When I grew into my teens, he stopped having me strip down to use his belt and switched to his fists to the point of causing black/blue bruises about the shoulders, upper back, the upper arms, the face along with black eyes, bloody fat lips, bleeding noses, lumps about the head and often the loss of the use of an arm or two for a couple of hours or so because it was too damned sore to be moved.

<u>Welts</u>: red, swollen marks left on flesh by a blow or pressure; and

<u>Bruises:</u> A contusion, commonly known as a bruise, is a type of hematoma of tissue in which capillaries and sometimes venules are damaged by <u>trauma</u>, allowing blood to seep, hemorrhage, or extravasate into the surrounding interstitial tissues. The bruise then remains visible until the blood is either absorbed by tissues or cleared by immune system action. I had a damaged immune system as it was so, not only did I bruise easily, I stayed bruised longer because I took longer to heal than most people, but then we've already established the fact that I ain't like most people. Google these images sometime, that is if you have the stomach for it. Go on, I dare you! No, in fact, I double dog dare you!

A few times I had to have stiches or was hospitalized courtesy of his brutality.

Over the corner of one eye, I have a scar which he claimed I "fell against the windowsill." A scare over the other eye because "the clumsy kid fell up the stairs." Wrong on both counts. His wedding ring cut open one eye when he back handed me in the face and knocked my thoughts into the middle of the next week when I was only five. His belt opened up the other eye when I was five as well and I have very few eyebrow hairs in those areas still today, but at least I have a matching set. A couple times he asked…

Cousin It: "have you been plucking your eyebrows or something? They look stupid"

Me: "ah, no, they're thin at the ends because of the scars you gave me"

Smack! Across the face with a backhand.

Well, you asked! I guess the truth hurts, doesn't it? Asshole!

Talk about a bully, today's bullies could have taken lessons from this piece of shit. I know the Bible says to honour your parents, but how could I honour anything or anyone of such character? Oh, I honoured him to his face or I'd be bloodied for not doing so, but not under my breath or behind his back that's for sure. When we moved to a new neighborhood I always told the kids that the scars and bruises were from playing goalie and that's why I refused to defend the net anymore when we'd play road hockey. If they wouldn't let me play any other position, that was okay too. I always enjoyed my own company better anyway. Friends, as a child; who needed them? I always had me, myself and I, who were my closest companions all of my life and still are today, so why should anything change?

What is your earliest childhood memory of one of these beatings?

There were several of them all pretty close together that I don't remember which one came first [the chicken or the egg] so I'll explain all 4 of them [why? because I ca, that's why]. Eeny, meeny, miny, moe, catch a tiger by the toe... you're it!

When I was perhaps 4 or 5 [before the youngest child was born into our family], we lived in an apartment above a retail store on King Street in downtown Waterloo. I accidently broke a basement window of the store [with my ball] and I tried to run away. I don't know where I thought I was going but the squire waited for me to come around the bank at the far end of the block. He grabbed my arm and lifted me up off of my feet, whipped down my garments and used his belt to deliver multiple wacks on my bare buttocks right there on the street for all the world to see. I couldn't run anywhere because he was holding me so tight I thought he was going to break my arm while my entire weight was being held up by him pulling my shoulder out of its socket. No one came to rescue this poor kid who was being brutalized by this savage beast. I suppose back then it was a perfectly normal occurrence, highly recommended if not encouraged to keep your kids in line. "Somebody call the cops, I'm being tortured again! Help!" "Ya, that's right, keep on walking, you prick, you don't see anything out of the ordinary over here, nothing to see at all. That's it, look away and keep going, you Coward!" I'm thinking as a man walks out of the bank and witnesses this spectacle but makes an abrupt U-turn and scurries off.

One of his sisters was just as mean as he was, cut from the same cloth I suppose. My female cousin and I (ages 4 and 5) [while living in the same apartment], were playing outside and we both had to go to the bathroom, well of course we thought nothing of it and went in together.

What was the big deal? Mom use to bathe us boys and girls together so why can't we use the toilet at the same time? I don't know? My aunt heard us talking in the bathroom and came in with a BIG, Huge, no, I mean, Ginormous, wooden spoon. I think it was the gigantist wooden spoon I had ever seen in all of my 5 years. I didn't even know we owned one that big [as it turned out, we didn't own one that big. She carried it with her wherever she went just in case the witch had to discipline her children and those who weren't too, apparently] and... SHE... LOCKED... THE... DOOR! Holy Shit Patgirl! We're in for it now! We both got a look at that spoon and started crying [as if that would fend off the inevitable or something]. The problem was, we had no idea what we had done wrong for that monstrosity to make an appearance from the hags' handbag where she stashed it away. I guess we were about to find out... weren't we?

We knew what was coming and I could feel the pain on my ass just looking at that thing. If I hadn't already had gone pee, I think that I would have let it go right then and there I was that petrified. And you thought I was afraid of the old man? I remember her calling my cousin a slut and me a pervert. Huh?

While wailing upon my cousin's bare bottom, my aunt was yelling "You're a little girl, not a little slut, [what's a slut?] and little girls, don't go to the bathroom with little boys. Your private parts are to remain private! That's why we wear clothes, is to cover them up and don't you ever let me catch you showing little boys your p-p ever again!" Her bum was so red, I don't think I've ever seen that colour before.

But that's because I could never see my own butt. However; I saw the bruises and welts form upon her little bum and legs right there in front of my eyes. Oh shit... I just realized something... I was next.

I leaned over the tub, she stood behind me, pulled my shorts and my underwear down to my ankles. Why, how thoughtful of you. She held onto my arm so I couldn't get away, I suppose? "Where the hell was I going? You locked the damn door!" I was given the same speech. "And you, you little pervert, [it was the first time I had ever heard that word... what's a pervert?] little boys don't go to the bathroom with little girls, our private parts are to remain private, that's why we wear clothes is to keep them covered up and don't you let me ever catch you showing little girls your p-p ever again!"

Yes, damn... is another word I heard in our house on a regular basis.

I'm sure I got a smack or two for every word she said, which would make it 44 wacks or more. I don't know which raised more welts, the spoon or the belt? Needless to say, we both ate our dinner standing up that night and for a couple of nights there after. Man, did that ever hurt. We showed each other our bare butts a couple of days later to see if the sores were going away. That was the first time I do believe I've seen such sickening colours that just didn't look right on a person's body.

Hold it!

Stop the presses!

Rewind the tape... put Humpty Dumpty back on that wall!

I just thought of something as I recalled this beating which had never occurred to me before, until now that is...

Huh? What did I miss?

How could I have been so dense?

What did I miss?

Oh, you're going to love this...

Just picture this... here are two little kids of the opposite sex at a very young age going to the bathroom together exposing themselves to one another and thinking nothing of it because we don't know any better. Along comes auntie who is beating the living daylights out of us while giving us her version of an education.

Okay?

So, what does auntie do in the process of this beating?

I don't know, what does she do?

She pulls down our under garments right in front of the other, which naturally exposes our "private parts" once again to the other of the opposite sex, which was the reason for her beating our asses in the first place. She just did, exactly what she said we should never do. It's not like I was sent out of the room while my cousin received her beating and I went in alone to get mine. No, she beat our bare asses in front of each other, which of course, meant exposing our "private parts" [I know, scratched record, right?] "which are to remain private" once again to the other of the opposite sex. Does any of this make any sense to any of you? Or, am I the only one who's crazy here? Double standards eh? "Do as I say, not as I do!" [monster's voice again]

Adults? Damn them, Damn them all! These people are sicker than I am... no wonder I all grew up confused.

Interjection: Now that you've had a taste of how I was raised... double check one of the 'Risk Factors' presumed to be a cause of bipolar disorder... Periods of High stress, such as the death of a love one ... or, another traumatic event, drug or alcohol abuse [which we will get too]. How about a life time of 'periods of high stress' combined with constant 'traumatic events'? But this wouldn't count in the least... why would it? Nor would it be enough trauma to cause PTSD because kids can't suffer from any such ailment, can they? But, what do I know, I'm not the expert here, am I?

The thing is, when mom looked after my cousin and her other siblings, we still bathed together. Oh, and to let you in on a little secret dear auntie... that beating didn't stop us from going to the bathroom together, when you weren't around that is. Psst, yet another secret... and you'll love this one... sometimes we even had the pleasure of sleeping together when we were older children. More often than not, when we were together, we were inseparable. I remember chasing her around the yard, "Kiss me, kiss me" how did we know cousins weren't suppose to do that? I know I said I didn't know what love was, but there was just something special about this girl and I wanted to be with her all of the time from a very early age. It broke our hearts though when they finally [and to their amusement too I'm sure] broke the news to us about how cousins were not allowed to marry each other. It wasn't until many years later, after I was married and had a couple of children of my own did I find out that 'He' was not my biological father but my step-dad, which meant 'she' wasn't my biological aunt, which also meant that 'her daughter' wasn't my biological 'cousin' after-all. "You lying bastards, Why? You broke our hearts". Talk about your childhood sweat hearts, two peas in a pod had nothing on us two. I often wondered what it would have been like, had we gotten married? Well, we'll never know now, will we? Oh, I'm sure with my crazy antics though, she would have kicked my sorry ass to the curb… and I wouldn't be able to blame her either. Or, would we have caught a lot of this and sought help sooner? It could have gone either way. Wherever you are, and if you are reading this… you need to know that I have never stopped loving you. You may not have been my last and only love, but you were my first. And I don't care whose reading this and knows of whom I am speaking of. What a bunch of pricks. Eh?

On with the show… Will someone change the bulb in the projector?

I can't remember if my older brother was involved in these shenanigans or not but I do remember when my younger brother and I, (ages 4 and 5) drew on the wall of that same apartment [yes, the very one where I broke the glass window and had the wooden spoon taken to my ass] with our crayons. Mom was probably busy with our younger sister and wasn't keeping an eye on us, but what else was new? I'm pretty sure my older brother was at school. Anyway, I remember the two of us standing there stark naked, scrubbing the crayon scribbles off of the wall while he beat us repeatedly with 'the belt'. The problem with that was that he paused going back and forth between the two of us so we never knew when to prepare for the wack [as if I could prepare for something of that nature anyway]. He hit me on my bare legs, butt, back and if I dare moved, that's where the next strike would catch me… on the arm, in the stomach, across the face, in the groin. It didn't matter to him where he hit me because flesh was flesh and he was after his pound of it no matter where he took it from. Come to think of it, if he was aiming for my ass, he wasn't a very good shot. Should I fall to the floor, well that was okay too… I recall during this beating I had done just that… I was lying there on the floor in the fetal position covering my head and the belt hitting my little arms as I tried to protect my face. I already had one eye ripped open by this time and desired not to have a reoccurrence but it was during this beating that he ripped open the other one which required about five or six stitches to close up. Lucky me, I now have a matching pair, aren't I special? I think someone once said that the best things in life come in pairs, didn't they? So, now he drew blood, but so what? He continued until he was satisfied that I had learned my lesson or that he had done his worse. And, it was usually the later satisfaction of course. The most severe one at that early age though was getting a beating from both my parents on the same day and the only time that I remember mom ever taking the belt to me.

"A Beating from Both of them? Come on, how did you manage that?"

"Yes, I'm serious, from each of them." Did I not just say that this was going to get gruesome or do you just like hearing me talk for the hell of it?" "Nuts eh?"

Wait a minute… I just realized that I should have explained The Corn Flakes War after this… oh well, I put the cart before the horse again, sorry.

"Welcome to my Nightmare!" by Alice Cooper 1975. Alice had no idea he was singing about my life. But, that song was really a pansy ass rendition of what my living hell was all about. Alice had no clue as to what a 'nightmare' really was/is. He should have asked me to write the lyrics, it probably would have been a number one hit from the start.

"A Beating, From both of Them!" "Oh, you're going to love this, I promise."

Still in the same apartment… I was playing outside with a friend [I did have those once upon a time, when I didn't know any better that is], the parking lot for an auto glass repair shop was across the alley and all gravel. One of us got the stupid-ass idea of putting sand and gravel into a gas tank of one of the parked cars. Of course, I'm going to blame him, he was older, it was his fault because he should have known better.

The parents had to split the bill for the repairs. But, when the police officer informed mom of what I had done, she didn't hesitate for a split second and reached over to the counter [wait a second, why was the belt on the kitchen counter? I always thought it came off of the step-dad's pants] and took the belt to me right then and there, yes, right in front of the policeman. At least she permitted me to keep my clothes on [as if that made a difference]. That was the one and only time I remember mom ever hitting me with a belt. At one point I do remember the officer reaching out to stay her hand and telling her "that's enough." Where was he going to be when the old man got home? "Sir, can you come back later in the day when my daddy gets home?" "Why son?" "Because all hell is going to break loose on my sorry ass, and I want you here to protect me when it does, that's why?" Oh, shit! Wouldn't even begin to express how I was feeling... waiting, waiting... just sitting there waiting. "Has eternity passed me by yet?" I had to spend the rest of the day on my bed waiting for step-brute to come home from work which was a living hell in and of itself. I was only permitted to climb down from my bunk to use the bathroom, then I had to run back to my bed. I wasn't allowed any toys, a colouring book or anything at all to play with to help pass the time. All I could do was lay on my top bunk [supposedly thinking about what I had done wrong] while looking out of the window, down onto busy King Street. I suppose I past the time watching the cars and the people below... "help, somebody, anybody, help!" I do remember looking for a way to escape. But I didn't know how I'd make it all the way down to the sidewalk below from our balcony and run away. I even tried the front door but the safety lock was too high for me to unlatch. I couldn't even reach it while standing on a chair... I told you, I was a tiny thing.

I know I was crying even before he arrived home, and it wasn't from the beating that I had received earlier. That had to have been an hour or so ago at least. No, I was crying because I was so scared "how scared were you?" I was scared to death that I'm sure I was whiter than a ghost. I even wet my pants on one of my trips to the bathroom because I heard a noise... out... in the hallway... outside our apartment door. I froze right then and there on the spot and the warm wetness trickled down my leg. I thought "OH NO! he's home!" Talk about being terror stricken. These actors on the television horror shows could have taken a lesson or two from me I tell you. Well, I had wet my pants so I may as well take the rest of my clothes off. They were going to come off when shithead arrived home anyway. Not too long after that I was told to 'adopt the position' which was nothing more than more psychological torture. This way, I was readily available and waiting for him to pounce upon my trembling body at his earliest convenience and it was always convenient for him to tare into me. Adopting the position meant laying over the edge of the bed, a chair or a couch which ever was the most convenient apparatus handy in the room, naked as a jay-bird exposing my bare ass to the world which of course made for an easy target for him to wail upon. As was already discussed... painting a bullseye on it wouldn't have matter though, his target was anywhere and everywhere on my person.

When he heard the news, all I heard was the sound of his belt coming off of his pants and me screaming bloody murder.

Screaming Bloody Murder: Screaming much more intense then normal screaming, close to an insane breakout of rage.

If he was yelling at me I couldn't hear him over my blood curdling cries for mercy.

Mercy of course wasn't even a word found within the pages of his dictionary for which because he had no concept of its meaning as he never had any compassion or the capabilities of extending it towards myself.

Bloodcurdling screams: arousing from fright or horror.

Mercy: noun; compassion or forgiveness shown toward someone whom it is within one's power to punish or harm.

I'm sure the neighbours thought that someone was being murdered in our humble abode but no one came pounding on the door to investigate, so, I didn't matter to anyone, not then, not now, not ever. Where was that cop when I needed him? I know that I have a good imagination, but even I can make this shit up... I ate a few meals standing up over the next few days... again. I must have like eating horsey style or something, I don't know… it always seemed to me that I was too sore to sit down and eat like a 'normal' kid. Not to mention the fact that I wasn't allowed to play outside for awhile. I was stuck in that damn apartment for what seemed like a life time to a little kid because it was summer. I know kids today are different but back then, what kid wanted to be indoors during the summer time? Not me, that was for sure! Especially with the park just a short ½ block away.

Interjection: 0912-18-07-2018; I don't know about these sleeping pills. I took one at 1900hrs last night, went to bed for 2300hrs and laid there for a couple of hours before finally falling asleep only to wake up at 0900 not wanting to get out of bed. But, what's the alternative? Not sleeping at all? I don't know, I still maintain the fact that sleep is over rated and so are chemical aides.

"Oh! Oh! Mr. Kotter! Mr. Kotter!"

I just remembered my very first cut… while we were living in this afore mentioned apartment, Waterloo park was at the end of the short ½ block and just inside the park was the kid's playground. In this playground they had a circular monkey bar apparatus we use to climb up all of the time. "Last one to the top is a rotten egg" and with that, I ran ahead and scrambled up that thing faster than the 'Flash'.

I dropped down into the center for another go around and OH SHIT! "Waaaaah," I was 5, give me a break… I hadn't seen the broken glass pop bottle [Ya, imagine, small glass pop bottles, I think they're making a come back] in the sand and a large piece went right through my running shoe and deep into my foot. My younger brother was only four and he was upset that we had to leave the park so soon. I guess I was always spoiling another person's fun too. Oh well, a trip to the hospital, and you know the rest of the story… I got a beating again, because mom told me to wait for her but I hadn't listened, ran ahead and ended up getting hurt. So, of course, it was my fault and I deserved it for being a stupid-ass. Not to mention that he had to buy me a new pair of shoes and more meds. Gulp, gulp, gulp… goes his beer money into my body again…

<u>The Flash</u>: the original Flash first appeared in Flash Comics #1 (cover date January 1940/release month November 1939 https://en.wikipedia. org/wiki/Flash_(comics)

I never did like comic books [and still don't] and I have never ever read one from cover to cover... in my opinion, they aren't interesting nor are they funny... in fact, they're rather quite boring actually and could never hold my interest long enough to read beyond a couple of pages never mind progressing all the way to the end. Come to think of it, I've never read a magazine or a news paper from start to finish either. Huh... oh, speaking of which, the comics in the papers are just as stupid.

Oh yes, I also learned at an early age [probably about 6 or 7] that talking to a school nurse or any school official for that matter, was never a good idea and didn't do me any favours either. I was sent to see the nurse one day because I was complaining to my teacher of having a sore stomach. I think she noticed a couple of bruises on my arm so she asked me to lift up my shirt. After a quick visual inspection, she sent me to the see the nurse, the teacher was on the phone as I made my way out... The nurse closed the door behind me and asked me to take off my clothes... since when did school nurses beat on little kids? I didn't know what I did wrong but I was scared and started crying. Of course, she caught all of that and calmed me down. I'm pretty sure that was the first time any 'official' at school had seen what the troll was capable of dishing out. Then she started to spread some sort of ointment on my welts. When she was finished she sent me back to class. Now the problem with all of that is quite evident if you've been paying any attention whatsoever... Yup, the school nurse called step-monster at work that day and questioned him about the bruises and how they came to be about my entire body? So, why didn't she call the 'Children's Aide Society' whoever they were to come and take me away? Now, that's a very good question that I just thought of. [Oops, is a minor booboo, her calling the tyrant was a major catastrophe] Needless to say, he was waiting for me when I got home from school... I remember seeing his car in the parking stall, and I wanted to pee my pants again. My heart? Not bloody likely, my testicles climbed up and joined my heart in my throat I was that petrified. How petrified were you? I was so petrified that I really did have to urinate, but I knew I wouldn't have made it past him to use the washroom so I used the flower bed by the back door before I went into the house. He almost never came home from work early, not even if there was an emergency with one of us kids but for some reason, I knew he was there for me that day. Yup, I was right... he came home early to beat upon my sorry ass because he enjoyed it so much... not to mention to get an ahead start on his other favorite pastime, next to beating upon me. I still remember the stern warning; "what happens in this house, stays in this house, [and you thought that only pertained to Vegas] and now I'm going to make sure you remember that!" Once again, the clothes came off [they came off so often I may as well have waked around the house in the buff] and I was the object of his amusement for opening my big mouth. And that my friends, is another way that I had welts on welts and bruises upon bruises. Because I was beat so bloody often and usually for a minor offense or because he didn't know who the guilty party was, so the 3 of us boys usually got it for some reason or other... as if he ever needed a reason.

Have you heard Bill Cosby's skit: To my brother Russell whom I slept with?

January 1968; https://en.wikipedia.org/wiki/To_Russell,_My_Brother,_Whom_I_Slept_With

Well, Bill's description of his dad's belt went something like this... the belt was 9' long, 8' wide, and it had hooks on it, and it would rip the meat off of your body when it hit you. My ignoramus' belt may not have matched that exact description but he sure knew how to swing that thing so that it felt as if the flesh was being torn from my body when it connected. For those of you who aren't familiar with the word <u>welts</u> or have no idea what I'm talking about nor what they even look like; they are red, swollen marks left on the flesh caused by a <u>heavy</u>, <u>hard</u> <u>blow</u>. Google that one too just for shits and giggles.

If you've ever seen anyone flogged on television, [I know, that's only pretend and make-up, but they do a bang-up job of making it look so bloody real, believe me] then you have an idea of what I endured... and yes, he would almost inevitably break the skin and drawn blood and no, I'm not exaggerating! I'm sure that bastard was never satisfied until he drew blood. I swear that man was half vampire or something, hence again referring to him as 'monster'… monsters eat little children, don't they? If he liked drawing blood so much, why wasn't he working at the blood bank or for the Red Cross? I received many <u>floggings</u> when I was a child. I sometimes wondered if he was a reincarnated Roman Centurion or something he did it so well and so often and I know he was sick enough to enjoy it each and every time.

How good is your imagination… it should be pretty good by now with all the descriptions I've been overloading you with?

Now, picture this if you are able to… many of these long nasty red swollen marks layered upon each other across my bum because I was hit numerous times [without number so it seemed] in one area. Oh, but that would have been a blessing, just being hit in one area that is, I was never so fortunate. No, I'd have welts all over the surface of my ass, my upper legs, perhaps my lower back and that is if I managed to stay in one place. Which in itself was a feat to be sure.

"Bullshit!"

"No one can endure what you're describing, especially at such a young age".

"Well, let me tell you, to go… '! @#$%^' okay, I won't… but you weren't there. And of course, I don't have the doctor's reports to prove it. You're only calling foul because your pansy asses had never seen the broad side of a hand never mind a wooden spoon or 'the belt', so you're not in any position to be calling me a liar. Parents can't use corporal punishment today because it's against the law… check the laws back in the 1960's, children were nothing more than property I'm sure. Go further back into history and check out what our African-Canadian or African-American neighbour's ancestors endured and then come back and call, Bullshit! I'm telling you it happened. Seriously, No one can make this shit up. Well, they probably could but they would have to have been exposed to it somewhere first and then expand upon what they have seen.

Well, you did warn us that it would get gruesome, I can't even imagine anything remotely coming close to something like that.

Do you remember the last beating you ever took before you left home for good?

Yes, I do remember. How could I ever forget Friday January 30th 1976 about 1545hrs? I remember it as if were yesterday! It was exactly a week after my 17th birthday. I came home from school with just about enough time to quickly change, grab a bite to eat and head out the door to be at work with maybe 10 minutes to spare and that was if I ate a sandwich or something while I walked to work. I entered through the back door as it were a typical day. I greeted my mom who was in the kitchen. Nothing unusual so far. She promptly asked me to run to the convenience store for her. It was about 2 ½ blocks away... being that I never said 'no' to her, off I went without hesitation [which of course meant I wouldn't have time to eat and would have to grab something at work]. When I returned I put the bag on the counter, quickly took off my boots, mitts, hat, coat and started to head for my room so I could change before going to work. She met me at the doorway to the dinning room, something was wrong but I didn't know what, nor did I care because I was in a hurry. She informed me that she had forgotten something and asked if I would mind going back to the store for her. "**No**, I can't, I have to get to work, ask my brother to go." I think that was the first time past the age of 3 that I had ever said 'NO' to her [unless it had to do with eating something that I wasn't going to eat that is]. Well, what I didn't realize was that the atrocity incarnate himself was home early from work [why? I don't really know why, does it matter? He was home, Fuck! I can't catch a break]. I swear all he heard was the word "**NO**" and he flew out of the den through the dinning room like Superman and laid a beating on me once again. He pounded me about the face, head, and shoulders. My head bounced off of the doorway, the fridge [how come the word 'refrigerator' is spelled without the letter 'd' but we put the letter 'd' in the word fridge?] and the counter. When I tried to duck from one of his swings, he followed through with an upper cut and split both of my lips. Blood splattered on the wall, the fridge, the counter top and spilled onto the floor, not to mention all over my clothes. He also ripped my shirt when he grabbed a hold of me and lifted me up so he could punch me in the face again. He then grabbed me by the throat, escorted me, walking backwards, out of the house, threw me down the 4 steps off of the deck and into the snow bank. "As long as you live in my house, you'll damn well do as you're bloody well told!"

Off I went, back to the store in late January in my sock feet… without my boots, mitts, hat or winter coat, scooping up snow as I walked along in attempts to stop my nose from bleeding and my eye from swelling. There I was, walking on the road like some drunkard staggering all over the place, with one handful of snow on my nose and the other handful over my eye while still seeing stars. I didn't even worry about the split fat lips until my nose had stopped bleeding, nor the fact that I was in my stocking feet or the fact that it was late January and I didn't have a coat on… none of that mattered at that point. I arrived back at the store, still dripping blood, which was getting all over the floor of the store. Oh well. The clerk had asked what had happened, and if I wanted him to call the cops? I told him that it wouldn't do any good, made my purchase and returned home. Mom was in the kitchen and said thank you. I whispered a "fuck you" as I hastily put on my boots, grabbed my winter coat [leaving my hat and mitts behind] and stormed back out of the house [without closing the interior door] hoping that the bastard hadn't heard me swear at her. I do believe that was the first and only time I ever swore at mom [to her face], but at that point, I'm sure I felt as though she had it coming. After all, it was her fault I took a beating. She knew I had to go to work and I didn't enjoy being late. On the way to work I was still scooping up snow to place upon my wounds. I didn't change my clothes and arrived at the restaurant late with a ripped, bloodied shirt, which I threw into the garbage, bloodied pants and in wet socks. My boss asked what had happened to me… I guess I gave him 'a look' "never mind, I think I can guess" he said. He knew the old man all too well and handed me a Vodka and Orange Juice and a wet towel, suggesting that I take a few minutes to clean up before starting. I think he gave me 5 or 6 drinks throughout the evening. Later on, I told him what had happened. My story didn't surprise him in the least. The heartbreak of this story is that I took a beating of that magnitude over a $0.39 can of Ocean Spray Cranberry Sauce for that bastard's chicken dinner and what did get to eat? Multiple knuckle sandwiches, that's what! "Yummy!" And you wonder why I hate the wanker so much today or have no respect for him? Well, wonder no more! I vowed that night that would be the last beating I ever took from that man. I didn't know how, I didn't know when, but I wouldn't be living in "his house" any longer than necessary and I started making plans to leave that year. I left in October of 1976 and never looked back.

How did you make your escape?

Sorry younglings, but it was everyone for themselves at that point. I had mentioned that I was in Cadets. Every year for the past four years I had been applying to multiple summer camps because I didn't know which ones I'd be accept to. In February, I went to the recruiting centre for the Canadian Armed Forces... Hey, I've seen these applications before. I took the CF application form to Cadets and compared them to the camp applications which would be coming out in March. Then I got the most cunning, awesome, wonderful idea that I have ever had in my life... They were exactly a like, a perfect match in fact... well what good fortune is this? There just might be a God in heaven after all? The next month I filled out 3 Cadet applications and 1 CF application and presented them to the asshole in my life. Okay, here you go... "What are you applying for this year?" [like he really cared] "One is for the US Exchange program, and the other three are for various programs at Cornwallis, band and leadership stuff mostly." But, we all know the application for the Canadian Armed Forces was in the mix, and Boot Camp was being conducted at Cornwallis Nova Scotia and it is a 'leadership' style of training, sort of, so technically, it was a half truth? That's it! Right there, on the dotted line if you please and he signed all 4 applications without taking a second looking at them... just like I knew he would... see Ya, you bastard, have a nice fucking life! I'm out of here! Victory, at last! Who's your daddy? Come on! High Five! And the crowd enthusiastically applauds the ingenuity of this maneuver... A standing ovation in fact, "oh, you're too kind, thank you... Thank you, Thank you very much!" Pretty smart eh?

I must say, that was very clever of you.

Earlier you mentioned being hospitalized: what happened there?

I was hospitalized several times by that man because he went overboard with the belt [but, when didn't he?], but there were two severe beatings that I remember without even having to think about them.

Let me guess, as if they just happened yesterday.

How did you know? You must be a quick study as well.

Other than the stitches already mentioned, I think I was about 7 and not really sure why he was smacking me on the bare hands with the belt for [sometimes he'd switch things up between my hands and my behind. I suppose it depended upon what I did and how mad he was I guess]. Either way, being hit on the hand or the behind was never a treat that's a for sure. I was to stretch out my arms in front of me one at a time about shoulder high. I had to hold my hand open with the palm facing the ceiling to allow him to come down on it with the belt. I was to switch hands from left to right and back again as he wacked away. Sometimes he'd make things interesting and say "faster, faster" as if he were a captain on a rowing team or something. If I didn't raise my arms up fast enough he'd smack me in the face with the belt and I'd get a second chance to comply as he called out the cadence. Sometimes he'd count, and if he had to break rhythm for whatever reason, you bet he had to start the count right back at 1. Then he'd lose count [because he's stupid] and stop counting altogether and just keep going anyway so, why bother counting at all? It's not as if he was going to stop at some mythical or magical number only he knew of. And they weren't love taps either, that fucking hurt, more than I can describe. I don't remember how many times he had hit me but both hands were beginning to bleed, and they were sore to the point where I could barely open them anymore and I had, had enough. However, for some reason that day I wouldn't give him the satisfaction of crying out. I remember biting my tongue to stop myself from making more than a whimper. I bit so hard that my tongue bled. As the tears rolled down my face... like I said, I had enough... and without even thinking about it, I then made a big mistake, almost a fatal one really. For some 'stupid-ass' reason [impulsivity kicking in again] I pulled my hand away at the last second as that belt came down and he wacked himself in the leg, [Yes! He scores! How does that feel asshole? Hurts, doesn't it?] to which I then laughed... Oh shit! My 2nd worse mistake of my young life! I'm half laughing now reminiscing here, but what followed was no laughing matter, I assure you. Oh man, that was the first time I thought he was going to kill me and almost wishing he had of and the first time I remember mom ever coming to my rescue. He beat me so hard and hit me so many times that I was black and blue from the top of my head to my feet and that was with my clothes on. I shit you not, I had welts on my head, my neck and everywhere else that I can think of. I was in the hospital for over 2 weeks doped up on pain killers and what not. I couldn't sit, stand, lay down or even go to the bathroom without something hurting somewhere. I don't think there was a spot on my body except the soles of my feet that wasn't in pain. I had to take ice bathes to reduce the body swelling because he beat me that badly. I have no idea how mom explained that one to the medical staff… if they even cared that is… so who or where was this 'Children's Aide Society' and what was there mandate? I had no idea because I never saw them.

The other time I remember was when I was about 12 and the three middle kids were getting it for some reason or other [as if he ever required a reason]. We were made strip down naked as usual… 2 boys and 1 girl in front of each other. It wasn't the first time I had seen my sister naked or a female body for that matter, but it was the first time I remember ever experiencing an erection… [talk about abnormal excitement… again, what was one of the symptoms?] unless I was holding back having to urinate that is. Oh Damn, what's this? Where did you come from? Not now, I have no idea what you're about, but I don't think that now is a good time to make your appearance. Oh shit, not now! Butt naked right there in the living room and I experience a hard-on, needless to say it wasn't hard for very long. Oh Shit, again doesn't even begin to describe the whirlwind that was unleashed upon my tiny naked body that afternoon. Well, it was game over for me to say the least when he noticed it. And, notice it he did… my little soldier was standing straight out and all of sudden his complete attention was focused on poor little ole me and my 'manhood' at that point and the other 2 got away without a beat down. But I'm sure they were just as traumatized by what they had to witness that day. All I heard was "you little <u>pervert</u>" [I'm going to have to look that word up because it was the 2nd time now someone had called me that and I still have no idea what it meant] and out of nowhere, without warning, he hit me so hard in the testicles with that belt that I doubled over, collapsed to the floor while puking. He wailed on me so many times and so hard that mom thought he was going to kill me. I had the same thoughts running through my head. Just before I blacked out

I heard mom call out "Stop it, you're going to kill him!" No, leave him alone, let him finally do it and put me out of my fucking misery all ready. The last thing I remember was his foot in my face and I blacked out. My brother informed me later [after I returned from the hospital that is] that mom came to my rescue and he hit her with the belt a couple of times for interfering then stormed out of the house. He had slammed the storm door so hard that he broke the glass. He went to the Legion no doubt for more beer and to cool off [as if that were ever possible]. I remember waking up in the ambulance naked underneath the sheet with a catheter in. I had an ice pack on my boys, and one over my face. I had the taste of blood and vomit mixture in my mouth and down my throat. The blood of course was from the fat lips and the flow going down the back of my throat because he broke my nose when he had kicked me. Not to mention being unable to see out of one eye because it was swollen shut and I'm sure that I urinated blood off and on for a day or two afterwards. The embarrassing part about being a pre-teen was having the nurses taking me for ice baths and replacing the ice packs on my scrotum. A couple of years later, remembering that beating, I asked mom if I'd be able to have children? She assured me that everything would be okay. That was the last beating I remember where I took my clothes off. From that point on he hadn't used the belt either, he switched to beating me with his fists.

For the ladies out there and the gentlemen who have never experienced such a traumatic injury to the groin region: Groin kicks (injuries) are **horrendously** painful. The nausea, tears, and collapse might seem like overkill, but they are actually ways your body is trying to improve the situation. "This is essentially a defense mechanism by the body to reduce the painful sensation," says Dr. Muhammad A. Mirza, founder of erectiledoctor.com. Signals are sent to the abdominal region because that area shares pain receptors with the groin. Some of these signals are what make you want to grab your stomach, bend over, or lie on the ground in the fetal position. The abdominal pain, paired with possible nausea and dizziness, can sometimes cause vomiting. Increased heart rate, sweating, and higher body temperature are other common responses to this kind of injury. Basically, your body is going insane, all probably an attempt to tell you to never get hurt like that again.

https://www.mensjournal.com/health-fitness/what-really-happens-after-a-kick-to-the-groin-20140528/

I don't think even <u>Muhammad Ali</u> ever beat an opponent as bad as the beating I took that day. I never understood why that man was never arrested or why he hated me so much to do something like that to a kid.

<u>Muhammad Ali</u>: Born Cassius Marcellus Clay Jr. January 17, 1942 Louisville, Kentucky, USA. Died June 3, 2016 (aged 74) Scottsdale, Az.

He was, in my opinion the greatest boxer who ever stepped into the ring.

https://en.wikipedia.org/wiki/Muhammad_Ali

<u>Pervert</u>: noun; a person whose sexual behavior is regarded as abnormal and unacceptable.

So, I finally knew what a pervert was. What the hell does a kid at 5 years of age, let alone a 12-year-old [who has had no formal sex-ed] know to be called something like that?

<u>Slut</u>: noun; a woman who has many casual sexual partners. And to call your daughter something of that nature at the age of 4?

These people are sicker than I am. How more disgusting can you get?

And they wonder why I never wanted anything to do with them, especially after I left the house.

<u>Interjection</u>: 0123-30-06-2018: I didn't take the sleeping pill last night. I forgot… now I'm paying the price. I had been in bed for the past 2 hrs trying to go to sleep. What a joke, why do I even bother? So, I got up and am continuing to write.

I guess you are lucky to be alive today to talk about all of this.

How does it feel to recall these memories and to talk about it now after all these years?

I don't think it will put me back into a depressive state or anything like that if that's what you're concerned about. Presently, I'm in the coasting phase I was talking about earlier and while in this phase, I can't say that I really give a shit about anyone or anything… so, thanks Eeyore! He's actually been my only real companion over all of theses years. I'm fine… [FINE… Feelings Inside Not Expressed, Felling Inadequate Need Encouragement, fucked up, Insecure, Neurotic, Emotional or Feeling Insecure Neurotic and Emotional, Frantic, Insane, Nuts, Egotistical… there are actually 50 acronyms for 'F-I-N-E', so take your pick, almost any one would just about fit the bill] for now, I think? I can't change what was, so there's no sense in crying over spilt milk. I can only deal with it and continue going forward. I have enough crap going on right now without worrying about the past. It does open old wounds, it brings back hatred, loathing, disgust, shame, pity, anger, and I'm sure an entire host of other feelings that I've managed to bury for so long… I know there is an intellectual disconnect though and that's how I am able to say… "who gives a rat's ass?" The thing that upsets me is that I've even tried to reach out to the prick to make amends, as if I have anything to make up for a wrong doing. I only forgave and tried to reach out because Christ compels me too. Okay, I've researched this forgiveness aspect and it briefly goes something like this: I have to forgive or I won't be forgiven but nowhere does it say that forgiveness means that we have to be friends or that I have to continue to subject myself to his verbal abuse. We are to love our enemies, so I'll love him enough to pray for him as an enemy, but I don't have to extend my hand in friendship with him. I don't have to give that man the time of day really… so, I won't!

You said shame?

Yes.

What do you have to be ashamed of, you never caused any of this, you can't hold yourself responsible for the actions of your parents, nor anyone else for that matter.

True, I think its more shame and embarrassment for perhaps telling these stories to the world, and people knowing what I had to endure I guess… it's also humiliating in some respects, but, I have to deal with my demons and this is one way for the healing process to take affect, so the shrink told me. The other part would be that it's a 'crying shame' really, that no one did anything to lift a finger to save me. It's also a shame that the bastard was never arrested for his cruelty and I'd really like to know why. People were arrested back then for cruelty to animals but beating a kid within an inch of his life was acceptable behaviour or what?

Again, you have nothing to be ashamed or embarrassed about.

Yes, I know… but it's difficult to explain what I'm truly feeling about all of this.

I often feel as though I've danced with the devil and lived to tell about it but I'm still battling with his demons and one always figures, or thinks about the 'if only'… if only I wasn't so sick, if only I had been a better student, if only I didn't get into mischief, stuff like that.

You also said pity, what's that all about?

Well, in some respects I pity the poor soul. I'm sure he had his own demons to deal with. It's a pity that no one has ever helped him either. But then again, I'm sure he never asked for any and I'm pretty sure it was because he probably thought that all of that crap was normal behaviour, who knows? It was all pretty sick shit if you ask me or any other intelligent person on the planet. Unless of course they to are a fellow abuser, controller and a down right evil person. I've heard stories about how his old man use to beat him. But, one would think that it would stand to reason, if you didn't like it, why would you continue the pattern and become what you loathed the most? Did he have some sort of mental deficiency himself that I'm not aware of? If so, why didn't he get help? Oh, I know… if he had gotten help, he'd have to pay for any medications that they told him would be necessary and go for therapy, which again would take away from his beloved drinking money. Oh, I'm sure he was even told to stop drinking, and we all know how well that would have gone over. He just enjoyed his drinking which of course fed his demons until they were finally unleased upon my poor sickly physical being. Don't get me wrong, it's not as if I'm going to be holding out a Kleenex box for the under-lord and master should he happen to purchase this book and actually read it and become weepy or anything. No doubt he would deny it all anyway and call me a liar because ½ of the time he was either too drunk, extremely pissed or too busy thinking about drinking to remember. How the hell would he know what the truth was? He was so mean, miserable and drunk most of the time I even wonder how he managed to keep down the same job for twenty-six years. I don't think that man has a remorseful bone in his entire body. So, I can't see any water works coming from him. And it's not like I'm going to weep for him at his funeral because his soul is going to hell. I tried to share Christ with him on several occasions but he told me to keep that shit to myself… so, he has made his choice, hasn't he? So now, I refuse to give that man the time of day. Like mom use to say… "you made your bed, now you have to lie in it." Well, he's made his.

You mentioned name calling, what type of names would they call you?

Sometimes on the rarest of occasions mind you, he would get my name right. Wayne, my name is **WAYNE**! Asshole! Besides, I like my name… But usually not before calling out the other two boys names first, then he'd forget about the names all together, while pointing at me, he'd say: "you, stupid-ass, get over here." Then out of the blue, Whack! I'd get smacked across the head for not coming when I was called the first time. Huh? "You never called me, how was I suppose to know you were talking to me?" and I'd get another smack for talking back. Oh, Ya… I'm the 'stupid-ass', how could I have been so stupid as to forget? ["Which way did I go George?"] The other names were little bastard, asshole, retard. But his favourite which I heard more often than not and I'm sure was reserved just for little ole me was; "stupid-ass." I actually don't recall him calling the other siblings that, but I could be mistaken, but usually not. If I had never left the house and heard my 'real name', I swear I would have grown up thinking my name was 'stupid-ass'. He'd call me a "cry baby" and tell me to stop crying or he'd give me something to cry about. Meanwhile, he had just back-handed me or smacked me across the face with the belt, as if that wasn't something to cry about? I remember thinking on numerous occasions; "let me do that to you and see if it doesn't bring tears to your eyes, asshole." He started calling me 'momma's boy' because he picked that up from my brothers and thought it was funny. He found out that I'd do anything for mom and that I was her 'favorite' so everyone thought. It wasn't that I was her favourite, it's because I was born sickly so she had to protect me more than the others but she hadn't done a very poor job at that just as everything else in life. Plus, as was already mentioned... Wayne would do things for her the others wouldn't. My siblings made up names over the years besides mama's boy... little man, pecker head, pipsqueak, fuck-nuts, and wiener man. I'm sure there were a few more, but I can't remember them at this particular moment. They were just as mean as he was for that. Come to think of it, my youngest sister was the only one of them who used my real name and never called me names or made fun of me.

Thanks Sis!

Then there were the other put downs, such as; "you'll never amount to anything," "I didn't expect anything out of you anyway," When I'd surrender my report cards... "a, 'C' again, typical" "why can't you do anything right?" "You'll never learn," "why can't you learn from his mistakes?" "How many times do I have to tell you?" "Don't you ever listen?" "Do as I say, not as I do" and then his favorite was... "as long as you live in my house, you'll..." whatever came after that was usually... "do as you're told." Generally followed up with a punch or a smack across the head. He was always smacking me across the head, YES ALWAYS! Oh, how I hated that. But there were so many put-downs that I swear he made a few up just for me. The put-downs were constant but the one I remember hearing the most was that "you'll never amount to anything."

Well, I guess the joke is on him now, isn't it? Mr. who barely accomplished grade 9...

Mom usually called me a little bugger [actually, I don't recall her calling me anything else] or she'd tell me that I was just like my father [meaning step-dad]. Which of course was a real insult because I always thought he was the biggest asshole God ever permitted to walk the face of this earth. Who'd want to be associated with, or be referred to as being like him? [When it was parent's day at school or he happened to do something with the Cadets and the kids asked who my dad was... I'd always say that he wasn't there]. Mom mostly yelled a lot, stop this or that, stop fighting, be quiet, go to your room, and so forth. One time she did beat me about the head with a telephone receiver though. She was always threatening us children with calling the Children's Aide Society [which would amount to calling Family and Community Social Services today] who would take us away and we'd never see each other again if we didn't behave. More often than not I'd answer back, "good, I hope they do, I hate you and I hate it here" and I'd run away before she could smack me. Funny thing is, she never ran after me. Being the 'stupid-ass' that he always said that I was, one day [impulsivity kicking in] I looked up the number for the Children's Society in the phone book... he, he, for those who don't know what a phone book is, it's a hard copy of a telephone directory: https://en.wikipedia.org/wiki/Telephone_directory

and I dialed the phone [without thinking about the consequences of this insanity].

Me: "Mom, [calling out above the racket] there's a lady on the phone who wants to talk to you" I said holding out the receiver.

Mom: "What lady? I didn't hear the phone ring."

Me: "It didn't ring, I called the Children's Aide Society for you so you wouldn't have too" [Ha, ha, hilarious, 'stupid-ass'].

I believe I was 9 at the time.

Another big mistake... she ripped that receiver out of my hand "you little bugger" and hit me so hard about the head that she actually broke the thing and gave me a concussion. How do I know? Because I started vomiting and she had no choice but to take me to the hospital, that's how I know. Not to mention my seeing stars and having a headache for a week. Oh, and yup, as if a trip to the hospital wasn't bad enough... you guessed it, Beelzebub wailed upon my body when it arrived home because he had to replace the telephone and it was all my fault. But, then again, when wasn't it my fault? More precious beer money out the window because of yours truly, ain't I a stinker? It's funny now, but it sure as hell wasn't funny while I was getting hit over the head or the belt across my bare ass.

My older brother thought it was a classic 'stupid-ass' maneuver though when I told him about it when he had asked what I had gotten it for this time? We've reminisced over the years, we still get a good laugh over that one. Even he took to calling me 'stupid-ass', they all did actually, all except for little sis. "Why did you get the belt this time, 'stupid-ass'? It seemed like I was always, YES, ALWAYS! getting it for one reason or another… but like I said before "as if he needed a reason." Besides, the beating for the stone in the gas tank, Mom took the wooden spoon to me one other time but those are the only times I remember her ever hitting me. That's another one of the reasons why the kids always called me 'mamma's boy' because I was never in any trouble from her. Not that I hadn't ever caused her any grief mind you, it's just that I wouldn't get in trouble for it. I could get away with things the others could not. I'd apologize, do something for her and all was good again… Oh well, sucked to be them. Besides, anytime mom asked any of us to do something, I was always the first one up and, on my way, to accomplish said task… hence, being called 'mamma's boy'. Wayne would never say "No", <u>no matter</u> <u>what</u>, it was she had asked of me.

Not matter what? What does that mean?

I'll explain that later.

When was the first time you ever remember being in a state of what you now know to be in a 'depressive state'?

Oh God, when was I ever not in some varying state of depression?

Growing up with that <u>monster</u> was enough to make me depressed just waking up in the morning wishing, hoping, praying that it would be my or his last day on earth and either way suited me just fine most of the time. The childhood prayer we were forced to recite I'm sure was a standard prayer for most kids: "Now I lay me down to sleep, I pray the Lord my soul to keep, if I should die before I wake, I pray the Lord my soul to take. God, bless mommy and daddy, aunts and uncles, grandma and grandpa, brothers and sisters and cousins. Amen?" Well, during this I would add, to myself… "yes, please, take my soul because I do not want to wake to another day." Some times I'd ask this mystical God to take away the monster, but he didn't do that either. But, like I said, God never answered my childhood prayers.

A monster is a creature which produces fear or physical harm by its appearance or its actions. Derived from the Latin monstrum, the word usually connotes something wrong or **evil**; a monster is generally morally objectionable, physically or psychologically hideous, or a freak of nature. They are usually composites of different creatures, or hybrids of humans and animals, but the term can also be applied figuratively to describe someone with similar characteristics, such as a person who does cruel or horrific things.

https://en.wikipedia.org/wiki/Monster

And, that pretty much sums him up if you ask me. Oh, you didn't ask, Okay, well this one's a freebie then. No matter how you slice that pie, you can not argue the fact that the man is/was a monster to a child. I often wondered if he was the devil himself, he was that evil because to me, he was a personification of pure evil.

Interjection: 0401-24-07-2018; been awake from 1122 yesterday. Been trying to sleep without the sleeping pills without success. I took one the other night at midnight, slept until 1122, but went to bed at midnight last night and I've been lying in bed now for 4 hrs, enough already. So, here I am, continuing with my final edit. I believe the book is finally completed, containing all that I think I should say. There is obviously more to this hellish nightmare, but you have more than enough to get an idea of what it's like to be me.

As previously mentioned, I don't remember too much of school because I was always venturing in/out of the hospital… I liked being in the hospital, no one picked on me in there. I believe it was while I was in grade 2 that a couple of the bigger kids pulled my pants down while we were out in the play ground and were putting stones into my anal cavity. One time while I was in grade 3, the bastards caught me in the boy's room… they stripped me naked, shoved a carrot up my rectum, pushed/ pulled me out into the hall for all to see. The biggest one wouldn't let me back into the bathroom, but what did it matter at that point? When the teach came out of a classroom to see what the loud laughter was all about, she found me encircled by a group of boys and girls having a grand old time at my expense. Yes, these were some of the same bullies from grade 2.

In grades 3 and 4, I have no idea how many times they took my bike away and would leave it in the middle of the road down the block somewhere so I'd have to fetch after it. Or they'd hang it up on the chain link fence by the handle bars. I was a small kid, so it was difficult for me to climb up the fence and fetch my bike down from up there and they knew it, that's why the did it. In grade 4, this one kid punched me in the eye, which knocked me down to the ground... he and another fellow opened my pants and put a heavy string around Mr. Wiener and my scrotum. They dragged me about the playground by pulling on the string of course. They got the strap from the principal for that one but that never stopped any of them from picking on me. One other time, this same kid pulled down a girl's panties and was putting stones in her vagina. I came to her rescue and got the crap beat out of me from 3 others for interfering. One of them kicked me in the nuts and I spent a couple of days in the hospital once again. After that incident, this same kid hung a cat in the play ground, then set a fire in the laundry room of his apartment building all in the same week and we never saw him again... maybe the Children's Aide Society does take children away after all?

Another time in grade 6 [I was just coming out of the shower] one of the bullies ripped my towel away while another flicked my dick with his towel... that didn't hurt as much as the belt in the groin, but it still stung. Then a bunch of them continuously snapped my naked body with their towels... The only way I could escape was by running out into the gym butt naked [well of course the girls laughed] to get the teacher. I didn't care at that point who saw me, I wasn't taking a whipping. It was my only escape route to safety and to fetch someone in authority. The boys received the strap and were awarded detentions for it, [oh, big deal] they got me back later, trust me. How did they get me back? A couple of them dragged me up the stairs to the roof and locked me out there. I had no choice but to find a way down or jump. Well, lucky for me, I saw a guy climb up a drain pipe in the movies. I figured if he could climb up, then, I could climb down and that's how I made my escape. It was shortly after that, that we had moved again so I finished grade 6 at another school. I didn't meet up with some of these kids again until grade 10. I'm not sure if they recognized me or not, they never picked on me but I stayed clear of them anyway thank you very much.

The problem was, that it was never just 1 on 1 or I would have cleaned a clock or 2 because I didn't normally display fear nor would I back down, not even from 3 or more of them. I could take what these pansy asses could dish out. Trust me, their punishments were never anything compared to what the monster doled out. I remember a few times getting even though. I'd get beaten up during the morning recess, go home for lunch, have a couple shots of mom's liquid courage and return to school to beat the crap out of them one at a time. I was usually sent to the office but getting the strap was worth it. Oh, but it didn't matter that they had beat me up during the morning recess, this was an entirely different incident. Compared to the old man, the principle hit like a girl... no offense again ladies. Getting blamed for stuff my brother would get into at school and getting the strap because of it though was never worth it. No one dared squeal on him because then he'd beat the crap out of them. So, they always blamed me. When I'd say that I wasn't involved, no one believed me because it was always 2 or 3 against 1, and the majority always won out against little ole me. Who wouldn't be <u>depressed</u> all the time if they were in my shoes? I often felt as though I were a professional punching bag or something.

<u>Depressed</u>: a person in a state of general unhappiness or <u>despondency</u>.

I told you that I didn't know what happiness was.

<u>Despondency</u>: a state of low spirits caused by loss of hope or courage.

That's more like it, not this pansy-ass 'depressive' state crap.

<u>Interjection</u>: 0415-24-07-2018; speaking of despondency, I've been down and out for the last several days, can't seem to shake the doom and gloom. I spent 2 hours in the hospital reception area for no other reason than because I felt safe there. Then I spent several hours on the beach just walking in the surf. I finally got cold and came home.

Okay, seriously... the first time I was in a state of 'despondency' was when I was 6 years old, which <u>coincidentally</u>, was the first time I tried to kill myself. I just wanted the beatings to end.

You tried to kill yourself at the tender age of 6?

Yes!

How did you attempt to kill yourself at 6 yrs old?

I drank a little bit of whisky and then a fair amount of bleach.

<u>Coincidentally</u>: in a way that results from chance despite being very unlikely.

I don't believe in coincidences, shit happens for a reason, usually unknown ones, but shit always happens to me just the same...

"You drank straight whisky at 6 years old?"

"Yup, I sure did."

"Unbelievable"

"I know, right?"

"How did you know to drink whisky straight up?"

I saw my mom do it a time or two after taking a beating from her husband. This one time after downing the whiskey I asked her why she just did that, "don't you usually mix it with coke or ginger ale?" "Yes, I do, but this numbs me faster" and she explained what being 'numb' meant. So, I guess I figured if I were 'numb', I wouldn't feel myself dying. I keep telling you; I'm pretty smart and a quick learner but no one gives me credit for it. Especially those who should.

Attempt #1: I don't know how much I drank before mom saw me and knocked the bottle out of my hand, then called 911. If 911 had public stock options, I'm sure we'd make a good dollar for every time we called that number over the years. Back then, bleach was colourless, odourless and tasteless, but it sure burned in both directions, but here I was <u>chugging</u> it at 6 years old.

How did you know that drinking bleach would kill you?

All in good time kind Sir, all in good time...

Today these kids and their 'Tide Pod' challenges... what a bunch of idiots.

Why idiot?

Because they're old enough to know better for one thing and it's not like they're trying to kill themselves or anything. It's all for fun and games and on a dare, that's why. I mean seriously, how stupid can you get? There are other things one can do for a 'rush' and to challenge each other than that.

While at the hospital I recall a conversation, I had with one of the nurses that went something like this... speaking of course was a struggle. I managed a whisper, more than anything because my throat was burnt from the Bleach going down, and coming back up when mom made me vomit... which I'm sure is one of the things they tell you... not to do.

Nurse: "did mommy ever tell you not to drink that stuff?"
Me: "yes."
Nurse: "and did she tell you what would happen to you if you did?"
Me: "yes."
Nurse: "what did she tell you?"
Me: "that I would die."
Nurse: "and do you know what it means to die?"
Me: "yes, mommy told me"
Nurse: "so, why did you drink it?"
Me: "I want to go to heaven"
Nurse: "why do you want to go to heaven?"

Y's a crooked letter... gee lady, you ask a lot of questions, you writing a book or something?

Me: "to be with the angels."
Nurse: "why do you want to be with the angels?"
Me: "because they'll keep me safe from the monster."
Nurse: "who's the monster?"
Me: "my daddy"
Nurse: "why is your daddy a monster?"

Talk about the 3rd degree, add a whip or chains and you'd be right up there the SS goons.

Me: "because monsters are mean, they hurt people and they eat little kids."
Nurse: "does your daddy hurt people?"
Me: "yes"
Nurse: "who does he hurt?"
Me: "my mommy, and me and the other kids."
Nurse: "well, you're safe now honey."

Ya, right... by who's stretch of the imagination was I safe lady? But of course, nothing ever became of that conversation and I lived at home for another 11 years being brutalized, tortured and tormented every chance he got. There were many periods over my life it felt as thought I were brutalized on a daily basis.

"Why hadn't she called the Children's Aide Society, I'll never know?"

Drinking Bleach: The active ingredient in bleach is a salt-based chemical compound called sodium hypochlorite, a relatively clear liquid that's diluted with water and used to kill fungi, bacteria and viruses, and helps you make it through flu season in one piece. But sodium hypochlorite is also corrosive, meaning it can destroy human tissue. "What if I popped the cap and start guzzling away?" You're in for a world of hurt. Symptoms range from gagging, pain and irritation in the mouth and throat; pain and possible burns in the esophagus and stomach; vomiting; and shock can appear right away to within a few hours. If you don't treat the symptoms immediately, you can permanently damage your gastrointestinal tract and internal organs -- and, depending on how much you drink, you could **die**.

That's the ticket, that's what I was looking for! I like Dragon Lilies, thank you.

You said that you were only 6 years old the first time you tried to kill yourself; there were other times then obviously?

No, that was the one and only time…

Seriously?

There were several other times throughout my life, but whose counting? But, then again, the 'so-called experts' never listened to my troubles. So, who cared? They didn't and neither had I, obviously.

We're listening, now, please continue.

It's about bloody time, I'd say.

After the bleach incident I didn't have to worry about killing myself for a little while because there were a couple of times I thought he'd do that for me, but no such luck there either. If it weren't for bad luck, I'd have no luck at all! But then, what's luck got to do with it? Damn Him! I often wished he had finished the job so that he'd finally end up in jail where he belonged.

Attempt #2: I was in in grade 3 [about 8 yrs old] when I was riding my bike home from school. I was zipping along Weber Street and detoured to the intersection [which was past our street] where Weber Street intersects with King Street in Waterloo [which are 2 major thoroughfares] I waited on the hill by the church and when I saw a bus coming, I pedaled as fast as I could, jumped the curb right in front it. I remember hearing the squealing of tires and the blast of the horn. I guess I was going faster than I had thought because the bus only caught my leg and the rear portion of my bike which spun me out and I sprawled onto the roadway into the next lane… I suppose I was lucky [depending on how you want to look at it] that there wasn't a car traveling in that lane [but then, I was trying to kill myself, no success this time either I guess]. The bus driver picked me up and sent me on my way with a few colourful expletives naturally. On my way home, I put my bike by the dumpster because the back tire was wrecked and said that the bullies had stolen it [how was I suppose to know all he had to do was buy a new rim and tire?] I explained that I was all scratched up because I was riding fast to get away from the other kids, but they caught up to me and knocked me off of my bike and took off with it. I was all scraped up, had a goose-egg on my head. We had to wait for the albatross to get home from work but then they [both parents, because mom didn't give meeny a choice] took me to the hospital to get checked out and yes, another tetanus shot and a minor concussion. My left leg, left arm swelled up and I stayed home from school for a few days. Oh well, better luck next time. Oh, and of course, more antibiotics so you know what that meant…. He, he, he… Say good-bye beer $$! Of course, I didn't say anything about the bus or wanting to kill myself. It didn't work with the bleach incident, why would it work now?

Was this after another beating from the monster?

No, from the bullies at school. Remember the carrot incident a few pages back? It was at the end of that day. I laugh actually at this cyber bullying crap… What a bunch of Cowards! And the stupid kids that put up with it… give me a break… don't they know that all they have to do is ignore them, block them, find different social media sites, or even disconnect! But, heaven forbid they can't 'connect' with their other friends… Dah, it's called getting up off of your lazy ass and getting out of the house and meeting them in person! You might want to try it sometime. Try getting away from them at school or in the hood, its an entirely different matter! But I never really had any friends who were on my side to help me out so I was always on my own. I was always a loner. The only way to get away from them was to stay in the house or in my own yard. If I ventured out beyond my yard, I never knew where they'd be and I didn't want to be caught out in the open and too far away that I couldn't return to safety. It's kind of like that mouse who scurries against the wall. I suppose that lends to a false sense of security… but then, hey, he doesn't want to get caught out in the open either, does he? Well, neither did I!

Attempt #3: In grade 4, I had been in the hospital for a while again due to the illness and I was down and out. We lived across the street from a high school and would often climb up onto the roof and play up there.

Why up on the roof?

I don't know, Why not? Just because we could I guess. We'd go up there all the time and collect the balls that the high school kids would kick up. The school had multiple levels to it's roofing system and the highest part was off to one end which had a paved parking lot below. Well, I had been thinking about death for a while now because when I was in the hospital I thought for sure that this time the illness would take me out and that would be the end, finally it would be all over, and I was okay with that. But it didn't happen then either and I'd continue to live in misery. I remember walking to the edge, looking over and backing up... okay, on the count of 3... and I'd run as fast as I could and just keep on keeping on... look ma, I can fly! "1-2-3" ... counting out loud. "Okay, this time... 1 – 2 – 3" ... Psyching myself up... "What's the matter, you chicken?" "No, I'm not chicken." "Are too, you're a little scardie cat." Still talking to myself... "Hey, stupid-ass" it's my big brother, "What are you doing?" "Nothing" "Then do nothing over here, it's time to go." So much for that. If you can call that an attempt that is. Half-hearted effort, perhaps? "Weren't going to jump anyway" "was too" "was not".

Misery: noun

1. wretchedness of condition or circumstances.
2. distress or suffering caused by need, privation, or poverty.
3. great mental or emotional distress; extreme unhappiness.
4. a cause or source of distress.

I suppose that would sum up my miserable life while living a hellish nightmare, wouldn't it?

Attempt #4, grade 6, about 12 years old I guess... before we moved again and I finished grade 6 at the new school... remember the towel snapping episode? Well, of course, everyone was laughing at me for days afterwards... some of the girls were even calling me "little wiener" and of course everyone would laugh harder. Well, that's just great! Put 2 + 2 together and it immediately put me in another depressive state. I went into the boy's washroom and broke the mirror. I took a piece of the mirror, slit my wrist with it and just my luck… a kid came in, ran out, fetched a teacher and I went back to the nurses' office who bandaged me up and took me to the hospital… well of course I got the crap beat out of me from the evil overlord. Who do you think had to pay for the broken mirror? Not to mention more meds, and again the loss of an allowance and extra chores to pay for it all. Who cared that I tried to kill myself? No one, that's who? Nobody even mentioned it while I was getting the flesh ripped from my body with his belt…

Attempt #5 Again during my grade 6th year.

Twice in one year, this just might be a new record? But, I doubt it.

In the new house…. my younger brother and I were in the kitchen and were going at it for some reason. He clobbered me so I picked up a shoe. I don't know why I hesitated, but then I threw the shoe at him as he was laughing and running away from me. He ran out of the kitchen, past the basement door, down a short hallway and instead of dodging up the stairs to his left or into the living room to his right, he went out the storm door just as the shoe hit the glass… which of course caused the glass to shatter. A large piece fell and sliced his hand causing 11 stitches [did I mention that I liked to throw things when I got mad? I had a lot of practice at both actually, being mad and throwing things. Because of it I managed to develop a good arm and a great aim]. It seemed as though I was always mad, or irritated and I was always… Yes… always… throwing something. Oh shit! Oh shit! Oh shit! Other than the pain in his hand of course, he was laughing because he knew I was in for it and off they went to the hospital to stitch him up… which was a switch, because it was usually myself going to the emergency room. Perhaps I thought I'd switch things up a little, I don't know? I don't remember all of the details about this one, but I do remember getting a beating when the old man got a hold of me. As if that wasn't bad enough I was awarded extra chores [again] to pay for the damages. Not to mention, going without an allowance [again] for several months for the same reason and I'm sure he took more than his fair share as well.

<u>The very next day</u>

Even though I was grounded and wasn't suppose to leave the yard, I hopped onto my bike with my empty school pack on my back. I went to the lake in Waterloo park and filled my pack up with rocks. It was so heavy… how heavy was it? it was so heavy that I barely managed to get it onto my back. I walked out into the lake in hopes of being weighted down so that I would drown… someone saw me going under and pulled me out, while someone else ran to the pay phone and dialed 911…

<u>Pay phone?</u> What's that?

Right, eh? I don't think there are anymore to be found.

<u>Pay Phone</u>: is typically a coin-operated public telephone, often located in a telephone booth or a privacy hood, with pre-payment by inserting money (usually coins) or by billing a credit or debit card, or a telephone card. Calling the Operator or 911 was always free.

https://en.wikipedia.org/wiki/Payphone

I stayed for another week at what was appearing to becoming my third home, [the mental health unit at the hospital] hell, I practically lived at the hospital as it was anyway, may as well make it permanent, right? Needless to say, my parents had to collect me at the hospital a week later and I got another beating… for leaving the yard while I was grounded which meant that I was disobedient of course. And, for swimming in the lake when it's against the bi-laws and for trying to kill myself. Well, talk about your slow learners he was ½ of the reason why I was trying to kill myself in the first place. Here's your sign! But had anyone looked at taking this kid to therapy for the attempted suicides or for any other reason? Of course not! Were any medications prescribed? Not to my knowledge.

"You stupid-ass, what's the matter with you?" I remember him saying while delivering the belt to my bare ass [once again, that's how I got welts and bruises upon welts and bruises].

I'm not sure if they paid for ambulance rides back then, but wouldn't that have been a bitch? My older brother had only caught part of what was going on, so he asked me what I was doing in the lake and why my pack was soaking wet. I told him and all he did was call me a 'stupid-ass' while laughing at me. Why do I bother answering his dumbass questions anyway? He always just laughs at me... well I'm so glad I'm your source of amusement big brother...

Attempt #6: When I was 14? I don't remember a significant beating but I do recall being so down and out for some time that I didn't care about anyone or anything anymore and of course, not even myself [which seemed to be my normal state of mind, didn't it?]. I had been drinking a little more than usual, cutting classes, not doing my homework [as if I ever did that anyway], making excuses for not going to Cadets [and I loved going to Cadets] or going out at all for that matter. Not even my girlfriends [yes plural] could cheer me up. I normally made any excuse to be out of the house away from the monster, but I remember not caring if I lived or died for a few weeks at that point and had thoughts of killing myself. I had been sneaking more drinks off and, on that week, but this day [impulsively] I took a brand-new bottle of rye from the cabinet, went into the bathroom and mixed it with a bunch of their pills. It didn't matter to me which ones, because I was determined to take them all and drink that entire bottle. I didn't even know what I was taking, how many pills I was taking, or even how many bottles I had emptied. I didn't stop until I cleaned out the entire medicine cabinet. I just opened a pill bottle one at a time, emptied the contents into my mouth [or as many pills that would fit] and washed them down with mom's rye... one bottle of pills and a chug or two at a time. That combination only made me throw up so much so that mother heard me making all that noise in the bathroom. I don't know anyone who can vomit quietly, do you?

Mom: "who's in there?"
Me: "Wayne"
Mom: "what's the matter?"
Me: "nothing, go away"
Mom: "don't tell me nothing, are you being sick in there?"
Me: "no, go away" Liar!

The door was locked, but I guess that didn't matter or slow her down.

Mom: "no, I'm not going away"

When she came into the bathroom, even after me telling her to 'go away', [several times] she saw the bottle of rye on the floor beside me and the empty pill bottles in the sink "damn you" she said and dialed 911. Damn, again?

Why is it that people figure they have to keep saving my sorry ass? I didn't ask them to do that you know. Just leave me the hell alone, already will you? But no, people have to be fucking hero's and butt into things that aren't any of their business. So, why is it that people don't leave me alone after me telling them to do so? I'll never know because it still happens today. Go figure. Except of course when a poor 5-year-old is being brutalized in broad day light on the main street in downtown Waterloo.... or the Nurse at the hospital who interrogates me about drinking bleach... or the school nurse who sees bruises all about my body... or the med staff at the hospital after the few times he put me there from another one of his beatings... no one cared then.

After another week or so at my favourite vacation resort, I returned home only to receive yet another beat down because he had to spend his prized beer money on replacing all the medications that I took. Once again, I was doing extra chores and going without an allowance to pay for everything. So, I always paid for my mistakes in more ways than one. I remember him laughing at me, [he was usually laughing when he beat on me... I told you, he enjoyed it] while beating on me with his fists. "You can't even kill yourself properly, can you? You stupid-ass! How bloody stupid can you be?" Oh, I'm sure he enjoyed dishing out that one just as much I enjoyed taking it. Another fat lip, another black eye later, and not to mention sore arms that I couldn't move them for a day or 2 without wincing. Ya, that really taught me a lesson, thanks for the educational update, asshole. I went on to try it a few more times, so his schooling never hit home now, did it? I never did like school, in fact, I still don't like schools or hospitals either. More than a week on the inside and I've gone batshit again.

Attempt #7: The next time I was 16, [impulsively] I had changed the price tags on some goods at K-Mart so that my 'first' paycheck would stretch a little further. [I should point out the fact that the old man said he wouldn't be buying any more clothes for me because I was now working. He cut off my allowance as well but I was still expected to pull my weight around the house and put 10% of my take-home pay into a savings account. That part was okay though because it did help me to purchase my first car]. Needless to say, security caught me, I had my day in court and I was charged with fraud, sentenced to 6 months probation and 6 months community service. A letter went home to the old man [the return address was the Kitchener Court House, so I knew what it was] but I found it first and got rid of it rather quickly. My older brother had brought in the mail and saw the envelope. He also saw me get ride of it and had asked what that was all about. I told him what it was and he laughed at me, calling me a 'stupid-ass' once again, "wait until the old man finds out about this one… hey, do me a favour… let me know when he does find out will you, so I'll make sure that I'm not home when all hell breaks loose on your stupid ass". Then he just shook his head and walked away laughing. What I didn't know was that a response was required and the court clerk sent a second letter… after which… I received a beat down… 'A', for not telling him about it in the first place and 'B', for destroying the first letter because it was addressed to him. Just in case you were wondering… my older brother was not at home that day when shit hit the fan on my ass. Why yes, I had sore arms, bruises and another black eye, thanks for asking. I went out to King Street and stepped off the curb in front of a big-truck. I didn't know they could stop that fast, he must have been empty. I'm yelling and swearing at the driver [from under the cab] for stopping. The driver gets out of the truck, yanks me out from underneath, picks me up off of the pavement, spins me around and kicks my ass off of the road and back onto the grass. He called me a few names, jumped back into his truck and carried on his way. You have to remember, I was a scrawny-ass little kid, probably not even 98lbs soaking wet. I was a skinny rat right up until the age of 40… so anyone could have kicked my sorry ass. I'm sure even my little sister could have if she had half the mind to do so. I was banged up pretty good from that one. Head bumps and stuff, I thought I had another broken arm as well. So, yes, another trip to the hospital was in order. As it turned out I had a severe concussion, scraped up arms, the road ripped up my jeans and tore my legs up pretty bad. You have to know, I didn't go to the hospital by choice... another couple had witnessed the entire incident and wouldn't take no for an answer. Church people, go figure? I do remember speaking with a shrink that time, and I saw him at the mental health unit at the hospital a few times... no one was going to take care of the dragon-man for me, so what good was talking to someone going to do for me? They hadn't picked up on the bipolar thing then either... all everyone wanted to talk about was my depression, why was I so depressed? Blah, blah, blah... what was the point? I told them about the beatings, about the bullies, nothing was done so I was wasting my breath. I was given a prescription for antidepressants but the old man wouldn't pay for them. I was working, remember... if I wanted meds, I had to pay for them myself. Yet, he had the medical coverage through his work, I hadn't. So again, another example of his love and care which continued to promote an atmosphere of happiness. What was the point? No one in authority had informed me that I was now an adult and could have him charged. But, if I had, and he didn't go to jail, I'd be in even a bigger world of hurt, wouldn't I? You know the rest of the story... Okay, I'll spell it out for you. I got another beating once again for trying to kill myself. Hell man, why don't you just do it for me and save me all of this trouble already? You're the reason why I want to kill myself in the first place, old man. Speak about being a slow learner... what part of all of this was he just not understanding?

Attempt #8: I was living in Halifax when I was in the Navy. It was May 1978, I was 19 years old. Upon my release from the crowbar hotel, they took me over to the dentist to have all of my wisdom teeth taken out [yes, it was a prearranged appointment]. I was supposed to have someone drive me home but there was no one coming for my sorry self because I hadn't any friends then either. I was still higher than a kite and walked out of the office, out the back gate of Stadacona and turned left to go across the Angus L. Macdonald Bridge, or better known as 'the old bridge'. I didn't even think of taking the bus or calling a taxi I guess. It was only a couple of miles or so across, and a couple more to where I was living once I reached the other side. If I made it to the other side that is... not a big deal really, I've walked further drunker than a skunk, I can do this... so, off I went. As I was stumbling across the bridge, I kept hearing a voice in my head that kept repeating itself... "Jump! Go ahead and jump! Jump! Go ahead and jump! You can do it, Just, Jump!" I waited until I got out in the middle of the bridge, climbed up onto the top rail... just as I got one foot up there, I felt a sudden jerk and I was slammed to the ground and the handcuffs were locking in place... Damn! Not again! "Damn You!" I probably cried out... I had no idea where the cops had come from or even if they were following me... had someone seen me staggering and called them or something? One would have thought they'd put me into some sort of program or something, but no! I spoke with a Shrink for about 45 minutes and they turned around and stationed me to a little backwater town called Shelburne Nova Scotia and I was on the bus the following Saturday. What I didn't know, was that this Shrink, had done up the paperwork to start a medical release. [While my mouth was still swollen and sore, I had to do an out-clearance from the Ship, and the Base... that was fun!] I guess they figured I wouldn't get into any trouble down there... or would I? Those are other stories.

"Go Ahead and Jump" Song release in 1983 by Van Halen; https://en.wikipedia.org/wiki/Jump_(Van_Halen_song)

Attempt #9: The next time I remember was when I was 23, [our daughter would have been almost 3] and it was a week after my first son was born. I had just lost 2 part-time jobs [from impulsivity and my own stupidity, naturally]. The week before I went on a bender and was sick for 3 days afterwards. I didn't show up for work, let alone calling in sick. I'm sure I was still under the influence when I was in the delivery room with my wife while she delivered our son. I had been mentally down for a while now, but this week I was in rough shape. I wasn't drinking because that last hangover wasn't finished kicking the shit out of me as of yet. I remember having thoughts about how my family would be better off without me, that I was no good for them or to anyone, blah, blah, blah... Boo, fucking hoo! I was on my way to the other part-time job [that I hadn't lost] at about 2215hrs when I impulsively [there's that word again, what is this action or reaction that keeps popping up out of nowhere, time and again? I'm going to have to look that up as well] decided to drive the Westbound lane heading Eastward with my headlights out, hoping to run smack head-on into a tractor-trailer, instead of showing up for work. I was intercepted by the police once again… where are these guys when you really need them? I spent a night in jail and another week at club 'MH'. I can't remember all the details but I do remember being 'ordered' by a judge to go for counselling for which I couldn't afford. That was the first time I had ever received proper counseling and was diagnosed with 'Clinical Depression' instead of 'just being depressed'. Is that all? Just clinical depression? I'm no psychiatrist, but even I could have told you that. There has to be more to it! But, okay, it's a start…. Clinical Depression it is, no shit Sherlock, what took you geniuses this long to figure something out? I don't remember how long I went to see this guy, but I'm sure it wasn't very long before I had moved again. So, back out on my own… without medications or counseling and we know how far that always got me.

Sherlock Holmes: famous private detective: https://en.wikipedia.org/wiki/Sherlock_Holmes

Impulse: adverb; without forethought;

Well no kidding!

Here's the longer more interesting version: In psychology, impulsivity (or Impulsiveness) is a tendency to act on a whim, displaying behavior characterized by little or no forethought, reflection, or consideration of the consequences. Impulsive actions are typically "poorly conceived, prematurely expressed, unduly risky, or inappropriate to the situation that often result in undesirable consequences," which imperil long-term goals and strategies for success. Impulsivity can be classified as a multifactorial construct. A functional variety of impulsivity has also been suggested, which involves action without much forethought in appropriate situations that can and does result in desirable consequences. "When such actions have positive outcomes, they tend not to be seen as signs of impulsivity, but as indicators of boldness, quickness, spontaneity, courageousness, or unconventionality" thus, the construct of impulsivity includes at least two independent components: first, acting without an appropriate amount of deliberation, which may or may not be functional; and second, choosing short-term gains over long-term ones. Impulsivity is both a facet of personality and a major component of various disorders, including ADHD, substance use disorders, <u>bipolar disorder</u>, <u>antisocial personality disorder</u>, and_borderline personality disorder. Impulsiveness may also be a factor in procrastination. Abnormal patterns of impulsivity have also been noted instances of acquired brain injury and neurodegenerative diseases. Neurobiological findings suggest that there are specific brain regions involved in impulsive behavior, although different brain networks may contribute to different manifestations of impulsivity, and that genetics may play a role.

Now this is more like it and something that I can understand.

So, I constantly lived out the Nike slogan over and over, Ya, baby... **'Just Do It**!"

Just Do It: a trade mark of the Nike shoe company: https://en.wikipedia.org/wiki/Just_Do_It

Hold up a minute… SIDE BAR

You mentioned 3 part-time jobs here?

Yes, yes, I did.

You had 3 part-time jobs all at the same time?

Yes, for the second time… I had 3… part-time positions.

How did you manage that?

Looking back, actually quite well during my maniac phase to be honest with you and I even took on extra shifts from time to time as well.

I worked as part-time cook 3 <u>days</u> a week; Sunday, Monday and Tuesday

I worked as a bartender 3 <u>evenings</u> a week; Monday, Friday and Saturday

I worked as a driver's helper 3 <u>nights</u> a week; Tuesday, Wednesday and Thursday.

<u>Sunday</u> I'd work all day… 9:00-1900hrs. = 10 hours

<u>Monday</u> I'd get up, prep for opening, open the restaurant and I worked form 8:30am until about 1500 = 6.5 hrs.

I was at the bar by 1600hrs and we closed at 01:00, I'd get home about 2:00 or 2:30 = 9 hrs for a total of 15.5

I'd get up <u>Tuesday</u> morning and go to the restaurant and work again from 8:30-1500, = 6.5 hrs go home for awhile and report to the warehouse for 10:30 and we'd generally return by 7:00 the next morning… = 8.5 hrs = 15 hrs

<u>Wednesday</u> morning… I'd go home shower and go to bed. I'd be back at the warehouse by 10:30 again and work until about 7:00am = 8.5 hrs

<u>Thursday</u> morning and be back at the warehouse for 10:30 until about 7:00 Friday morning. I'd go home, get some sleep, spend time with the family = 8.5 hrs

<u>Friday</u> afternoon, I'm back at the bar for 1530, close about 2:30 a.m. because we had to count cash, restock, and stuff like that. It was generally 3:30am by the time I'd get home = 11 hrs

<u>Saturday</u> I'd be back at the bar for 1530, [that is if I wasn't asked to open at 1300hrs] work again until 2:30am = 11 hrs I'd get a few hours sleep and be back at the Restaurant <u>Sunday</u> morning for 8:30am and my week would start all over again…

So that's what? Somewhere in the neighbourhood of about 80 hours a week?

It wasn't so easy when I was depressed, but that's what I had to do to pay the bills, and so we could eat… I just couldn't find a full-time position. It is from here that I went into Poultry Farming.

How long did this go on for?

About 2 years or so, I think.

And you said that you were fired from 2 of them?

Yes, I went out drinking on Good Friday instead of going to work at the bar. I lied and told my Mrs. and told her that I had the night off. I wanted to go drinking instead of going to work, I needed a break. I asked for the night off the week before but the boss said no… oh well. I was fired from the restaurant and the bar at the same time because I didn't show up nor had I called in sick at either location. The restaurant was a small fish 'n' chip joint so Easter weekend was their busiest time of the year and there were only 2 cooks, myself and the owner. Him being upset that I hadn't showed up would be an understatement. It was also Easter weekend April 1982… our second child was due <u>any day</u>… the sisters and husbands went to the Jr Ranks Mess… brother-in-law was RCR and the sister-in-law was also 9 months pregnant… Every time brother-in-law and I went up to the bar, we downed a shot of Yaeger and got blitzed to say the least. We called a cab but they said it would be over an hour or so because of the weather. The ladies didn't want to wait that long so, sister-in-law decided she was going to drive. Part of this problem with this is the fact that neither of our wives had their license, nor even knew how to drive a car. Here's my sister-in-law, behind the wheel, 9 months pregnant, never driven a car a day in her life and trying to drive in a snow storm [which had come up while we were in the bar]. It's a good thing they only lived a few short blocks away. We arrived safely, the boys passed out in the living room… me on the floor and the brother-in-law on the couch. Mrs. didn't even bother to bring me a pillow or a blanket, needless to say that I hadn't received any sympathy from her. I was sicker than a dog for 3 days, our son was born on Easter Monday. I was still sick and hungover while in the delivery room. Needless to say, my wife was extremely pissed. To this day I have not touched a drop of Yaeger and it's been over 36 years. Even the smell of it still makes me gag and want to hurl.

Attempt #10: I was in my mid 20's somewhere and took the family up to the Tobermory area for a camping weekend. Remember that 100' cliff I told you I had jumped off of earlier?

Yes, I do.

Well, it was no accident that I had jumped… [yes of course it was on an impulse… but opportunity presented itself once again. The thing is that I was neither depressed nor maniac at the time, I just did it!] I thought that I would hit the water on a weird angle or something and perhaps split myself open some how and drown and I'd be fish food. I successfully landed the first time so I walked back up the path to the top and jumped off the second time. An almost a perfect entry, rats! I did hurt my back though on that one so I didn't jump the 3rd time.

I told you I could fly! Okay, maybe I can't, but that was a long way down it sure felt as if I was flying. The first time I was scared for about a second but I was really hoping to make a big splash, if you know what I mean.

Attempt #11: It was shortly after our 3rd child was born [9 years after child #2]. I was 32 and had been unemployed for almost a year. [What's with my cycling through a deep depressive state after my kids were born?] Another mouth to feed and no way to take care of the ones already have I suppose, I don't know? I had lost my last job in the usual manner… by my own stupidity of course…

Not another job?

Yup, another one… I had an affair with a younger, single co-worker [torn between 2 lovers, feeling like a fool comes to mind]. We were caught together by another co-worker who blew the whistle and we were both fired on the spot. Of course, I had to tell my wife why we were being let go [she worked on the farm as well] it was difficult for her to say the least and I went for counseling but again, it had nothing to do with the bipolar stuff. The counseling was short lived because I didn't feel that it was helping as I just kept sinking lower and lower to the point of being suicidal. One night, with no hope insight, blind to the future I guess… what? like you can see into yours? My late wife found me sitting on the living room floor in the dark with my back up against an inside wall with a loaded double barrel 12 gauge shot gun in my lap and a half empty [or half full, I suppose it all depends on how you want look at it now doesn't it?] bottle of Scotch in my right hand. I might have been waiting to finish the bottle I suppose. I don't know, but I can only imagine what would have happened had I reached the end of that bottle and she hadn't woken up and realized I wasn't in bed beside her and came looking for me. Needless to say, she made me sell all of my guns the next day, I had 3 of them. Saved again, what can I say?

Attempt # 12: At 35? I was working as a Meat Inspector for Agriculture Canada and there were lay-offs across the country thanks to the Conservative Party and their dirty cutbacks which created a huge downsizing. I drove to the tallest parking garage in downtown Kitchener, parked the car, and sat on the ledge for what seemed like an extremely long time, just watching the world pass me by.

Were you drinking?

Of course, I was drinking, why do you ask?

A natural question, given your history...

Which is probably the first and only time I've sat that long and still in one spot my entire life [except as of late doing my school work and writing this book]. A fellow came by, I believe he was in his mid 50's and asked "do you mind if I join you?" "Nope, it's a free country, ain't it?" "oh wait, yes, it is because I did my part to help keep it that way" [as if I'd ever been to war or anything]. He ignored that remark and climbed up onto the ledge and we just sat there awhile sharing my bottle without saying a word. He finally spoke and we had a long conversation about life, family, work, the city, other people, etc., while just sitting out there on that ledge. The thing that has just occurred to me... no one else came by and asked what us two clowns were doing just sitting out there on that ledge... there were no police, no fire trucks, or anyone down below, and no one approached us from up top either. Huh? After awhile, we climbed down, shook hands, slipped into our vehicles and went our separate ways. So, if you don't believe in Angels, maybe you do now? Well of course I was contemplating on jumping over the edge, that's why I chose the highest parking garage in the city and was sitting up there out on the ledge in the first place.

So, this one obviously wasn't an impulse attempt?

No, I had been thinking about doing myself in for a while and just decided to act on my thoughts. I chose a parking garage because of the easy access. I don't recall the fellow's name or the exact conversation, but somehow, he had convinced me not to jump. Why do people keep interfering with something that isn't any of their business? I guess "God isn't finished with him yet." I told you I hear things... I hadn't heard those words in years. Huh?

Attempt #13: Okay, here we go... lucky 13, right? Ya, no! It was another crap shoot. Later that same year I had left my late wife a note that simply read: "I'll see you on the other side" and walked out. She woke up, found the note and phoned the police, who, not too long there after, found me sitting on the rails of an overpass across Hwy 86 [The Conestoga Expressway] in Kitchener. I don't even remember how I got out there because I left the car in its parking stall outside of our townhouse. Nor do I remember how long I was sitting there. I didn't even know who or where I was when the police talked me down off of the rail and questioned me, nor had I any ID on me. I'm sure I walked there though because it wasn't all that far from where we were living. But was I up there for 5 minutes or 30 minutes? I hadn't a clue because I don't even remember leaving the house. I don't know? Did I have a thought of self preservation? Nonetheless, I was found, cuffed and brought to my favorite resort for another week or so. And all they ever treated me for was the 'clinical depression.' Thanks again folks... see you next time.

Attempt # 14: If you can even call it an attempt, not sure, you tell me.

However; shortly after my 40ᵗʰ birthday [Tuesday February 9 at 5:21am actually, 16 days after my 40ᵗʰ birthday... happy fucking birthday! On January 22ⁿᵈ we were in the Oncologist's office being informed that my wife may have 3 days, 3 weeks or 3 months to live, they didn't know] my first wife had died from a cancerous brain tumor they called a mixed glioma [there's something else for you to Google]. My life as I knew it was all over... my entire world had been shattered... tell me, what the hell was I suppose to do now? The older two children were out of the house and I took the youngest to live with his maternal grandparents because I didn't think I'd make it through another day let alone another week while trying to look after the both of us. I just lost my wife, people at church were giving me a hard time about being there…

Hold up here a minute: People at church were giving you a hard time… are you serious?

Yes, I'm dead serious!

My wife had died on Tuesday morning, we had the service at the Church Thursday morning, the minister rode with the body in the Herse as a few of us drove up to London Ontario from Port Colborne to lay her to rest in the city where she was born and always called home. We buried her Thursday afternoon, I arrived at church on Sunday morning about 15 minutes prior to the beginning of the service as per usual and the conversation was <u>exactly</u> this:

Elder: "Hi Wayne, what are you doing here?"

[Half blocking my way into the sanctuary and he wouldn't even shake my hand. His wife was standing beside him].

Me: "It's Sunday morning, where else am I suppose to be?"
Elder: "Anywhere but here" he said…
Me: "Are you serious?"
Elder: "Yes, I'm serious"
Me: "What?"

I was shocked when he said that, paused a moment and asked…

Me: "What do you mean anywhere but here? If I can't find solace in the house of God, after just burring my wife, where am I suppose to find it?"
Elder: He repeated himself… "**Anywhere but here!**" rather sternly too I might add.
Me: "**Fuck You too!**" I said

Loud enough for any number of people to hear me. I turned around, walked out the front door never to darken the doorway of that church again and it's been almost 20 years. What the hell was that? We had been attending that church for about four years or so. We gave of our tithes and offerings, helped out with the youth and children's ministries, assisted with weddings and funerals, did street ministry with them and now all of a sudden, "I was to be anywhere but here"?

What the bloody hell?

Just who did he think he was? Needless to say, that I was extremely pissed! I don't remember the last time I had been so insulted nor so upset in my life.

The Pastor had the nerve to show up at my door the next day with a cheque to assist with the funeral expenses. I told him exactly what he could do with their money, ripped up the check and threw it at him as he stood on my step and I closed the door in his face. How's that for impulsivity? I was so mad he's lucky I didn't punch him or something while I was at it. I don't even know how much the check was for because I hadn't opened the envelope to look at it, and I didn't really care either. I didn't need nor want their money after being treated like that. Then a couple of weeks later, I lost my job because I couldn't return to work mostly because I had no one to look after my young son [so, yes, I was depressed]. A company rep came by and asked me for the keys to the transport I was driving, my uniform and handed me my last pay check. Great! Fucking-fun-tastic. I went to see a social worker at welfare who gave me a hard time about 'quitting' my job and they were debating as to whether or not they were going authorize financial assistance and would inform me of their decision in about a week or so.

Recap: I lost… my wife, I wasn't permitted to attend Church, my job and Holy Shit Batman… what's wrong with this picture?

So… you wonder why I say that I don't want friends and that I don't need them… well, there's another good reason. Here's another one; because people continuously hurt me… let me down, beat the crap out of me, or I'm bullied more verbally now but same difference and I'm ignored, that's why! As if that wasn't bad enough, the grief counselor they assigned me too was a close look alike to my late wife that she could have passed for her sister. I showed her a picture of my wife and even she agreed that we wouldn't be a good fit. Take a step back for a second. Between the Thursday afternoon service and Sunday morning, no one from the church bothered to bring meals over, they weren't calling to invite me out for coffee, so it would appear that I had been abandoned by everyone, and I do mean EVERYONE! Fuck You too! I guess without my wife, I was truly a nobody, or had they only tolerated me because they liked her and the children? I had no idea what their problem was. So much for brotherly love, care and compassion when your brother in Christ was hurting. The thing that really got my goat was when that an older lady in the church lost her husband the year before in a drowning accident… she had children who lived right there in town near by and she was surrounded by family, church members and friends alike… I had no family in the area, my older daughter had moved away, my older son was in high school and working so I couldn't burden him with my responsibilities and I had just lost my wife… I had a young child at home, so, where was my surrounding? I was treated like a leper. I may as well had walked around town repeating out loud… "unclean, unclean", so that people could scatter when they heard me coming. Of course, I questioned again whether or not there was a God in heaven. But I learned that you can't question or judge Christ by his people because people aren't perfect and they will hurt you. So, no, I don't and won't trust anyone enough to have friends.

I believe it was the beginning of March when I called a few of my wife's friends who lived out of town that she kept in touch with and informed them of her death. One friend who lived on Vancouver Island had invited my son and I out to her place. She had a lovely spot right on the shore of the straight. I hadn't slept all night and I remember sitting on her picnic table [drinking] looking out into the straight. Suddenly, a small pod of killer whales appeared… I walked into the water to go swimming with the them… if they ate me, all the better. My friend said that she called out for me but I didn't hear her and kept walking out into the cold water… she came in after me of course… took me into the shower then into her bed to warm me up… I was despondent again and just wanted to die.

Attempt 15: After all of that went down I was back home, son was at his grandparents and I was drinking, [after her death, when wasn't I?] I was trying to the fill the void anyway I knew how. It had been raining a fair bit and I still like walking out in the rain. All I could think about was doing myself in. Who was I without her? How was I to go on living without her? I was totally lost without her.

Without You, Song by Harry Nilsson; 1972

Lyrics: https://genius.com/Harry-nilsson-without-you-lyrics

Became my theme song, I played it over and over and over again, while drinking and wishing I could just curl up into a ball and die. The song was playing for the umpteenth time and I remember grabbing the open bottle of Scotch. I walked out into the rain without footwear or a rain coat, leaving the front door open… it was dark because it was somewhere in the middle of the evening, and the ice was just coming off of the lake. I decided to go down to the beach and take a long walk off of the short peer. I can't remember if it was the beginning or the middle of April but you'd have thought that the water would have brought me to my senses… but it hadn't. I don't remember passing out, but I do recall someone performing CPR on me. Oh joy! She's back? No, lucky Me, some dumb ass is saving my life once again… I can't even kill myself properly… Back to club MH I go. Yippee! How many times does that make now? I don't know, nor do I really care. Who's counting anyway? A few days later and back at home, all alone, I put on some tunes, but not 'Without You' a couple of my other favourites were:

Three Times a Lady by The Commodores released in 1978 https://www.youtube.com/watch?v=fjfq0Fr85Yg

I guess we had come to the end of our rainbow, hadn't we?

And: The Dance by Garth Brooks https://www.youtube.com/watch?v=bpwdwbO1uvM

Which were obviously just as bud, but… I could have missed the pain, but I'd have to have missed the dance… I guess the King had fallen, once again but he really fell hard this time. It still hurts to hear these songs almost 20 years later but I still like them.

<u>Interjection</u>: 1459-28-06-2018: Looking back over my life… I guess that's how I'm feeling right now, I've come to the end of another rainbow only to discover there is not a pot of gold… they lied about that all of these years too. What don't people lie about? Not that I ever believed it, but hey, it would have been nice to find. We lie about Santa Clause, the Easter Bunny, the Tooth Fairy, where we've been, who we're dating, how we're doing… what are we doing?

It's been so fucking difficult and once again, I have nothing accept an wife who still loves me for reasons only she and God knows, my children and my grandchildren. I'm starting all over once more because of my own impulsivity, stupidity, which keeps sabotaging myself… will I ever learn? I highly doubt it because in many situations I don't understand the word **<u>No</u>**! Then I ask myself another question; Why bother? Answer: I really don't know? I just want to walk away again and I don't really know what's keeping me here… do I just want to leave everything, or just go off somewhere by myself for a while? I can't answer that question either. So, again, what's wrong with me? Why are things so bloody difficult all of the time?

<u>NO</u>:

1. a negative used to express dissent, denial, or refusal, as in response to a question or request;
2. used to emphasize or introduce a negative statement;
3. not in any degree or manner; not at all!

And there you have it! Impulsivity always means the opposite… which of course is YES! And/or Why not? And… Just Do It! And that my friends, is my life. At that point, I had nothing left to lose except for myself. Silly me, I thought I could drink myself to death or something and I set out to do just that. That didn't work either. No Kidding! Of course, who's thinking straight under those circumstances? I guess you can't really call this a suicide attempt, so I won't. I suppose what I didn't realize was that at the end of every bottle the memories remained, and the whiskey was suppose to drown her memory, only her memories drowned the whisky and I had to open another one to drown my sorrows in. But, that hadn't worked either so I'd open another one… perhaps I thought I would die of alcohol poisoning or something, I don't know, all it ever did was make me pass out for awhile, I'd wake up and start over again. But it didn't work, why wasn't it working? Every time I woke up, I was still alive. About a month or so later, I have no idea… a dear friend of hers [who had a key to the house] finally came by to see how I was and she sorted me out. I cleaned up, went to another church, went to AA, found another grief counselor and received some much-needed help for a short time but then I moved again and was on my own once more… he, he, he… we all know how well that goes for me, don't we? I had asked my daughter to return home for a while to help me look after the little one so I could find work and get caught up on the bills. Which didn't last long because she could only stay for a short period of time and I couldn't get anyone to look after him with the crazy shifts of a trucker. Well, it appeared as though my trucking days were now gone too, so I tried going back to a farm, but that didn't work out very well either… which is another story, but an interesting one I'd say. Hint: Rats and Snakes…

Attempt #16: I believe I was 51 when I had made another attempt upon my life. I was diagnosed with <u>Hepatitis C</u>. I just can't catch a break, can I? The doctors figured it finally materialized after the blood transfusions I received as a child. Before I could start treatment for the Hep C, they had to bring my iron count down because it was dangerously high… they were wondering if I also had <u>Hemochromatosis</u>. I had a phlebotomy every week for 10 weeks where they drew an entire pint of blood. I then started the Hep C treatment [which alone was enough to kill me]. All hell had been breaking loose at work for sometime now because of my illness, I was shifted to another department to assist them part-time instead of being put on sick leave like I was requesting. My specialist had suggested the same, but the doctor wouldn't let me off fulltime for whatever reason. I had a situation go sideways with my step son, the Mrs. was away and not returning my phone calls, I had been depressed for sometime but not drinking because I wasn't allowed alcohol while on the medications for the Hep C, but I drank that night anyway. I took a straight edge steak knife and cut my left wrist. I didn't cut very deep apparently but it hurt like hell. I didn't remember it hurting this much when I was a kid and cut my right wrist. I don't know how much I had to drink but it obviously wasn't enough. Well, I suppose the pain and the blood woke me up and I chucked the steak knife through the screen and out the open kitchen window. I called the duty Padre, who called the MP's [Military Police]. They arrived at the house about the same time, one of the MP's bandaged me up, they took me to the hospital to get stitched-up and escorted me back home. The Padre and I chatted for quite some time. One of the MP's sat with me the rest of the night, a co-worker was called in to sit with me during the day [that was embarrassing], but they had placed me on a 'suicide watch' so he hadn't a choice. My wife arrived home later that day and took over. But of course, there was nothing wrong with me... all of this was just another way to get some much-needed, desired and deserved attention, right? Right! Poor little me, I have Hepatitis C... boo, hoo, hoo! Cried the <u>Grinch</u> with elation because he had just stolen all of the Who pudding and all of the Who hash... So, now what? Not much, that's what. We start all over again. Out on sick leave, then the counseling started [they focused only on the depression once more... same old merry-go-round], continue with the meds, not drinking again, life on the hellish roller coaster continued. I was off on sick leave for 48 weeks while undergoing treatment... that was fun! The biggest problem was, I had received treatment for the depression but no one asked any of the questions listed above to dig deeper into my life to see if there was anything else going on and through it all... I only saw a shrink on 2 occasions. What good was that? Not to mention the fact that he too was an ass... he was the one I told you about who had me write the autobiography but hadn't opened it. I was cycling out again and felt on top of the world and wanted... no, needed to get back to work so bad I was going stir crazy. That was not a good scene either, I can tell you that. Come to think of it, I should get my iron count checked again. I saw a counsellor though for quite some time and she hadn't picked up on the bipolar thing either... huh? A really nice lady and she did help, but she missed the mark. The <u>Pegasus Treatment</u> was rough, I had felt as though I went a few rounds with Muhammad Ali himself.

https://www.gene.com/patients/medicines/pegasys

<u>Hepatitis C</u>: Another interesting disease... which can eventually kill you.

https://www.webmd.com/hepatitis/digestive-diseases-hepatitis-c

Phlebotomy:

http://hemochromatosishelp.com/therapeutic-phlebotomy/

Hereditary hemochromatosis (he-moe-kroe-muh-TOE-sis) causes your body to absorb too much iron from the food you eat. Excess iron is stored in your organs, especially your liver, heart and pancreas. Too much iron can lead to life-threatening conditions, such as liver disease, heart problems and diabetes. The genes that cause hemochromatosis are inherited, but only a minority of people who have the genes ever develop serious problems. Signs and symptoms of hereditary hemochromatosis usually appear in midlife. Treatment includes regularly removing blood from your body. Because much of the body's iron is contained in red blood cells, this treatment lowers iron levels.

How the Grinch Stole Christmas: A Classic Book and Movie [the original animation that is]

https://en.wikipedia.org/wiki/How_the_Grinch_Stole_Christmas!

Attempt #17 Age 59, you'd think I'd get it right by now? Well, apparently not!

Life went sideways again [when isn't it sideways, backwards or upside down, or all around? When I'm a maniac, of course, but then that has problems of its own too, doesn't it?] Looking back; I would have to say that the slippery slope started with the death of my son, almost 2 years ago… I hadn't allowed myself the time to grieve properly and I buried myself into my studies and my volunteer activities… I was 'fine' and we all know what that means. Things at the church weren't the greatest, but I won't talk about that. I was receiving rejection letters, or no replies from various positions I was applying for. I even looked into switching denominations but many people had a problem with the fact that I married a divorced woman. Other people had a problem with my son's activities which got him killed. Just when are we no longer accountable for the actions of another adult, adult children or not? I went back to drinking not too long ago for whatever stupid-ass reason, which as we know is a dangerous activity for me to be participating in. The decline had been so gradual this time and I thought that I had it under control not realizing how far I had fallen until I actually hit bottom once again... but this pit had been deeper than that previous 2. Thanks to my buddy Eeyore... I didn't give a shit about anything, anyone, or what I did to others or to myself but wasn't aware of it, until I'm now looking back that is. Hindsight is always 20/20, isn't it? I was receiving these rejection letters, see... what a fool... no one wants you... why even bother? Here were go again. I was a stupid-ass, play it again Sam... had impulsively submitted my resignation and called a couple of people I know who hunted and asked them if I could borrow a rifle to go out to the woods and pop off a few rounds... I don't have a fire arms safety certificate so both of them said "no". Damn... but there was a minor difference this time... something in my tool box jumped out at me and I went looking for counseling at the Family Community Social Services...

Me: "I'm in need of some counseling and I need it as soon as possible." Not telling her the crises situation for which I had found myself to be in, nor had she asked.
Receptionist: "I'm sorry Sir, we don't have an opening until October".
Me: "Wow, that's a long waiting list".
Receptionist: "Are you a veteran by any chance?"
Me: "Yes, I am."
Receptionist: "You may have coverage through Veteran Affairs, try that route, you may get in to see someone sooner elsewhere".
Me: "Thank you".

Off I went, up to the Base. I spoke with a VAC representative, Nope, no coverage because my current crisis has not been attributed to my military service... I even told her that I was suicidal and to my amazement she hadn't batted an eye or offered any suggestions or displayed any type of concern whatsoever. Hmmm? I guess I was shit out of luck there as well, wasn't I? Still on Base... I went over to the CANEX building and upstairs to the walk-in medical unit, Closed! From there I drove next door to the Family Resource Centre. No one available there either... Well, I'm doing everything I'm suppose to be doing and continuously striking out.

I'm using the tools that I was trained to use during the Suicide Prevention classes, but no one else seems to be co-operating. I completely forgot about the 1-800 # though and the VAC lady hadn't offered it up either...

"See, no one cares... no one will help you... you truly are all alone!"

Voices in my head... shaking that off, my next thought was going to the walk-in clinics at the hospital... there are actually 2 of them there on the 2nd floor.

I left the Base and started making my way to the North side of town, which is probably a 10 – 15-minute drive depending on the lights and the traffic.

However; those words in my voice, continue to haunt me... nagging, somehow beginning to take control.

About half way there... Fuck-it-all kicks in and I [impulsively] parked my car at the bank along the main highway. But I had the forethought to sit on the grass beside the road waiting for a big truck of any kind to come along as those voices continued in my head... I guess I like trucks, if/when they hit you properly, they'd finish the job where as being hit by a car, they may just badly bang me up... who wants that? Hwy 28 can be a busy street so I didn't have to wait long and I stepped off of the curb. I closed my eyes and heard the screaming tires, smelt the burning rubber and the vehicle came to a sudden stop with me underneath it... after being knocked off of my feet of course and sprawling a few feet. I was knocked to the ground but without much force to cause the severe injury of death that I was so desiring. Other than banging my head against the ash fault, which did give me a headache and a slight concussion, I scrapped my arm up a little and my back but I was still breathing... I was yanked out [once again] from underneath the cab and the driver helped me to my feet... needless to say he was not a happy camper... and people came out from Timmies by this time. No, I didn't tell my wife all of this... I didn't give a shit about myself remember?

Driver: "what the fuck are you doing? Are you crazy?"

Me: "Why, Yes, I do believe I am" I said, cool as a cucumber.

Haven't we been here before?

Why, Yes, I do believe we have!

Driver: "I could have killed you"
Me: "that was the whole point of stepping off the curb, asshole"
Driver: "get the fuck out of here and get some help"

With that, he shoved me towards the grass, I fell over the curb and yelled a "Fuck You" as he got back into his cab. I have no idea how many people were standing around at this point, nor did I hear anyone ask me if I was okay… my mind was a total blank and I hadn't heard anyone but the truck driver. Perhaps no one spoke at all? Obviously, no one in the crowd knew who I was either or I'm sure they would have woken me the hell up. Well… so much for that… I guess I have no other choice but to get some help. I sort of shook it off, got back into my truck and went to the hospital, up to the 2nd floor to the walk-in clinics… both of them were full and not taking any more patients for the day. Can't really catch a break today can I… I do everything my tools suggest I do but I guess they're all faulty too so what good had those classes done me? None! Now what? On my way back to the elevator I noticed a sign which read: 'Mental Health Department'. I'm not sure I've ever noticed that sign before… Okay, last call!

Make mine a double Scotch please, just 1 ice cube!

Me: "I'd like to see a psychiatrist or a counselor or someone, anyone, please!"
Receptionist: "no one is available right now. But if you don't have a referral or an appointment, there isn't much I can do for you today" the nice lady said.
Me: "Well, I just made another attempt on my life and if I don't get some help immediately, I probably won't be alive by the end of the day."
Receptionist: "Oh, in that case, I think you had better come with me"

She escorted me downstairs to the main receptionist and stayed with me while I registered. She walked me to the Emergency department and retrieved a nurse for immediate assistance. I was triaged and taken to the back and put in a room all by myself... needless to say it took a few hours for the doctor to come by. But while I was waiting in that little room, I think they alerted security because he checked on me a couple of times and I saw him by the main entrance a couple of more times when I went to the washroom. A nurse kept dropping by but I was by myself that whole time. I finally saw the doctor, met with someone from mental health and the doc referred me to the nut house in St. Paul.

I was transferred at 2200hrs Thursday evening. I was checked into the ICU for observation overnight and for the next day (Friday). I had a young lady babysit me all day Friday who practically stuck to me like glue... except when I went into the shower and to use the toilet. But, she was right outside the door to make sure I didn't make a run for it. I must say though, she was pleasant to chat with, very patient and understanding. By 1500hrs that day they had me in the secured mental health ward on the main floor. Yeeha, another stint at my favorite resort. Trust me, this has been the worst place I've ever stayed. Oh well, beggars can't be choosy, can we?

I count what, 17 attempts? Did you realize that you've made that many attempts on your life?

No, I've never bothered to recall my entire history nor had the occasion to count them all before now, because no one has ever asked. Oh wait, I was asked... the fellow from the hospital who came down from mental health department and interviewed me in the Emergency department had asked if this was the first time I've tried to harm myself... I had said no, it wasn't the first time, but he didn't press further either and I didn't think that was the right time or place to be digging up my history. He asked if it was the first time I'd ever been hospitalized... I lied and said yes, it was the first time... why? I don't know, perhaps I didn't trust him, that's why. I've seen him since and have come clean... he has a pre-empted copy of this book you're now reading. I'm sure I've missed 1 or 2 attempts along life's highway, but oh well. So, I've tried to kill myself at least 17 times... as if anyone gives a damn? Will I ever see the light or will I just keep trying to kill myself until the night closes in? I'm not suicidal now nor have I been for awhile now, but I think I've come to learn one thing… God mustn't be finished with me yet or he'd let me succeed, now wouldn't he? I've been asked a couple of times if I've ever had a plan or have made an attempt in the past, my usual answer was yes, a time or two… but why bother going into the history, the so-called 'experts' never really pried beyond that, which proves they were never really listening or interested anyway and had no intentions of helping me… they've proved that over and over so what makes me think that this time will be any different? I've found that over the years, people ask questions they don't really care to hear the answer too. It's like passing a co-worker or a friend… "Hey, how's it going?" and they keep walking on, not pausing to hear your answer… why? Because no one really gives a shit, that's why? So, why bother asking in the first place? I had gotten to the point where I never answered the question and totally ignore them. But then I thought, what if I told them exactly how I feel, how would they react? All answers were met with the same or similar responses which told me 2 things; they either weren't listening or they didn't really care… so, again, why do people ask if they aren't going to actually listen for a response?

Several times a conversation went just like this:

Person: "Hey, how are you?"
Me: "I feel like killing myself today, how are you?"
Person: "Well, that's good, have a nice day"
Me: "Ya, you too."

OR

Person: "Hi, how's it going?"
Me: "I fell like shit"
Person: "Great, see you later"
Me: "Maybe."

And even

Person: "Hi! What's up?"

Me: "Oh, nothing much, I just tried to kill myself again!"

Person: "Awe, that's too bad, have a nice day."

Thinking... Awe, that's too bad? What's too bad, that I tried, or too bad that I hadn't succeeded? What was that? Do they even hear a word I say? More than likely not, because they aren't listening! Am I invisible here? No, they had acknowledged my presence which means they can see me... so, what gives? And, yes... that was a demonstration of a few real live conversations I had with co-workers... no one slows down long enough to hear what anyone says, not just me... Why?

NO ONE IS LISTENING BECAUSE, NO ONE GIVES A SHIT ABOUT THE OTHER PERSON! Everyone is too hung up on their own crap.

And you can't tell me that I'm the only one it happens too so I won't take those seriously. But seriously people, somewhere we have to start to give a shit about our fellow human beings and give each other the time of day. We just have too!

Or do we?

And, no one assumed that you had any major mental incapacities?

Well, Obviously not. Here I am, still undiagnosed, still untreated, still without medication. The demonstration above tells us that people are only interested in themselves and their little world... the so-called 'experts' well, I have no idea what they focus on but it sure wasn't listening to me and my raggedy ass story, that's for damn sure. For the most part, all they had focused on were the depression, mood disorders and the alcohol abuse. Which should have been clues to many underlying issues if you ask me.

Back tracking a bit... that's quite a few attempts on your life though wouldn't you say?

Now that I've had the occasion to recalled them, and I'm sure I've missed one or two, yes, that's quite a few. To be honest with you, it's bloody embarrassing and scary actually.

Why is it embarrassing?

Well, it just proves that I am a stupid-ass just like the old man says and that I can't do anything right. I can't even successfully kill myself. Well, lets do the math here... I'm 59, I've made 17 attempts [that I can remember] so that equals 1 attempt every 3.5 years... and no one has bothered to find out if I was seriously troubled or not in anyway, shape or form... other than the diagnoses I have already mentioned... which they didn't bother to attempt to connect the dots to either. So, I can't help but wonder, what makes me think that anything will be any different this time? We all know what the definition of insanity is, don't we? Well, this feels exactly like that... doing the same thing over and over again while expecting different results. What makes me want to believe anyone is going to take me seriously and give me the help that I truly need and have been begging for all of my life? Fuck, what is their problem anyway? Am I the only one smart enough to think outside the box? I know I'm not, but it sure as hell feels as though I am. I truly do feel all alone! Meaning that no one understands! Therefore, I am alone, aren't I? I know I have all the tools, I know that I'm suppose to be doing this or that or another thing, yes, I'm a very smart guy, but when I get to a certain point or into certain situations... or come face to face with whatever demon that plagues me at that particular moment... it's flight or fight and I don't know which way I'm going until I make my move at that split second and it's usually on impulse and it usually doesn't turn out to be a good move. I don't plan these things out ahead of time. Shit just keeps happening, over and over. There are no stoppages and I don't know why! But I often don't give a shit! And, that's part of the problem... I just do what I want too and when I want to do it no matter what that is, which I want to do! They say in AA that it truly is 'one day at a time' or another 24'... well... right now, it's more like 1 second at a time. When enough seconds have gone by, it's a minute. When I collect enough minutes, I have an hour. But I can't look that far ahead... I could explode and do God only knows what a minute from now... so, when I say 'leave me a lone' that's what you need to do... is leave me the hell alone! I'm irritated and I may explode in a <u>New York Minute</u>, it takes a long time to come back down as it is, but with every irritation, I'm back to the top and it takes even longer to come back down. Does the phrase... Bang, zoom straight to the Moon, mean anything to you? How about: 1 of these days Alice? If not, look up the Honeymooners and Jackie Gleason. Unfortunately, that's what I feel like when people keep bothering me when I've asked to be left alone.

A <u>New York minute</u> is a quick instant. Or as Johnny Carson once said, it's the interval between a Manhattan traffic light turning green and the guy behind you honking his horn. It appears to have originated in Texas around 1967. It is a reference to the frenzied and hectic pace of New Yorkers' lives. A New Yorker does in an instant what a Texan would take a minute to do.

https://www.urbandictionary.com/define.php?term=New%20 York%20Minute

<u>The Honeymooners</u>:https://en.wikipedia.org/wiki/The_Honeymooners

Surely your suicidal attempts are more than a cry for attention, they're really a cry for help, I would think.

Like I said… "NOBODY WAS/IS LISTENING!" all they saw was the clinical depression, or a couple of other things, toss a prescription at me for more meds and send me on my way. And when my moods changed for the better, the medications were stopped. So, when the meds ran out I didn't get a refill because we were always moving, or I couldn't afford them. Or, I hadn't needed them because I was fine again. Sure Roy! Many places where we lived, we didn't even have a family physician and they don't bother retrieving medical records between walk-in clinics, especially from out of province… everywhere I went I had to start over with my history… it got to the point where I quickly realized that no one was listening so I stopped offering the information in its entirety.

Do you think that with all those failed attempts there must have been some self preservation in you somewhere? Or, if I may, suggest that "God wasn't finished with you yet?"

I suppose, I never looked at it that way. There must have been. As far as God, not being finished with me? I suppose he still has plans for me but I don't know what they are and really wish that he would share them.

Beside the attempts, you mentioned that you often 'thought' about ending it all. There were other times then when you had thoughts or had even made plans to harm yourself or someone else but you didn't carry them out. Tell us what you can remember about those thoughts and/or plans.

Sorry about the seemingly fascination with death, but, that was my life…

When haven't I thought about doing myself in during my depressive state or while I was somewhere in between? Please tell me when? I even had thoughts and have tried it during a manic episode, so, suicide is a regular thought of mine. Has there ever been more than 2 months in a row where I've not had thoughts about calling it quits? I don't think so, but then, if some of my reckless behaviours went sideways during my maniac phases, I may have ended up dead or crippled for life, which would suck even worse than being dead I think. When I was growing up there were many times, no, let me correct that; how many times am I allowed to use the word 'many' in succession and still be somewhat grammatically correct? Let's just say… that 'countless' might be more of an accurate word to describe the 'many' times I had thoughts about killing myself. There were countless times that I wanted to kill the old man as well so that everyone would finally be safe and then kill myself immediately afterwards because I didn't want to go to juvey hall. I heard all sorts of nasty things that happened to little boys like me in there. I had enough nasty things happening to me in life as it were, I didn't need any more misery added to it, thank you very much. When I got older, I was afraid to kill him for the same reason… I didn't want to go to jail, so I was going to have to take out the booth of us, or it would be just me who would be looking at grass roots. Most of the time I didn't care which way I went, but there was no way it would have been just him should I have ever acted on my thoughts and my hearts' desires. I have a saying: "I'd rather be on the outside looking in than on the inside looking out, thank you very much."

There were countless times when I couldn't sleep [insomnia is another situation that has plagued me my entire life. But again... no body's listening] and I'd quietly make my way to the kitchen, over to the drawer, pull out a butcher knife and just stand outside of my parent's bedroom door. Sometimes, I'd be sipping on a whiskey, sometimes I would not. But I would be thinking; "if only... why don't I just do it and get it over with?" All the while wondering what was stopping me? I could just go nuts and it would be all over with in a New York Minute. The bastard wouldn't even know what had hit him, then I'd slit my own throat, just like I've seen numerous times in the movies and I'd go down in a blaze of glory, I'd be a hero! The headline would read; "6-year-old drenches bed with gasoline and burns his father to death in his sleep." "7-year-old finally had enough and took out his abuser!" "8-year-old stabs the old man to death then takes his own life!" "9-year-old goes berserk and beats the old man to death with a baseball bat before taking himself out." "10-year-old finally cracked under pressure and beats his father to death with a tire-iron." "11-year-old locks his old man in the bathroom then burns the house down around him." It would have been so easy, but why hadn't I ever followed through? Fuck, how many times do I have to say it... "There is something seriously wrong with me!" before I get the required help that I need?

General applause please... "thank you, thank you, oh, you're welcome, no, thank you." Somewhat freakishly creepy, and disturbing all at the same time, isn't it?

Generally, when I was depressed, and again there weren't too many times when I wasn't in some state of depression... mild, middle-of-the-road, severe, or completely off the rails, is all being in a state of depression to me. I'm sad to say that there were times, like this past week for instance and even more so today; I would think about doing myself in almost every minute. They say an average healthy man thinks about sex every 7 seconds throughout the day... which has been proven to be false by the way... but that would be about the same frequency in which I would be thinking of killing myself. That's 8.6 times per minute, 516 times per hour and an average day for a kid would be about 12 hours? That comes out to 6,192 'thoughts' about killing myself in a single day. Of course, many of those 7 second thoughts turned into pondering moments which lasted far longer than the 7 seconds. But still, that's pretty morbid for a child between the ages of 6 to 16. Not only did I have thoughts about how I would do it, I'd go over my funeral service as well… what it would be like, who would be in attendance and perhaps who would weep for me? One of these day dreams was how my siblings were complaining about how they 'had' to be in attendance and my older brother saying: "he was nothing but a stupid-ass anyway" oh well.

Who will weep for You, when your time comes?

These feelings would go on for a week or two, stop for a week or two then start up all over again just like the flickering of a light switch and watching the light come on and go off. Thoughts… no thoughts… thoughts… no thoughts… thoughts… no thoughts… you get the picture.

I remember thinking [many times] while walking to school all I had to do was go down Weber Street and step out in front of a car, a bus or maybe a truck [as we know, I tried that]. One house we lived in was near the train tracks and I could sit by the rails waiting for the train and at the last-minute I could jump in front of it. A train can't stop as fast as a vehicle can. Or perhaps, I'd just sit in the middle of the tracks playing cards or something totally ignoring the train as it barrelled down on top of me and I'd be nothing but a mess for them to clean up. Many times, we'd jump a train and ride it to the park, but we had to jump off at a certain point or it would be going too fast to jump off safely. I often thought… what would happen if I hadn't jump when the other kids had and just kept on riding along to see where it would take me [not to kill myself but to run away], other times I thought of jumping off when it was going extremely fast in hopes of tumbling head over heels in hopes of breaking my neck and meeting certain death. But then I'd have visions of being crippled up and in a wheel chair for the rest of my life and again, I'd chicken out and jump off with the other kids. While playing on the roof of the school all I had to do was pretend I could fly and take a running leap of off the highest section and over the edge… I'd go down, down, down, letting gravity do its thing while I'd sail through the air for a few seconds and it would all come to an end with that sudden stop as I splattered all over that parking lot below [I almost carried that one out too, well, sort of]. I'm sure I've seen that in the movies 100 times as well, it looked easy enough, all they did was just 'step off,' why couldn't I just 'step off?' Or… 1 – 2 – 3… wee…. Nothing to it. All I had to do was pretend that there was water down below, then run and jump! But, it wasn't as easy as it sounds or as I envisioned it. I couldn't muster up the courage to do it. Does the word 'chicken,' mean anything to you? And my big brother interrupted me. So much for that… "Ah, you weren't going to jump anyways, big baby." "Was too." "Was not." "Well, I was thinking about it." "Sure Roy!" A few times I thought about biking to the lake in Waterloo park, filling my school pack with rocks and wading out into the water. I thought of jumping from the top of the oak tree I use to climb in our back yard as well, hoping to hit my head on a few branches on the way down. With my luck, I'd end up with some sort of brain damage and crippled or some other thing besides dead, so, I hadn't tried that one either. I even thought of jumping off of the roof of the house a couple of times. The second time I thought that, I actually managed to get myself up there but I just sat on the peek of the roof looking around. A neighbour saw me and yelled at me to get down, so, I climbed down never to venture up again. The next house we lived in was a ranch style house so it wasn't high enough to do any real damage had I found the courage to jump.

What about thoughts of suicide as an adult?

When I was in the Navy the first time I thought about just pulling the trigger on the riffle while on the weapons range or jumping overboard while out in the middle of the Atlantic Ocean had occurred to me many times to get away from the perceived abuse there in hopes I would drown but I was afraid of being eaten by sharks first. While driving the transport I remember thinking… if I just turned the wheel sharp enough, I'd go over the cliff and it would be all over, or I could just cruise into the on-coming traffic doing 105 kms and hour. A head on collision when both vehicles meet doing the same speed would double the intensity of the impact… but then you add the weight of the goods I was hauling… now that would make for a really big mess, don't you think? Yes, that would do it! Or maybe, I just might not make that next bend in the road and drive straight on through into whatever was out there. While on the ranch in Southern Alberta I had even walked into the bull pen in hopes that one of them would go nuts and trample me to death… but nothing happened, they obviously didn't feel threatened by my scrawny ass so they paid no attention to me. Typical. While in the military the 2nd and 3rd time... Deja Vu hit me... on the range I often had thoughts of just turning the gun on myself and with one quick squeeze of that trigger my brains would be splattered all over the place just like that guy in Platoon, or was it Full Metal Jacket? Either way, wouldn't that be a hoot? But, I scared the hell out of myself and from then on, I hadn't enjoyed going to the range and found every excuse not to go. I thought of jumping off of the bridge in Halifax on more then one occasion, and the one in Burlington Ontario and again in St. Catharines. I even wondered if I turned the wheel of the truck hard enough would I be able to go through the rails of the bridge and it would be all over as I plunged into the waters below. The Garden City Skyway is about 130 ft at its tallest point... I'm sure that would do quit nicely. Many times, while visiting Niagara Falls I wondered how those other people had just climbed the rail and over they went... why couldn't I do the same? I stood there many times thinking about it, but again, I'd chicken out and hear the old man in my head again, laughing at me while laying a beating on me. I've also been on a few cruises where Deja Vu hit me all over again... but once more I was afraid of being shark bait so I hadn't jumped. I guess the movie 'Jaws' had impacted me more than I had realized.

Jaws: A series of movies about a man-eating shark. First one came out in 1975.

https://en.wikipedia.org/wiki/Jaws_(film)

I even thought of jumping into the canal locks there in Welland Ontario at the right moment as the ship was rising and I'd be squished between the ship and the concrete wall... fish food! It seems as though I've <u>always</u> thought about doing myself in one way or another. The funny thing is, when you have a medical in the military, they make you fill out these health questionnaires and they always asked if you had thoughts about suicide or hurting yourself or someone else... to which I would chuckle and answered; 'No'. If they only knew? I answered no, because they've proven on several occasions that I wouldn't receive 'real help' except perhaps being shown the door on a medical discharge like the first time... I really don't remember what I said to that psychiatrist for him to start the proceedings for a medical release… See, even the 'professionals' in the military didn't want to help me and he just tossed me aside. With that in mind one time, I answered 'yes' to those questions if for no other reason than to find out if someone, anyone, actually read those stupid cards. Wouldn't you know it, somebody did actually read those stupid questionnaires. They never took them seriously enough though because all that happened was me receiving an email notification that I was loaded on the next suicide prevention course. I found myself sitting in a classroom somewhere with 11 other people being put to sleep for 7.5 hours a day, for 2 days straight, participating in a [death by power point] lecture on suicide prevention. But that was it, no questions asked, no follow-up and no further counseling of any kind. Just as I anticipated. OMG! That was painful to say the least and I think in all my years I went through the same lectures 3 times… so, why bother answering their questions honestly, when NO ONE WAS PAYING ATTENTION! I know, I sound like a scratched record but what the hell is wrong with everyone?

And That's It? No counseling on a regular basis of any kind?

No, not really. I keep telling you 'No Body Is Listening!' and that proved my point once again, didn't it? So, play it again Sam, because they missed it the first few hundred times… why should I expect anything different? The system had constantly failed me because my cries for help kept falling upon deaf ears and now blind eyes. Okay, not entirely upon deaf ears… I did receive some counseling after I actually attempted suicide when we lived in Winnipeg. There was one person there and a couple here in Cold Lake who eventually did listen and they had helped out for a time, but it wasn't enough to keep me from cycling through depression and the maniac phases and not enough to get me some real help, else I wouldn't still be here in this mess today, now would I? Again, no one was thinking outside of the box because they missed the bipolar and other difficulties I was having.

The shrink here in Cold Lake is a nice guy but all he focused on was the PTSD. Great, more meds for depression, a minor mood disorder stabilizer tossed in for good measure, and regular check ups were every 6 – 8 weeks or so… whoopee! Like that was going to do me any good…

but it was better than nothing I suppose. Something about telling your therapist that everything was grandiose while your world was falling apart around you but I didn't know anything was wrong? Hmmm. Not very observant, was he? I'm not proud of this fact but the truth be told; there have been numerous times [again without number] throughout my life where I would lie awake at night, not being able to sleep because I couldn't stop thinking about anything else other than going 'postal' and taking my problems out with me…. whomever they may be. I haven't had any thoughts like that for years now. So, no one is in any danger. As insane as all of this sounds, there must have been some sanity in there somewhere tucked away in a deep dark corner which prevented me from carrying out these chilling fantasies. But then, I'd have to do myself in as well because I prefer to be on the outside looking in, as I've already alluded too, thank you. The most recent thoughts came about a couple of Saturdays ago when my wife and I were sitting in front of the camp fire and I was pissed off and I don't even remember why. I was wishing the fire was hot enough for me to step into it with hopes that I would be instantly incinerated or that by some strange events, the flames would leap out and consume me right there in my lawn chair. But we all know that campfires aren't that hot, so I stayed out looking in at the dancing flames, just wishing, hoping, praying. But again, nothing, my prayers are never answered. Typical. Eh?

You mentioned the nagging need to just get away, or 'running away', how often would you think about that or 'just do it' as you say, and then you'd get up walk or drive away?

In some respects, quitting a job or moving to a new location, even if it was just across town, may be considered in many respects to be a method of 'running away', would it not?

Yes, I suppose it would.

Well, then, with that in mind, how many times did I "**just do it**" as you put it?

Go back up many pages and we have the answer to this question, don't we?

Count the number of residences I was in after I left the Navy… Start with the Norton Cres address in London, Ontario and finish with that last one in Port Coulbourne before I met my current wift. Then there were all of those employment positions that we'll briefly touch on shortly. The problem was, and for me, there was always a problem and for some reason or other it took many years for me to realize that wherever 'I' went, and no matter where 'I'd' find 'myself' to be, 'I' was always right there with 'me', wasn't 'I'? Imagination that? Huh? It doesn't take a rocket scientist to figure that one out, but I guess that's where the 'stupid-ass' in me comes into affect. I couldn't run away from myself, so I suppose in retrospect, I knew that fact all along, hence the attempted suicides I guess… it was the only way to run away from myself now, wasn't it? Talk about baggage though, I have enough to fill a freight train of at least 100 cars in length I'm sure. How many skeletons have we played with thus far? I don't know if this is counts or not but the first time I tried to run was when I broke that store basement window.

I was running away so I wouldn't get clobbered. Even at 5 yrs old I had enough sense to know that I didn't want to get a spanking… so what does that tell you? It was an accident, I was a kid, but it didn't matter to him. He was going to make sure I learned from that 'accident' to never do it again. I had no idea where I thought I was going… I just 'instinctively' ran to get away from the monster. Other than that, the first 'real' attempt of running from home, I believe was at the young age 7. I packed a suitcase and headed off across the field to a friend's house. I couldn't understand why they didn't want me and called my parents. Good Lord! What did you do that for? Well naturally I got a beating when they finally dragged me back into the house kicking and screaming every step of the way.

Step-dad: "Why did you want to run away?"
Me: Shaking on my little legs… and dumber then a bedpost; I impulsively blurted out… "because I hate you, and I hate them [pointing to my siblings] and I hate it here and I hate school!"
Step-dad: "Is that so?
Me: "Yes"
Step-dad: "Take your clothes off and I'll teach you about running away and what hate is all about".

No thank you, I already know what hate is, why do you think I ran away? I just got finished telling you that I hated you. We can skip this lesson if you don't mind… Of course, I hated him even more at that moment for beating on me and I had other thoughts of killing him, but I didn't know how I could slay my dragon. The beatings were part of the reason why I ran away in the first place. Who's dumber than a bed post now? Stupid-ass. Needless to say, I never played with that kid again. I don't believe I ever ran away from home after that either. You'd have thought step-fiend would be ecstatic that I left the house… one less brat to put food on the table for, one less kid to be constantly purchasing medications for, which of course, would have meant more drinking money for him. I don't know about you, but maybe I would have celebrated if I were him? The way he treated me I'm sure he hated me anyway. So, why did he want me around? In retrospect, applying for so many Cadet Camps during the summer months was another way of wanting to run away if only for a short period of time. One summer, I managed to be selected for three separate camps which meant I was away for 8 weeks, yup, the entire summer… how fortuitous was that? Needless to say, I had a couple of girlfriends who weren't very happy… oh well, there were plenty of fish in the sea the way I looked at it. They weren't in my shoes so how could I expect them to understand. When I was stationed on board ship in Halifax I didn't want to go on another ocean adventure so I impulsively went <u>AWOL</u>. The morning the ship had set sail back across the Atlantic, I was on the highway hitch-hiking towards the ferry in Yarmouth to take me over to the States and beyond in the general direction of my girl-friend's house back in Waterloo [which was when I broke up with her, but hey, she's knows why]. I took my time returning but eventually reported to the MP's in Halifax. I was sentenced to 12 days in jail and fined a month's pay. The loss of pay hurt more than the 12 days in jail. Although I must say, the stay in the military jail was no pic-nic either and it was enough for me to realize why I liked being on the outside looking in.

<u>AWOL</u>: Away Without Leave. Leave is the proper term for holidays… to be away, I required a 'leave pass' which was my authority to be on said holidays.

If I wasn't thinking about doing myself in, then I was still thinking about how the family would be better off without me and I'd just get up early one day and walk away... or I'd drive down the highway after the evening shift instead of going home to bed. I always thought of myself as being useless, of being a loser, and/or good for nothing or to no one. I couldn't hold down a job, I couldn't love my wife and kids the way they deserved to be loved, I couldn't properly provide for them so what did they need me for? When we didn't have a car, I hitch hiked all the way to Thunder Bay one time and was gone for about 3 weeks or so. Another time I made it all the way down to North Carolina. I stayed there for several weeks living out of shelters or sleeping on the beach eating what I could steal or get money from begging. I'd soon tire of that and hitchhike back home. After I bought a car... countless times, I'd find myself driving down the highway after the evening shift just driving away, heading to who cared where? Sometimes I'd make it to the next town, pull into a bar, have a couple of drinks and go back home. Sometimes I'd just go for a drive with the intentions of not looking back but I'd make it to the US Border in Windsor when I'd turn the car around and return home. Sometimes I'd drive the other direction and find myself in Buffalo for a beer or 2 and head back home. Other times I'd be gone a couple of days, a couple of weeks or even a month or more [when I was unemployed] and she'd never know when or if I'd ever show up again. I didn't even have to be unemployed and I'd walk away... but then that was my way of quitting that job too, wasn't it? One time I was gone for a whole month I stayed at a friend's house in Hamilton while looking for work. Didn't find employment so I'd end up right back to where I had started... with the family, still unemployed, still depressed and still thinking they'd be better off without me and still wanting to kill myself.

Interjection: 1021-12-07-2018: this may be something small... but, isn't being easily distracted one of the symptoms? I just did it again... I walked to the Keurig, got the coffee going, went to the bathroom and returned to my writing... only to reach for my coffee, then realizing that I had left it in the kitchen on the coffee machine. I've been doing that a lot as of late, just so you know.

I didn't always have to be depressed to want to walk away. One time I was on a high and determined to head out to Alberta but I found this guy laying along side the 400 Hwy just North of Toronto at about 2300hrs. Of all things, he was sleeping right there on the shoulder of the road. I thought he was hit by a car or something and couldn't understand why everyone was just driving past him. I woke him up and asked if he needed help. I drove him to his sister's house in North Bay [4 hours away]. I stayed at their house over night then got a hotel room downtown for a few days with thoughts of maybe looking for work there [and not without incident, I might add]. I abandoned all notions of heading out west and returned home a few days later. There were many times I either had thoughts of leaving or would just get up and go. It didn't matter if I was depressed or maniac… I'd just suddenly get the notion and follow through because that's how I rolled. My maternal grandfather finally had enough, left the wife and 5 kids at home. He hopped a freight train there on Cape Breton Island and rode the rails all the way to Vancouver. He lived out the rest of his life in a boarding house where he finally drank himself to death in his mid 60's. May-be it's in my blood or something? May-be, I was a Gypsy in a previous life and cursed to wander the earth the rest of my natural days over and over again until I get something right [if you believe in that sort of thing]. Or may-be, just may-be mind you… I'm a descendant of Cain and the curse is still upon the family line and I'm left to be a vagabond and a wanderer all the days of my life… anything could be possible, couldn't it? Either way, I'm cursed in some respects because I've been a wanderer and a vagabond whose torment is living a hellish nightmare! Even after all these years, with my head full of knowledge, I still can't find wisdom because she is nowhere to be found. The only thing I know for certain is that my cycles will continue as long as I live and I'm getting tired of cleaning up the messes after the Maniac and Depressive phases and after each impulsive stunt. How many people have I hurt along the way? How many bridges have I burnt? How many people have I taken hostage? The worse thing is, What or Who's Next?

You've said that you couldn't hold down a job. What various positions have you held and do you even know how many jobs there have been over the years?

Oh God, that's an ever tougher one than my residences… I'm not exactly sure the number but it's up there I'm sure. There was always one stupid reason or another for walking off a job or just not going back. There were always odd things here and there as a kid to make or raise money for one thing or another but my first 'real' employment position was when I was 16. I worked part-time as a dishwasher at a steak house in Waterloo. From there I joined the Navy. Was kicked out of the Service and worked at various places as a waiter, bartender, a dishwasher, a line cook, a lead cook and even worked my way up to being offered a kitchen manager's position, which I turned down... I was already working too many hours as the lead cook. I've made deliveries around town in a couple of positions. I've sold cars, vacuums, frozen meats out of the back of a pick-up truck and I even tried selling insurance [sales positions have to be the worst, next to telemarketing] one time. I've driven taxi, a handy bus, transport trucks, dump trucks, a tow-truck, a water truck, worked as a shunter, tractors and other farm equipment. I even tried to haul cattle one time, but we know how that turned out. I once worked at a plumbing store in the shipping/receiving department, that was boring to say the least. I worked in a warehouse unloading and reloading retail goods into trailers, as a I driver's helper, and at a milk plant loading a transport trailer. I worked in a retail store as a stock boy during the Christmas season [that's all I could get]. I was even a professional paperboy or newspaper delivery man; however, you want to look at it and I delivered magazines, I even sold T.V. guides door to door when they first came out. I started out as a farm hand and worked my way up over the years to be a managing/owner. I've farmed broiler chickens, broiler-breeders, laying hens, turkeys, ducks, sheep and helped with cattle. I've even owned a couple of horses and a few milking goats and my own sheep along the way. I've been in and out of the military 3 times in total. I did house renos, painting, and installed fences, general labour for a construction company. I've worked for parks and recreation, and even a green house for a season. I worked on a gas line outside of Red Deer, that was dangerous work. I was a meat inspector for Agriculture Canada. I worked as a fabricator in 2 different shops. One place we made grain silos and the other fiberglass things such as boats and mailboxes, etc. I was allergic to the fiberglass and the I was laid off from the metal fabrication. At the present, I'm an unemployed minister because I've impulsively resigned from my last position as well. Then I'm diagnosed with this bipolar disorder and they pull my credentials. So, thank you very much for your love and support. I'm sure I've missed a few along the way. Considering that I've been in the work force now for 43 years, I can't be expected to remember them all, now can I?

And yes, some years doing my taxes were a nightmare.

I remember one job where I hadn't even made it through the shift. 2 or 3 hours into it, I walked over to the supervisor, thanked her for the opportunity but informed her I wasn't right for the position and walked out. Another job I was only there for 3 days, had a nervous breakdown right in the middle of the supper rush and absent mindedly walked out the back door with I'm sure, a blank stare on my face and my apron still on. I 'woke-up' if you will, because I started to walk across the street on a red light. Someone beeped their horn at me. The thing is, I had no idea how I got there or where I was and it took a few minutes for me to figure out just exactly where I was. Once the fog had cleared, I tossed the apron into a trash can and took a bus home. I retrieved my vehicle the following day.

Another place I was working in the kitchen, took my wife out for our anniversary dinner and spent something in the neighbourhood of $75.00 only to be informed by the owner on my next shift that the staff do not patronize the restaurant. I informed him that if I wasn't good enough to patronize the establishment, then I wasn't good enough to cook for its customers. I then took off my apron, handed it to him and walked out the front door.

I must have been in a maniac episode or something... but I'll explain the three-week stint for you, only because I thought it was funny at the time.

I've entitled this one: **TAKE THAT!** It's as good as the Corn Flakes Wars.

The three-week stint was on a farm outside of Dunville, Ontario. I accepted the job without seeing the house because the disgruntled employee wouldn't let me in. Had I the opportunity of seeing the house, I would never have accepted the position. After moving in, I realized it was over run with rats and corn snakes. I couldn't go down into the basement because of the floor was 'moving' and just about on every occasion, when I opened up the cupboard door, I found a rat helping himself to my son's Corn-pops or some other tasty morsel. I complained to the owner who promptly informed me that they had rats in Toronto where she lived and said that I could buy a cat or some traps, either way it wasn't her problem… Wasn't Your Problem? It's your house? But you're living in it she said… With that, I walked away fuming. I told my kid to get ready to move again. I don't know if he was happy about that, but he didn't like sharing his cereal with the rats either so I suppose we hadn't any other options. "Of course, you realize, this means war!"

Bugs Bunny and Merrie-Melodies

https://www.whosampled.com/tv/Merrie-Melodies/Of-Course,-You-Realize-This-Means-War/

The following morning, I called the health inspector and the child welfare agency who came out the very next day and early in the morning too, I might add. They weren't even in the house an hour and slapped a 'Condemnation Notice' on the back and front doors and informed me that we had 24 hours to move before they boarded up the house. Cool! Take that bitch! Fuck with me, will you? I called the owner and with a few colourful expletives, I left a voice message informing her of the condemnation of her residence and what she could do with her chickens, her job and her house. My son and I then lived into a motel room for a month until a place was available back in Port Colborne. We moved out and the owner had 30 days in which to demolish the building. Yes! Demolish, the building because it was in that bad of shape and they weren't permitting her to make repairs and no choice but to level it to the ground. LOL!

Demolish: verb; to pull or knock down a building.

Rock, Paper, Scissors… eh, Paper covers Rock… You Lose! Take That!
Rock, Paper, Scissors… eh, Scissors cut Paper… You Lose, again!
Rock, Paper, Scissors… eh, Rock smashes Scissors… You Lose, Again, Bitch!
It didn't matter how she sliced that Pie, I got the bigger slice.

10 years of military service was my longest running employment position, even that job had its ups and downs so much so that I would have probably quit 100 times over if it were that simple. Like they use to say; "there's no life like it" and I'll give them that. It had its moments but it also had its challenges as well and I'll leave it at that. I do believe there was only 1 job where I ever gave 2 weeks notice [besides being released from the military]. And that was only because I wouldn't receive a moving out allowance of $2,000.00 if I hadn't. That was the one where the general manager was yelling and swearing at my life and I put him on his ass on the floor. There have been multiple positions where I either quit on the spot or just didn't bother showing up for work the next day without notifying anyone one that I would not be returning… There were a few jobs that I was fired from. I guess supervisors don't like picking themselves up off of the floor after I've laid them out for being swore at. I've even informed a few supervisors that they couldn't do their job if their life depended upon it. Most of the reasons for quitting or being fired though was due to my impulsivity, arrogance or from depression… take your pick, it didn't matter to me. If I didn't want to be there, there was nothing to keep me there. I haven't learned how to curb that or learned to be content as of yet I guess. Not to mention the multiple times I've been unemployed for several months at a time. There was a couple of times there where I was unemployed for a year or more. I don't even know how many times I've been unemployed throughout my life time. Sometimes I'd find a 'better' job to start at on Monday so I'd quit the one I had on Friday. Other times, I'd walk off the job and I'd go for a year or more without work. It's not fun being unemployed for that long. And, I find myself unemployed once again… Go Team Wayne! I'm not sure when I'll ever learn.

How many jobs? I believe was your question…

To be honest, I really don't know and I'm not going to rack my brain trying to think of them all. I could come up with a number but it wouldn't be very accurate because I've tossed out my tax forms over the years. It too is pretty sickening when I think about it. Especially considering back in the day a lad would may-be change jobs 2 or 3 times or even be at 1 job for his entire career. According to 'Workopolis' though 'job hoping' is becoming the new norm.

https://careers.workopolis.com/advice/how-many-jobs-do-canadians-hold-in-a-lifetime/

Go ahead... Yes, you can say it... "**HOLY SHIT! YOU ARE CRAZY!**"

Right eh? That's what I've been trying to tell them all along, sort of.

What about education? Moving around obviously meant changing schools. For a man who quit high school, how on earth had you ever manage to earn a PhD?

I know eh?

That wasn't easy either, but I did it! I suppose that's another reason why I've never had any friends... moving around as a kid and as an adult. I never stayed in one place long enough to form any lasting 'real' relationships. But then I was also bullied, so with 'friends' like that, who needs enemies? Which brings me to never trusting anyone and right back around to; don't have them, don't need them, don't want them, you can have them, thank you very much. People are hurtful and a hypocritical species... if you don't fit into their scheme of things, then you don't fit in at all and they walk all over you. And, I've been walked over one too many times thanks. I'm only going to say this once, so keep up will you...

From K – 12, I believe there were 9 schools in 3 different cities.

<u>Brighton</u> in Waterloo: ½ of K

<u>Northdale</u> in Waterloo: ½ of K - ½ of 3

<u>Winston Churchill</u> in Waterloo: ½ of 3 up to and including ½ of my second year in grade 6... yes, I was kept back. I missed a fair bit from being sick and I was behind in all of my subjects... I'm surprised they hadn't kept me back in an earlier grade. I remember them saying that I had to bring up the core subjects or I'd have a tough time in grade 7. So, they kept me back in grade 6. The worst part about that was having to do French again... blah! At least the bullies moved on.

King Edward in Kitchener: ½ of 6

Margaret Avenue: 7 & 8

Kitchener Collegiate Institute: 9

Waterloo Collegiate Institute: 10

Beal in London: Summer School: 10 (English, Math, Geography)

Westminster in London: 11 & 12 [Core Subjects to graduate]

Central Baptist College and Seminary: 1st Semester, dropped out

Fanshawe College: 1st Semester, dropped out

Bethany Bible College: Completed 1st year, dropped out

Distance Learning: Animal Health and Science: Graduated 2 yr. program,

Bethany Bible College and Seminary: Completed Bachelor, Masters & PhD

I believe that's 13 in all… Now I aspire to complete a doctorate in Christian Counseling.

All through school I never achieved anything higher than a C average grading. With being in and out of the hospital so much, living in a monster's lair and with the never-ending bullying inside and outside of the home, not to mention the undiagnosed bipolar disorder, how could anyone achieve success?

I quit after grade 10… but hadn't passed all of my subjects because I was skipping so much. I went back [a few years later] and finished 10 at Beal in London [summer school], then completed 11-12 at Westminster in London ON. When I returned to finish grades 10-12, I managed that in one year which of course meant summer school, which also meant I was attending school from July right through to the following June while working part-time, with a wife and one child. Not to mention the fact that I was on the principle's list for achieving and maintaining an average above 95%. Now, how does a 'stupid-ass' go from a C average to straight A's to a 4.0 average? Huh? Not to mention being awarded the Spirit of Canada Award for top honours in his studies... take that...

I started and quit Bible college, I started and quit Fanshawe Community College, was accepted into a program in Hamilton, but didn't register because I realized a 'formal' education wasn't the best way for me to learn anything. It was too slow, tedious and boring! Emphasis on the boring! Shoot me now, I'd rather had been stabbed in the eye with a fork... Not to mention paying good money for someone to stand at the front of the class and lecture me to death with power-point presentations, or whatever, only to go home and read the text books for myself, when I could be in the comfort of my own home teaching myself at my pace, and in my pj's drinking my own coffee, using my own facilities, etc. I found that distance learning was more to my educational preferences. I earned an Animal Health and Science Certificate (98% average) when I was in my 20's which helped with the various farming positions. I started a Bachelor's Degree in Ministry but my late wife announced that she was not called to be a Pastor's wife at the end of my first year, so I quit that too. I had recently returned to finish what I had started. Being that I was medically releasing from the Military, they graciously paid for me to finish the Bachelor's Degree, so in a sense, I was accountable to them so it was actually pretty easy to complete really... I found that I enjoyed the research so I stuck with it even after my son was killed and went all the way to earn the PhD. I plan on continuing my education and earn a PhD in Christian Counseling. I once again have proven that it's never too late to do something that you desire... **Just Do It**! You never know what rewards might be waiting for you.

A second PhD will be easy when one gets to start at the Master's level which is only 10 months [or less] of study and the PhD another 10 months [or less] [the way I go at it that is] with time for the Thesis research. Piece of cake really, any 'stupid-ass' can accomplish that, especially in a maniac phase. But I plan on taking my time this go around.

Speaking of certificates and such; while in the military the first time I earned the most improved recruit award in Boot Camp and a couple of appreciation letters for excellent service. I was awarded several letters of appreciation during my 2nd and 3rd go around along with the 1 Canadian Air Division Chief's Collector's Coin for service above and beyond. I was also awarded the Canadian Decoration for long service. I have to give you both sides of the coin, now don't I? I was also reprimanded for poor conduct, bad attitude, tardiness and something about uttering threats, charged with physical violence when I pushed that fellow down the stairs oh, and not to mention the AWOL as well… shit happens! So, I guess things evened themselves out now, didn't they?

Oh, check this out: https://www.bethanybc.edu/the-canadian-connection/

2nd last name from the bottom. I think it's pretty cool… if they haven't taken me off of the list that is.

Like I said; "any 'stupid-ass' can do it." Especially in the maniac phase. I was only getting maybe 3 hours of sleep a night anyway, so why waste the hours away staring out into space? It wasn't easy during the depressive stages but because of my military training and my good study habits which I developed during my maniac phases, I adapted and overcame and just got her done. I'd study from dawn to dusk and dusk to dawn burning the candle at both ends. Or burning the midnight oil, if you prefer. I believe it was Thomas Jefferson who said: "If you want something you have never had, you must be willing to do something you have never done." I was willing and therefore, I accomplished! Churchill referred to his depression as the; "Black Dog" he was a great statesman who suffered from Manic Depression (Bipolar Disorder) but brought Britain to her finest hour. If he could do it, why couldn't I? I believe it was Julius Caesar who said: "I came, I saw, I conquered!" So, that's what I did instead of doing the same thing over and over again while expecting different results. Which we all know that to be the definition of insanity. Again; if it was going to be it was up to me! This saying is one of the 8 proven principles of positive thinking. How's that for 'tools' in the toolbox? Not to mention when I was a kid, it truly was up to me because no one was ever going to come to my rescue… the law of the jungle is survival of the fittest. I guess I was fitter than I could have ever imagined. Remember; No One Was Listening! And, they were always belittling me or beating me up. I had no one but myself.

But then... I came, I saw, and I conquered and brought myself to my finest hour!

Thank you, Doctor, no, thank you Doctor!

But, then I screwed everything up again, just like I always have... so, there you go!

Right back to square 1 which = Nothing! I'm now officially an educated bum, instead of just being a bum.

There were obviously other multiples in your life; what were they and how many if you can recall?

Okay, I'm not bragging or anything, okay, maybe a little but perhaps it was because they felt sorry for me or the fact that I was just so damn cute, I don't know. But... most guys have a few girlfriends growing up and on into high school then they get married and perhaps divorced and married again, I don't know. But after the age of 13, I didn't have any difficulty being with one or two or even 3 young ladies at a time [it was usually 2], sorry Girls! I was always coupled with someone and never and I do mean... I never, went without a significant other from the age of 13... on, until my wife died that is. I guess I was just an adorable fella that they couldn't resist. For example, when I was 14, I had 1 at Cadets, 1 at school and another 1 whom I met at the YMCA dances which neither went to Cadets or to my school, so I was home free wasn't I? Juggling the ladies on the weekends was tough though. Funny thing is, I still remember all of their names... but I said I wouldn't give out anyone's name so, my lips are sealed. And no, don't go there either... I never took advantage of any of them, I was a perfect gentleman, and never coerced or forced a young lady to do anything sexually that she didn't want to. I didn't have sex with all of them, only a couple, okay a few, but I'm not telling. I remember 1 girlfriend I had was a sick puppy though... we'd be kissing, I didn't have wandering hands or anything out of respect for her and because my mother raised me better than that, but of course my manhood would get excited and then out of nowhere... WHAM! She'd knee me in the groin and laugh her ass off while I was doubled over in pain on the ground. Needless to say, I didn't go out with her for very long. What kind of girl does that to a young guy? A sick one if you ask me. So, if you happen to be reading this book because you recalled the name or something; I hope someone finally got even with you! Oh yes, I still remember you… you were very memorable, how could I forget? I won't tell you her name but it was pretty close to Martini, and I'll leave it at that. She was a looker though, I'll give her that… and the way she kissed, um, if I didn't get excited then there was something wrong with me as a male, but that bad habit of hers I'm sure got her into trouble with more than one fellow along life's path.

I was engaged to a young lady just prior to meeting my first wife. I broke it up with her when I visited during my period of being AWOL and she knows why so, I won't go there either, but that's life I suppose. After my jail term I was then posted to Shelburne, NS where I met and married my first wife. She was in the military as well. I think her dad partially blamed me for making her quit. I did no such thing, it was totally her choice. She wanted to be a stay-at-home mom, so I did whatever I could to make that happen for her. I believe she only worked maybe 2 years of her life outside of the home. I don't believe in coincidences but the thing is… our folks new each other. Our dads were on board ship together. Problem with that was, her father didn't like my step-father [that makes 2 of us] but with that, he didn't like me much either and barely gave me the time of day the entire 20 years I was married to his daughter. Nor did his wife come to think of it… oh well, their loss. But they took to the kids though which was good. Her brother was a loner and rarely joined in on the family gatherings and I didn't like her younger sister much because she was nothing more than a cock tease at that time… traipsing around the house with nothing on. No shame or modesty whatsoever. She would come out of the shower and walk across the hall to her room butt naked and announce to me that "You can't have this" while baring all for me to see. My first wife and I had 3 children together and when I remarried she came to me with 2 so, that's make 5 children. My youngest was killed in 2016. We laid him to rest with his mother and in the same cemetery as his son. So, recap… I had 3 children, I have now 2 and 2 step-children. I have 6 grandchildren with one on the way and 4 step-grandchildren and one in the cemetery… Loosing a wife, a son and a grandchild have been the hardest experiences I've ever had to face in life. And of course, I have to ask; why me? Losing parents and grandparents is tough enough because we expect that to be the natural order of things. But, when one buries his grandson and then his son… it just doesn't seem right in anyone's books. And I'm not the only one who has experienced this and people wonder why we have a hard time believing in a loving God.

I think I've had about 17 various vehicles over the years. I've owned just about everything from a VW Beetle up to and including a ¾ ton Ford Crew-cab pick-up. I almost purchased a 1959 white Vet, one time… that certainly would have been an impulse buy [as if none of the others weren't]. I didn't fill out the paperwork after the test run though, guess I came to my senses or something?

I've owned 6 homes now mostly due to the military moves. I burnt one home to the ground [during a severe depressive episode and of course on impulse, sorry kids] and the volunteer fire department showed up in time to roast marshmallows, that's how fast it went up. We own a 23' travel trailer and I owned a 21' in previous years.

I've owned 2 horses, several sheep, goats, geese and a few turkeys along the way. Oh, I raised meat rabbits for awhile as well. God only knows how many farm cats and dogs we adopted over the years. When you live on a farm, I guess city folks like to just drop them off on the gravel road near the farm. I owned Zebra Finches for a time, they're neat birds. Not to mention multiples of fish, hamster, lizards, turtles, bunnies, and who knows what else for the children along the way. We currently own 2 cats and a dog.

There was a time when I wouldn't even wear a pair of sandals, now I own 4 pair which is a first for me. I wouldn't wear shorts unless it was a bathing suit, I have about 4 pair of those as well.

Who knows how many tents I've owned and sold over the years, along with lawn chairs, and other camping paraphernalia.

We've gone on multiple vacations to places such as multiple islands in the Caribbean, Hawaii and Mexico twice, and Alaska. Yes, a couple of them were last minute impulse traveling, like the last time we went to Hawaii, why? Why not?

I've purchased, sold or given away I don't know how much furniture over the years and don't really care because I've never attached myself to inanimate objects. I've never placed a 'sentimental value' on possessions. Oh, and books, same there… for some reason I'm fascinated with books. Gosh knows what else… mostly along the lines of clothing I suppose.

That's all very interesting… but now tell us about your impulsiveness.

Has it just been during your manic phase or during the depressive phase or would you say, both?

I would have to say it has definitely been during both phases but more prevalent during my maniac episodes though… I'd think of something out of the blue, next thing I know I'm elbow deep in whatever it was. As far back as I can remember I've always been impulsive… I can't remember a time when I haven't been. Unfortunately, 99% of everything I do, I'm sure were/are/have been done on an impulse. I don't think I've ever really planned much out and I certainly don't set goals. Even my education was impulsive… I've completed this, I may as well go for that… Set goals… Whatever for? What are they? I don't make New Year's Resolutions either… they're a waste of time considering most people break them the first couple of weeks or within the first couple of months for sure. I've always maintained that if I was going to do something, then I'd **'just do it!'** Let my Yes be Yes and my No be No… there isn't anything in between. Go big or stay home… Or don't, that's all there is to it. I'd impulsively decide to kill myself, get into a fight, steal something, throw something, drive down the highway just because it was there. I'd get up in the morning or go to bed on an impulse, I don't have a set schedule and never have, not even when I was in the military. Nor do I need an alarm clock, I can't ever remember a time when I had used one… I don't plan much, not even what time we're going to eat dinner. I might eat at 1630 tonight and 1800 tomorrow or 1730 the next day. Tonight, it was 1930… it's all the same to me. In fact, I ate at 11:25 yesterday and hadn't eaten again until 20:53 this evening for no other reason than the fact that I don't get hungry but have to stop whatever it is I'm doing and fix something to eat because the body requires nourishment. Not good I know and that's what my wives kept telling me. But, I keep saying "I'm not hungry" so I find myself constantly skipping meals.

I met my late wife on Saturday June 17, 1978 at approximately 2100 hrs. She had been reading all day and came late to Monti Carlo night at the Junior Ranks Mess. I saw this vision of loveliness and introduced myself. By Wednesday, I wanted to ask her to marry me. I went into Halifax that Saturday for something and while there I purchased a Diamond ring at People's because I had an account with them and for no other reason than, because I could. The following Saturday I proposed and we were married on Saturday December 16, 1978. Here, there was a mix of impulsiveness and planning. But for only knowing someone for all of 2 weeks, we lasted 20 years. Later she told me that I had her at "hello!"

Now, you have to realize that <u>I'm not proud of any of these things of which I have done</u> and I'm not bragging by any means... but you have to remember, I had a duplicity of disorders that weren't diagnosed nor treated, therefore; I wasn't on any medications nor in therapy and generally not in the right frame of mind either, apparently. I'm not using this as an excuse or anything, well, okay, perhaps a little. But, I'm just saying that I couldn't help myself in most respects even though I knew they weren't the right things to be doing. That, and the fact that I've never really planned anything in my life... shit just happens! Well there are the number of jobs I've walked out on which were mostly during a maniac episode. I figured I was smarter than this, I could do better and knew better and I'd just walk away. Some I quite due to boredom or the lack of advancement. There were a few that I quite while depressed too of course. Others I've walked out on after leaving the boss laying on the floor for insulting me for the last time or because he swore at me or for some other stupid reason which I thought was valid at that point in time. One really deserved it though. He was yelling and swearing at my wife and I don't think any man would stand for that. I don't know how many partial paychecks I've left behind through the years. Oh well. Then of course there were the times when I attempted Suicide and lost a position because of being in the hospital and or being deemed as mentally unstable and therefore I was a liability and the employer couldn't take the risk that I wouldn't hurt someone else.

<u>All</u> of them were due to my impulsivity and dumb actions I'm sure. Sure, I'd be thinking about death, thinking about doing myself in but the actual act was on an impulse. I don't think any of them were really planned out except for one that I can think of… like I've mentioned: I lived the 'Nike Slogan'. I suppose though when one is sitting on a ledge or a rail of a bridge and haven't jumped yet, that wouldn't be considered acting on impulse… but going up there in the first place sure was.

Both of my wives had mentioned that I spend too much on a regular basis but I can't/couldn't see it. I've started multiple businesses over the years during a maniac phase only to abandon them during a depressive state because I grew bored or just didn't care anymore. Or some person would piss me off again and I'd abandon the entire project. I have no idea how much money I've wasted on such foolishness over the years. I do remember spending… no, 'investing' $28,000.00 at one time on one such adventure. The problem is, I didn't even think twice about it until it wasn't returning anything and I had to tell my wife about it… it's a good thing I got every penny back. I've purchased a few suits over the years. I owned 4 of them at one time that I can recall. What does a guy, who isn't a businessman, need with 4 suits? I don't know, all purchased on impulse of course. When I was married the first time, I loaned my best man one of them for the day. I remember the days when I owned only 1 pair of each… dress shoes, running shoes, work boots, winter boots, rubber boots for the barn and that was it. Now I have no idea how may pairs of footwear I have. I think I have at least 3 pair of dress shoes, 4 pairs of sandals, 2 pair of running shoes, Western Boots, 2 pair of rubber boots, 3 pair of casual shoes, 2 pair of slippers [which I hardly wear], a pair of water shoes, a pair of flip-flops, but I don't own a pair of work boots. Just for shits and giggles, I went and counted my footwear: I have 19 pair of various footwear. Oh my! Ball hats, I use to have about 20 or so but I've recently gotten rid of a bunch and I think I'm down to 5 plus two casual summer hats. Winter hats? Probably about 4? I have no idea how many sets of lounge wear and short sleeved causal shirts, and yes, all purchased on an impulse. Huh?

Interjection: 2028-15-04-2018… I just realized while editing this that yesterday, I purchased another t-shirt and a hoodie because they were on sale at Mark's. **OMG**! May-be I am beginning to see what my wives meant that I spend too much on a regular basis. Well, I'll be darned.

Dress shirts and ties. I have about 17 dress shirts, 4 dress pants, no jackets but I'm down to only 1 suit. I have about 42 ties about 2 ½ dozen t-shirts, 4 pairs of jeans, many pairs of socks that I hardly wear, I go barefoot almost all summer, so who needs socks? When I was a kid, I'd be lucky if I owned 2 pair of jeans. One in the wash and the other on my bum. I think I own 5 or 6 pair now, along with 2 spring/fall jackets, 1 windbreaker, 1 rain jacket, 1 leather jacket, 1 winter coat and 1 long winter dress coat. Perhaps about 4 pair of mitts/gloves.

I've started several fights in my younger years because once I left home I vowed I just wasn't going to take crap from anyone, and I did mean 'not anyone.' I even took on 2 guys in the street in downtown London. One of them grabbed my wife's buttocks as we passed by them. Again, what man is going to tolerate that? I had to defend her honour, not to mention protecting my wife, not to mention having some fun while doing it. Without even thinking about it I laid one out cold. Then I fought with the other guy until the police arrived. Well, they had it coming... needless to say though, the one fellow did require a few stitches.

In Hamilton Bermuda I started a bar fight for $20.00 that was fun. I was given the money to punch a guy... I walked up to him and said; "hey mister" he looks up at me, "see that guy over there?" Pointing a few tables over... "Ya, what of him?" "This is from him" and I let him have it and walked right out the fight door without so much as a scratch on me... it was free drinking money, what did I care? Back then a can of beer on board ship was only $0.25, a shot was $0.10, a can of Coke was $0.15 and a bottle of wine was $2.00 [but only on steak night]. You either learned to stretch your Coke or you drank your liquor straight up. Well that's a no brainer, why waist money on Coke? $20.00, went a long way. Oh, and smokes were only $0.25 all of which was duty free of course, but we could only buy 1 pack of smokes a day and when we were out at Sea, the ranks couldn't have the hard stuff, only wine and beer. But the officers got whatever they wanted... oh, Ya, and guess where I worked? Yup, as a bartender for the officers, I had all the hard stuff whenever I wanted it.

My friend and I stole a few possessions from this one guy in Bermuda a few days after arrival. I think it was some jewelry, pot, and a bit of cash… wasn't much really… but it was still stealing. Well, that's a long story but we didn't have to break in because he gave me the key, [now who's the 'stupid-ass'?] but we took a few things and took off before he got home from work. Nope, not planned, just happened. Okay… okay, you win… My buddy and I were the only 2 in this bar in the downtown area of Hamilton, Bermuda. We were playing pool and you know how you get that feeling that someone is watching you. Creepy, right? Well, that's exactly what was happening. "Hey Wayne" my friend whispers… "Ya?" "When you make your next shot from the other end of the table so that's you butt is facing the bartender, wiggle your ass." "What? Why?" "Because, he's interested in you, that's why?" "No, way" "Yes, way." We laugh. "Okay." So, my friend set up the cue ball at that end on purpose. I bent over to line up my shot, looked over my shoulder at the bartender, smiled, winked at him, gave a little wiggle and made the shot. Apparently, he liked what he saw because he came over and asked if we'd like a steak dinner. Hell Ya, who's going to turn that down? We stayed for quit a while and my friend left us alone with plans to meet up later. A few more patrons came in so he couldn't close up as early as he had wanted to but he slipped me a piece of paper with his address on it and the key to his front door. He lived just down the street… Thank you very much, See Ya! I know, it was naughty but it was kind of fun playing with him… sick too, I know.

I've moved not only across town but across the country a few times just because I could and it seemed like a good idea at the time…

I don't know how many times I've hitched hiked around this country, down through the States, over in England, Scotland and in Bermuda over the years. One time I just grabbed my wallet and my coat. Didn't even bother to pack a few things nor take my house keys and walked out the front door. A couple of times I even left my wedding ring on her dresser. One time I left a note: "I love you, but you're better off without me" another time I left a note which read: "I'll see you on the other side." I walked out into the rain with thoughts of killing myself. She had the cops out looking for me.

Oh, during a depressive phase I burned our house down because everyone was bitching about the living conditions. Someone called the social workers who visited and threatened to take our children away. So, I made them find us more 'suitable' accommodations because we no longer had a place to live. I "accidently" set fire to the house, woke everyone up and got them out. I then kicked open the front door to get the cats but I couldn't find them. I grabbed the sewing machine and the rabbit on my way back out. I didn't have time to look for the cats because the flames were licking the ceiling and beginning to singe my hair. Yes, I had hair back then. I bought the 100 acres through a land broker for about $5,000.00 and sold it years later for only $7,000.00. I thought I should have received more for it, oh well. But that is one of the times I ran into the burning building when most people are running the other direction.

I broke into an employer's business one time because he withheld our paychecks for the 3rd week in a row. He complained that he couldn't afford to pay me but had no problem making me work my scheduled shifts or he'd threaten to fire me. I went in and got what was mine and then some. I was laid-off but I didn't care, I was going to quit anyways. I was compensated, thank you very much. I didn't like working there and went on a little trip to visit my younger brother in Vancouver.

I stole about $300.00 from another employer one time because I was being laid off so, the money came in handy for the move to the next job.

Another time I impulsively agreed to cover a couple of weeks worth of evening shifts for a co-worker. I didn't want to work the shifts but I wanted the $300.00 he offered. I was laid off at the end of the week without notice thank you very much. I didn't work the shifts nor had I returned the fellow's money. My attitude? Sucked to be him, didn't it? If he has purchased the book and reads it, he'll probably email me requesting his money… I don't blame him if he does and I'll gladly give it to him.

I've got behind the wheel I don't know how many times after drinking when I knew I shouldn't have. Thing is, I was never caught. Huh? I've drank alcohol on the job on many occasions but who hasn't? Have had a few cocktails in the morning to start the day with the attitude that I was on holidays and it was 5 o'clock somewhere, right?

We're still talking about impulsive behaviour, right?

I don't know, I'd grab an orange juice then add the Vodka without even thinking about it, so what? I've been doing that since I was a kid, besides, who hasn't done that to start off a Saturday morning or to start off their holidays? I drank many times as a kid out of impulse just because it was there, I wanted it, and for no other reason than, because I could. You know, looking back it seems like I've done a lot of shit for now other reason than; because I could!

My grandparents owned a restaurant at the beach. We would often sleep in the basement and sometimes I would sneak up into the restaurant and steal a chocolate bar... again, for no other reason than because I could. I can only imagine what would have happened to me should I ever be caught... hospital time again I'm sure, if not the morgue.

I'd often threw things at my siblings and other people, just because I could too, and because I was mad. I got the strap a few times for throwing the chalk brush back at the teacher... [those times were funny actually... well, the other kids laughed, so, they thought so too]. Well, he threw it at me first but that didn't matter according to the principal... there must have been a reason for getting your attention. Well, I got his then too, hadn't I? How come the teacher hadn't gotten into any trouble? Okay, he didn't bean me in the head, I'll give him that. But that's only because I was too quick for him... it's not my fault that he couldn't throw. Sissy! Thinking about this now, it's actually funny because I can see that chalk brush bouncing off of the back of his head. One time I caught the brush and whipped it right back at him and before he knew what hit him, I was picking him off right between the eyes... problem is, the stupid-ass never learned not to throw chalk brushes. Oh well... getting the strap was worth it. But getting it again when I got home wasn't. As long as that teacher threw brushes at me, I was going to throw them right back at him, and so I did. Why was he throwing brushes at me? I couldn't stay in my seat or I had some smart ass or other comment to say. Usually in a maniac phase [looking back] what did I care? Besides, the principle swung the strap like a pansy... not very hard... so, I barely felt it... I remember laughing at him one time. After our 'little talk' about behaving in class and the conversation was exactly like this...

Principal: "Hold out your hand"
Me: holding out my hand as if to get the belt from the old man.
Principal: Whack! He swung the strap... pansy...
Me: actually "Laughing"
Principal: "What's so funny?"
Me: "You hit like a girl"
Principal: "Is that so?"

Whack... he hit me a little harder

Me: "Is that all you've got, you should take lessons from my old man"

I said while still laughing.

Principal: "Get out of my office" fuming...
Me: "See you next time" still laughing and back to class I went.

It did sort of sting, but it wasn't anything that I wasn't use too. Besides, why should I tell him?

I broke up with a couple of girlfriends because I thought I had found someone more interesting and didn't think I could handle 4 of them at one time. The thing is, one of the one who I thought was more 'interesting', dumped me the following week and went out with one of my friends... like I said "friends, who needs them"? They are highly over-rated. So, in one foul swoop, I lost a girlfriend and a guy friend. Huh? Well, I hope they were happy together, who cared... next!

I bought and sold my first car impulsively. I was home on leave, walked into the Honda dealership instead of just passing by and walked out with a $4,000.00 hatchback. Ya, crazy huh... Honda Hatchbacks in 1978 were only $4,000.00. After leaving the military the first time, I sold it just as fast. Come to think of it, I've probably purchased all of my vehicles that way... 'just because.' On an impulse I purchased a Jeep

Patriot that was supposed to be a 'Northern Addition' [Yes, something else I 'just' had to have] which I though would be beneficial for living in Winnipeg. Boy was I wrong! There was nothing 'Northern' about it so I got rid of that piece of shit as soon as I could... yup, you guessed it... impulsively walking into a car dealership. I was driving home from work when I heard a commercial for Toyota's Red Tag Days, so I drove immediately to my nearest dealership in Winnipeg. Go directly to Jail, do not pass go, do not collect $200.00! And, in less than an hour I walked out the owner of 2 new Corolla's and $45,000.00 in debt. What, tell me you've never done that? Nothing to it! Everyone does it. Don't they?

I've drank more than I had planned too on many occasions. But who hasn't done that? Just about everyone who drinks alcohol has accomplished that feat.

We've taken a couple of last-minute vacations. On one of them we bought a time share that I just had to have for some 'stupid-ass' reason. We spent around $20,000.00 for this useless thing. We're now in the process of getting rid of it and I'm ashamed to tell you how little they're offering for it, so I won't tell you... tick-a-lock! What a load of crap.

I purchased a $215,000.00 home from just looking at pictures and floor plans over the internet. Everyone does that too, don't they?

I've gone to bed with a lady I had just met, even 2 of them on several occasions and didn't even bother to ask them their names, or if I had, I had forgotten. I use to climb up the outside of a 7-storey building, or was it 10? Oh, I've put dog crap in a paper bag, placed it at the front of a door, light it on fire, ring the door bell and run away. That was a big thing when we were kids.

I've hopped busses, trains and planes all for no other reason. I've stolen from grocery stores, fish markets, flowers at the famer's market... I don't know, gee, what haven't I done? I'm sure there's a lot of other crazy shit but I have no idea... I just can't remember all the impulsive things I've done. Oh, beginning to write this book is another one... I hadn't planned it, but now that I'm into it... try and stop me from finishing it!

Remember, I'm almost 60, so that's a life time of Just Doing It! For no other reason than… Because I could! No thought required.

What other things do you remember doing during your manic phases?

For some reason it's easier to remember the depressive phases. Why is that I wonder? Probably because I was depressed more often than I was a maniac I suppose?

I mentioned jumping off of the cliff. I did it twice, just to make sure the first time was no accident. On my second go around though my wife says "If you hurt yourself, I'm going to kill you". No problem sweetheart… to tell the truth, I had just that in mind… again, no such luck. I did hurt my back the second time, but I didn't tell her. I've ridden bare-back on several occasions but this one wild horse ended up throwing me over his shoulders and we spent the better part of an hour picking gravel out of my head, elbow, shoulder and upper back area. In my younger years, my cousin and I went out into the farmer's field and we were petting the horses… I jumped up unto one and was riding him around bareback. Cousin wanted a ride as well so I helped him onto the horse. He fell off and was hurt and I got a beating for helping him onto the horse in the first place. Here's one for you… if Jack helps you onto the horse, would you help Jack off the horse?

There's impulsivity for you… I just remembered that one… LOL!

Many times, when I was in my teen years, I would go to this apartment building not too far from our house and go skinny dipping in their pool. The situation was thus, I had to scale this 12' chain link fence, take my clothes off, swim for a bit, put my clothes back on and scale that fence again without getting caught, which, I never did, get caught that is. I would skinny dip at the beach, in my in-law's pool at night, I also would climb into this public pool and skinny dip there as well. I'd do pot, have a lot of sex, drink, take pain killers mixed with booze. Who doesn't do that? Come to think of it… all of these things could have fit up into my impulsivity as well… funny how maniac and impulsivity go together. Many times, we would play in the cemetery or take a short cut home from the girlfriends' house and while in the cemetery I'd scare people walking along the sidewalk on the other side of the fence... one time the buggers went and tied me to a tree in the middle of the cemetery and took off on me... not that I was scared or anything, the challenge was getting loose from the tree. Another time they [siblings and friends] tied me to a telephone post outside of our house. Sis went and got her make up, they put it all over my face and took off laughing... I got loose but the only person that I could catch was sis and I kicked her ass because it was her makeup... then the guys kicked mine for kicking hers... Like I've said; "who needs friends?" One time my brother stole my girlfriend from me but I got even by having sex with her... oh well, sucked to be him that night, didn't it? I drove a mini bike into a dug out on my uncle's farm. I went into a trailer with a stubborn steer because he wouldn't come out, already told that story. That was not fun, nor do I recommend it to anyone. One time when I was driving cab, I picked up this fare that was so drunk, it wasn't funny. I had to get her address from her purse. I took her home and luckily it was outside of the cab, she lost it all over the ground. I opened her front door, laid her on her couch, covered her up with a blanket, place a pot near her in case she had need of it. Left her purse and keys on the counter along with my business card, locked the front door knob and pulled the door too on my way out... now, had I been a total jerk, I could have done God only knows what to this young lady and she wouldn't have been the wiser... I hadn't even taken money for the fare out of her purse but I could have because I was entitled to it. She called the next morning, I went to see her and she rewarded me handsomely for taking such good care of her, a total stranger.

During the job as a driver's helper, we were at a small town in S.W. Ontario making our delivery. I kept telling my partner that I smelled smoke. He kept insisting that it was just someone's fire place, but it had a different aroma than just fire wood. When we were finished we drove to the end of the block, sure enough a store front was fully engulfed and there were apartments above the store. I didn't even wait until he had the transport to a complete stop and I hopped out and ran towards the burning building. He ran to the phone booth and called 911 while I went into the burning building and upstairs to make sure there was no one in those apartments on the second floor above the store saving 3 people's lives, thank you very fucking much. The thing that pissed me off was that he got all the recognition, a $500.00 cheque, a plaque from the company and a write up in the local paper...

Hold the presses! What's wrong with this fucking picture?

I'm the one who risked his life and he didn't even mention my involvement... the other thing is, our supervisor hadn't even asked where I was during all of this. Go figure. Huh? Again, friends? Highly overrated. Who fucking needs them?

I jumped trains many times, I hitched hiked a lot. I had several girlfriends at a time, I'd steal things just because I could. I'd start fights just because I could. I'd threaten to teach people either driving etiquette or manners, just because I could. I was often told that I didn't know when to shut up, even after being beat down, I'd just keep beaking off... my mouth got me into trouble plenty of times too. I'd never back down from anyone though, didn't matter how many of them there were, or how big the guy was, I wasn't going to show fear. Sometimes when I'd get a beating from the monster, I wouldn't make a sound... I'd be like that little grey mouse in the corner... seen but not heard. I wouldn't give the bastard the satisfaction of knowing he was hurting me. He'd keep going until I'd finally give in and cry out. Stubborn or what? Other times I'd scream bloody blue murder right at the beginning of the beating and he'd wack me across the mouth with the belt and tell me to shut the hell up, I've barely touched you yet. So, I couldn't win either way.

I'd threaten to pull people out of their vehicles and beat the shit out of them as well... what's surprised me over the years is that people have never called the cops on me... except this one time when this fellow was turning the corner and he didn't wait for me to get up onto the sidewalk and almost side-swiped me. I raised my foot and kicked backwards as hard as I could and dented his rear quarter panel. He had the audacity to stop his car, get out and start swearing at me... "why of all the nerve". I quickly moved upon him and got right up in his face and asked him if he had ever danced with the devil? Then I half beat him to a pulp and he ended up in the hospital and I ended up in jail with assault/battery charges against me... later though I ended up applying for 2 pardons, 1 for the fraud charges and for this 1, and both were granted. How I hadn't a rap sheet as long as my arm for uttering threats alone, I have no idea.

Often, I'd strap on my roller skates [yes skates, not blades, didn't have roller blades back then] and hang off the back of busses, cars, trucks and go for a ride. Often, I'd hang onto someone's bumper in the winter and go for a slide ride in my dress shoes, they were slick and I'd have no problem zipping along... until of course, I'd hit a dry patch and I'd go ass over tea kettle ending up right back in the hospital. But, that didn't stop me from doing it again. Nor did the numerous times I was caught by the cops. I even spent the night in jail a couple of time because I was a 'menace' to society... right? When wasn't I? A couple of times I did it with the intent of killing myself... but then, I was indestructible, remember, killing myself? Nah, wasn't about to happen. Not to mention working my way up the company and finishing my education.

I've taken a few vacations just because I could. I'd go for a drive down the highway heading to who cared where just because the highway was calling my name....pretty much like it is today. You haven't lived until the highway calls your name and you end up 5 days from home with barely two nickels to rub together. That's always fun. I've drank too much or had too much of a good time, if there is such a thing.

I'd drive really fast down the highway, over 230kms an hour fast... Got a speeding ticket one time for doing 200kms per hr. I almost was charged with reckless driving. I'd buy stuff I guess... I don't know... all sorts of stupid shit. I drove out to Vancouver to visit my younger brother on a couple of occasions for no reason at all. I went to the Halifax airport one time with just an overnight bag and hopped a on a plane to Toronto just for the weekend to visit mom or my girlfriend. I went to Bermuda several times from Halifax for the same reason... to visit a lady I knew there. I took a train to NYC a couple of times and ended up in a lady's booth instead of riding coach all the way. Oh, those Social Workers who threatened to take my kids away... I threatened them with a buckshot to the ass if they didn't hi-tail it off of my property.

Who needs broomsticks when you have bed knobs?

Another funny but most assuredly a true story… and this is only the half of it!

My favorite though was throwing things at my siblings when I was mad. I slept on the top bunk. My older brother had a habit of coming in after I was in bed. In the last house we were all at, my face was only a couple of feet away from the ceiling light, but when wasn't it? I slept on the top bunk for Pete's sake. Naturally, I finally wised up and took the light bulbs out. Out of nowhere, this desk lamp [which he still has today with the original shade undamaged, I might add] appeared on top of the television. That wasn't so bad, but I was a light sleeper and any form of light whatsoever would wake me up immediately. There were a few times he tried to illuminate his lighter only to be met with a barrage of verbal assault from me for waking me up. He would come into the room, turn on the desk lamp, go back out into the hallway and turn the hallway light off… come to think of it, I think he was afraid of the dark. But growing up in a monster's house, who wouldn't be? Well, on the four corners of my bed, where pins, and on these pins were little wooden decorative knobs that came off. Every night when I went to bed I'd grab a couple of them from the bottom of my bed and put them under my pillow… so now I had all four of these knobs at my disposal, just in case I missed or something, which was something I rarely did, miss that is. Okay, picture this… brother comes in turns on the desk lamp, Wayne wakes up and in a New York Minute grabs one of these knobs from under his pillow and hurls it at the desk lamp which generally broke a bulb and the light would go out and now big brother is left in the dark once more except for what is coming in from the hallway. So, with the hall light on, and with the door wide open, he gets ready for bed. He was now faced with a new dilemma… how dose he go from our room, back out into the hallway, turn off the light and return to his bed in the dark? Very good question indeed… which has an even simpler solution… he doesn't, and jumps into bed leaving the light on which of course pisses me off even further because now I have to get out of bed and turn the light off because he knows I can't go back to sleep with the light on… "Serves you right for breaking the bulb 'stupid-ass" he would say as I made my way out into the hallway. I could and can still walk throughout the house in the dark without bumping into things nor does it bother me. Sometimes, and more often than not, he'd smack me for breaking the light bulb… but that didn't stop me from throwing the bed knobs at the lamp or at him for that matter. I have no idea how many bulbs I broke over the 2 years I was in that house. More often than not, I was climbing out of bed, going out into the hallway, shutting off the light while beaking off at him the entire time for being a pussy… sometimes he'd get up and smack me again, sometimes he wouldn't. I do remember one time when I received a beating form both of my brothers. Remember I said my mouth got me into trouble… well, this was one of those times. Instead of hitting the lamp, I hit my older brother in the head with one of those wooden knobs, well of course it was on purpose… I told you, I have very good aim. Anyway, he pulled me out of the top bunk just like the old man had on countless occasions, pounded on me and went to bed leaving me on the floor and the lights on. I shut off the lights, I climbed back into my bunk while cursing him the entire time… well, younger brother slept in the bottom bunk and the light never bothered him as he generally slept through almost anything, especially if he had been drinking. Except my big mouth that is.

Younger brother "shut the fuck up, or I'm going to beat on you."

Not realizing that I had just been beat by our older brother. He thought I was lipping off because the light had woken me up again.

Me: "fuck you too." I said to him and still giving my older brother shit for beating on me.
Younger brother: "I said, shut up!" pushing on the bottom of the bed with his foot.
Me: Leaning over the edge for some stupid ass reason… as if he couldn't hear me or something, I don't know.
Me: "And I said: FUCK YOU!"

Next thing I knew, he reached up, grabbed a hold of me and I was flying to the floor once more. He gets out of bed, beats on the same shoulder the older brother had just pounded on so, now I'm doubly sore and had difficulties with that arm for a week, thank you very much. Not to mention the other arm was sore because I had landed on it not once but twice now. Meanwhile, older brother is almost pissing himself laughing.

Younger brother: to older brother… "What the fuck are you laughing at?"

Older brother: "I just got finished doing the same thing"

Younger brother, to me: "Oh, so you just can't learn, can you stupid-ass?" He says to me… And pounds me one more time for good measure. The only difference between the 2 brothers was that the younger one had the courtesy of throwing me back up into the bunk with such force that I bounced off of the back wall which I banged my head on and now I have a headache… all the while saying…

Younger brother: "Now shut the fuck up or you'll get some more you stupid-ass!"

Me: "Fuck You!" I told you I was stubborn…

Younger brother, jumps up, smacks me in the head this time… "No, I'm afraid it's Fuck You, now go back to sleep unless you want me to pull you out of there for the 3rd time."

Whimpering quietly into my pillow so not to make any more noise… I managed another "fuck you" once more for no one to hear but me. Unfortunately, this scenario played out more than I cared to remember, but, I did inform you that I was stubborn, and I still am. Some people just never learn either I suppose.

Another fight I started was on the school bus with my younger brother… Oh, I forgot to mention that by the time he was 5 years old, he was a couple of inches taller than me… and heavier as well. By the time I was in grade 3, he was in grade 2 but a few inches taller than me and at least 25-30lbs heavier… he still is quite heavy today in fact… 1 time I called him a refrigerator with a head, needless to say he didn't think that was as funny as I had and I got a beating for it. Okay, back to my story… We were in grade 7 and took a school bus all that year. For some reason my younger brother and I were squabbling at home [but then, when weren't we?] I continued it on the bus. I waited until we were almost at the school when I got out of my seat and gave him everything I had and punched him in the nose, which made it bleed… I'm surprised I hadn't broken it. But he was surprised for 2 reasons; 1, that I had actually just hit him in the nose and 2; the fact that I hit him hard enough to make it bleed. I quickly moved away back to the front of the bus so he couldn't hit me back… as soon as the bus driver opened the door, I took off like a bat out of hell and the other kids slowed him down so he couldn't run after me... Oh Ya, we were kicked off of the bus for 2 weeks too for fighting... but it wasn't him, just me and he was pissed... but then, when wasn't he pissed at me? During lunch time though he got even... "Come here pecker-head" I heard him yelling when he spotted me in the lunch room... as if I was going to go to him... I don't think so! I tried to get away but a couple of his buddies wouldn't let me through, he caught up with me... "You, stupid-ass, you got me kicked off of the school bus" and with that, he picked me up over his head and just like a wrestler being tossed out of the ring up and over the ropes... he picked me up over his head and I flew up and over 1 set of table and chairs and half way across the lunch room landing on a set of chairs about 15' or so away. He walks away leaving me lying there. I missed the table and bounced off of the tops of a couple of chairs which broke a couple of ribs... Damn did that ever hurt, but I'm invincible, remember? I didn't care, I ignored the pain and the other kids because come hell or high water, I was going to get even. I slowly picked myself up, made my way to his classroom, picked up a text book off of some kids' desk and I was gunning for him, but the teacher caught up with me before I could plant that text book into his face. I went down to the nurses' office and was taken to the hospital. The x-rays revealed 2 cracked ribs. He didn't bother getting even when he got home because I had already gotten the worse of it. "If you didn't already have a couple of broken ribs, I'd break them for you now, stupid-ass" he said and left me alone. When the old man found out what all took place...

Him: "maybe that'll teach you a lesson, you stupid-ass"
Me: "fuck you too" In my head of course.

Interjection: 1255-12-07-2018: I just did it again, I set up my coffee, went to the bathroom, only to return to my office without my coffee... damn. No problem with focussing issues today either.

Another time little brother had upset me and wouldn't leave me alone... he walked across the street... I picked up a rock... "hey bro!" I called out, he turns to look at me and as soon as he had, the rock caught him in the forehead giving him 3 stitches. Of course, he beat the crap out of me while his head was bleeding and dripping onto my face but that was okay. He went back home and had to be taken to the hospital, I went to school and received a good bruising when the old man got home... oh, well, shit happens.

Okay, one more... when we were at Band practice with Cadets this one time... he pissed me off for some reason or other, but then like I said, when wasn't he pissing me off? I picked up my drum stick to throw it at him as he was jogging away laughing... he looked back at me instead of looking where he was going... well, I didn't have to throw the stick that time because he ran smack into a steel girder... and we all had a good laugh... except for the officer that is who went to check on him. Oh well, sucked to be him that time. Come to think of it, for some reason, he didn't pound on me for that one... huh? Go figure. But you see... there is no irritation or violent streak in me when I'm maniac man... I'm no threat to anyone or myself, now am I?

Along the way I'd also help people out though, but I think I already mentioned some of that... on more than 1 occasion I'd help some poor soul or other stranded on the highway while others just passed them by. This one time I was heading to London on the 403. Just outside of Woodstock, in the winter, this family was stranded. I took them to the nearest Timmies, bought them all hot chocolate and took the fellow to the garage so he could have his car taken care of. That's the kind of guy I can be. More stories later on.

More often than not, substance abuse goes hand in hand with bipolar disorder and you've mentioned alcohol multiple times already.

Tell us about your illustrious career with alcohol.

I've been drinking as far back as I can remember. Mom had told me stories about putting brandy on my soother when I was teething. So... I suppose in a sense, it's her fault, right? Other than that, I was born an alcoholic I suppose. My earliest memory was when I was 5 years old.

5 Years Old?

Yes, 5!

I started everything early... had to get a jump on life after all, I never knew when the AIHA was going to kill me, or I'd do myself in, or the monster would beat me to it, so I had a lot of living to do before that happened, now didn't I?

We were moving out of the apartment above the store in downtown Waterloo to a 'rent-geared-to-income' townhouse complex which I referred to as 'the projects' further into Waterloo. That's where I first encountered the bullies. Anyway, step-dad had a bunch of friends helping and they drank beer while working away. My older brother and I would go around emptying the beer bottles. The problem with that was, in some of the bottles they would butt out their cigarettes and I was taken to the hospital with nicotine poisoning. I never drank beer again until I was 23 when I dropped by a co-worker's house on my way to the bar where we both had worked. He didn't have anything in his fridge except for Molson Export... Nothing, not even condiments for a hot dog, hell, he didn't even have a hot dog. He was as bad as the old man. "Here, lets have a brew before we head in" he said, handing me a cold one, "oh, okay" Molson Ex wasn't too bad but I preferred Canadian after that. That was the first beer I had ever touched since I was five years old.

I remember drinking wine from an early age as well. For some reason or other, my parents thought it necessary to share their wine at special meals. They'd pour us a small glass at Christmas, New Year's, Easter, our birthday and for whatever special occasion rolled around and more often than not, I'd help myself to more when no one was looking... I'm sure they never understood why they couldn't keep wine in the house. I've always preferred the red over the white and still do. I hate Rose and don't really have use for Champaign, even the good stuff. I've paid over $150.00 a bottle a couple of times back in the day and don't really care for it. My opinion is that Champaign is a waste of good money. I'll pay a $100.00 or more for a good bottle of Scotch or Kentucky Bourbon before I'd ever pay for Champaign again.

Black Label and Red Cap were the two beer I remember the parents drinking first. They moved up to Molson Export and Molson's 50, then on to the Canadian and eventually Labatt's Blue. God that's nasty stuff. I have no idea how anyone can drink that swill? He always drank the lagers while she drank the ales, and I wouldn't drink either because of the cigarette episode. When I did get back to drinking beer on a regular basis I mostly drank Canadian, but I was introduced to Guinness, now there's a brew worth paying good money for. I believe he drank the Rum, being a Navy man, but I can't remember and she liked her Rye, Vodka and Gin. I recall other stuff as well but that was usually for company, and it seemed as though they always had company over… so there was always and decent selection to choose from. I do recall drinking regularly from about the age of 7 on ward though. What do I mean by regularly? Weekly, if not twice a week or more often depending on how much I was bullied at school. After the bullies were done with me at morning recess, I'd go home at lunch time, down a couple of shots straight-up. I'd return to school and teach those guys a lesson. I wasn't always the smartest about it though when it came timing things out to take them down. That's another area where the impulsivity came in. One day, I walked into the class room just as the bell rang to sound the end of the lunch period. The teacher was waiting for us kids to take our seats. On my way, I detoured straight over to a kid who hit me during morning recess. I picked up his text book and wacked him right in the face and broke his nose. Needless to say, he never picked on me the rest of the time I was at that school and I got the strap from the principle and of course, I received a beating when the old man got home, but who cared, I got even. The Gremlin always did say that he didn't want us starting fights, but we were to do our best to finish them… so, I was finishing it, so I thought. I don't know what his problem was? There were many occasions when I'd go home for lunch only to have a shot or two of mom's liquid courage and give it to some kid or another after lunch. From grade 6 at the second school onward, I don't remember getting into anymore fights until I was 18 and onboard ship, unless I was fighting with my brothers that is. There was this fellow who didn't like me and the feeling was mutual. We got into trouble a few times for fighting. Well of course alcohol played a roll in most of those fights too. But he was a pig and had it coming on more than one occasion and the Master Seamen nor the Petty Officer would do anything about it… here we are, down in the Caribbean and he wouldn't shower or change his bedding and I slept right above him. He stank and I had enough of it… so, one day I dumped him onto the floor, ripped his sheets off of his be and threw them into the shower and turned the water on… he made the mistake of trying to stop me so I grabbed hold of a toilet brush and scrubbed him down while I was at it. Oh well, he could have showered himself but he wouldn't so I had to oblige him. Oh, I was working in the kitchen on board ship… there was this fat pig of a Master Seaman cook who use to like to sneak up behind me, grab my waist and pretend to dry hump my ass. I had a few belts before going into the galley this one night. He made the mistake of grabbing a hold of me, but just as he had, I pushed back with my butt, he let go of me and I turned around and hoofed him right where it hurts… he thudded to the floor, crying like a 2-year-old. The XO comes in, I'm laughing and informing him that he would get worse should he ever try that again. The cook is groaning the whole time and we were both charged with assault… as far as I was concern it was self defense on my part. When I saw him the next week, I grabbed a butcher knife, set it to his groin and threatened to cut them off if he ever did that to me again… Sorry, having trouble staying on track…

There was the odd occasion where I'd have to stay home from school because I had snuck too much, but that wasn't very often. I just liked taking a small shot and sipping it during the middle of the night when I couldn't sleep while contemplating on when I was going to go nuts and kill the old bugger while standing outside their bedroom door with a butcher knife in my hand.

This is the shit horror movies were made of. Well, where do you think I got my ideas from? The parents would go out and we'd often be downstairs watching good old Frankenstein, the Wolf Man, and all sorts of other crap on late night television that children weren't suppose to see… the only difference between me and Freddie is the fact that Freddie carried out his desires, I hadn't.

Over the years there were many parties at our house so the booze often flowed like water and I drank as much as I wanted. If the party wasn't at our house it was at the home of one of their friends and on the rarest of occasions the children were invited… with a stern warning of course… we were to be seen and not heard! We weren't supposed to speak unless spoken too, and if we were asked something or were given anything… it was yes please and thank you! I was too afraid to mess up at someone else's house because I knew what would happen as soon as we arrive back at our house. I didn't have a problem helping myself to their friends' booze either. Naturally I played the bartender and learned at an early age that is was a few for them and one for me. Later in life, it worked out to be 2 for you and 1 for me. It was December 1975 when I sat down and had my first 'real' drink and a heart to heart talk with my mother.

She was surprised that I was sipping my whiskey straight up with only one ice cube. "Where did you learn to drink like that?" she asked. "From you" I replied. She hadn't a clue, so I filled her in of my drinking over the years and of course, she had no idea except that one time I tried to do myself in. I informed her that I had been drinking for about steadily all of this time... she was clueless, which didn't surprise me. She then warns me to be careful because her dad had drunk himself to death. "Ya, Ya," I said, dismissing the notion that I'd ever develop any sort of a drinking problem. I had intercepted the RCMP phone call, remember? We were talking about the old man not being home much anymore and how I thought that he had a lady friend. I asked her when they were going to get a divorce. She denied my suspicions but, I knew that I was right. Part of the conversation was how she wanted me to be a Priest.

Mom: "I think you should be a priest when you grow up... I'm thinking of switching you to a Catholic School." She says...

Over my bloody dead body, I thought.

Me: "No way, I like sex too much" I told her, then added... "besides, I want to have a family someday."

Of course, I was lectured about sex, taking advantage of young ladies, making babies and then she continued with;

Mom: "Well, you could be a minister of another denomination then, you don't have to be a priest. But I think you'd make a good minister."
Me: "I'm not too sure about that."
Mom: "Why?"
Me: "Oh, I like helping people and all that, I just don't know about this invisible God who supposedly loves me yet permits the torture and tor-

ment that I've endured all of these years. I don't think I believe in him and I don't think I really believe in hell either."

Mom: "Why wouldn't you not believe in God or in hell?"

Me: "Because, if there were a living, loving God, how can he let me be sickly, and tortured all of the time... Not to mention that living with the old man is like I've been living in hell ever since I was born, how can anything or anyplace be worse than this?"

I guess she couldn't argue with that logic. So, we just stood there by the Christmas tree looking out at the freshly falling snow, finished our drinks and I went out for a midnight stroll.

New Year's Day 1976, was the day when they announced that they would be separating and filing for a divorce. "Yes," I was right! I knew it! I just looked at him and asked, "what the hell took you so long?" That was the first time I hadn't received a backhand hand for a smart-ass comment, question really but same difference. He couldn't argue with that, now could he? I couldn't have been happier and of course celebrated with not one glass of wine, but several. After they left the table and I cleaned up so that I could continue celebrating with more wine, I do believe I polished off a couple of bottles all by myself... I couldn't have been happier! Thanks again!

Then I joined the Navy and if there was one thing they taught us, it was how to drink and still do our job. I closed many a bar, curling clubs, junior ranks and officers' messes in my day and never had a problem at work because of alcohol in my younger days. Not that I recall anyways. Oh, of course, there was that very first day when I reported to the ship... I went back out with a friend because we were sailing to Bermuda the next day but we had just passed our seamanship course so we 'closed' the Junior Ranks Mess, went home with a lady and when I reported to the ship at 0500, I was still drunk as far as they were concerned. The duty watch wouldn't let me go to my rack. They made me stand at the brow for a couple of hours until I sobered up... what a bunch of jerks. They barely gave me enough time to shower, change, grab a bite to eat and report for duty. Yes, I've sobered up on the job, what of it? Many people have done that sometime in their life. While I was onboard I was introduced to luxuries such as Grand Marnier, Courvoisier, Bourbon, Port and a couple other fine delectable.

When I met my late wife, she was a Scotch drinker who introduced me to that intoxicating liquor which quickly became my new and favorite drink of choice. I do recall my first hang-over from Scotch though it wasn't a pleasant one. My fiancé was heading home to London on leave and I was to catch up with her in a week and had promised to ride the bus with her to Halifax then I had to ride back oh boy, that was the worse ride of my life. I then found out what "my head was like a football" was all about.

After the military; it was hit and miss, more leisurely than anything depending if I was employed or not and what I could afford. I vowed that I would never be like the old man when it came to my drinking though because my kids would always have food on the table. From time to time I drank excessively and usually ended up in one form of trouble or another. Things such as leaving home, wanting to kill myself, attempting to kill myself, messing with he ladies, the odd road rage, stealing, fighting, or some other dumb impulsive behaviour or another was generally mixed with alcohol. I often felt I was living up to my nickname but felt that I had little to no control over it. I'd just do stupid shit while drinking, just because I could, if for no other reason and because I didn't know what stop meant. Especially when I was feeling so good about myself.

When she died, I took to drinking quite a bit for awhile. Calmed down and controlled myself for many years, got out a hand a few times along the way, until my back pain worsened. I then drank to dull the ache and found myself addicted to alcohol and prescription pain killers. Generally, though, I'd drink to sleep because I always had a hard time sleeping.

So, now we have the Maniac-Depressive asshole mixed with Alcohol and Pain killers, a deadly combination to say the least. I told you, shaken and not stirred… nuts, eh? Go figure, because I can't.

I was eventually admitted to an inpatient rehab program and afterwards I was doing quite well for some time. Even after my son was killed, I thought I was doing okay. In fact, I was more than okay, I was 'fine'. Apparently not as 'fine' as I had thought. Then one day pretty close to a year ago, maybe, for no apparent reason, I cracked open a bottle and went back to drinking on a regular basis until the May long weekend 2018… I had been drinking all day Saturday, and before the night was over I was drinking and driving and I found myself once again in deep shit and in a world of hurt. I was in a deep, dark place I thought I'd never go again and wanted to kill myself… does "Play Again Sam" mean anything to me or am I just a broken record? Well, okay then let's "Play it Again Sam" because that week I impulsively quit my job and still had thoughts of killing myself and then attempted it as mentioned above. This of course is only the tip of the iceberg for my illustrious drinking career. Every pinnacle and every valley I've found myself to be on or in, and only by God's grace alone am I managing to crawl up out of another pit of despair… somewhere or somehow things appear to have always and I do mean always; involved the use of alcohol.

Be it a little or be it a lot, it's always been the other constant roller-coaster in my life. Oh, sure I've quit here and there, I've gone to AA meetings several times now. The other night I received my 30-day sobriety coin… probably for the 4th time. I don't believe I've ever made it to a full year as of yet, or have I? I can't remember. No, I don't believe I have. I'd drink, stop, drink, stop… kind of like the thoughts of killing myself… off and on like that light switch. What do I care? I'm wondering how long it will be this time before I crack another bottle open. I can't promise anything because it's "one day at a time." Well, this round didn't go long because here we are at Labour Day Weekend, and I'm drinking again. The difference is that I don't feel like killing anyone or myself.

You mentioned an addiction to pain killers, what were they and were there other drugs or substances involved?

I grew up with my parents and their friends smoking and back then everyone was allowed to smoke whenever/wherever so it was everywhere all the time. Naturally when I left home something was missing… oh Ya? So, I smoked for a couple of years but gave that up in 1978. I messed around with marijuana back in the day too but got my hands on some bad stuff one time that made me cough so much I ended up vomiting so, I stayed away from that as well. I also loved cigars until a couple of summers ago while I was enjoying one out on the deck, wham... out of nowhere I started hurling, so I gave those up. I smoked a pipe as well for awhile but could never keep the damn thing lit so I got rid of that too. Being that I grew up in and out of hospitals I had enough needles shoved into me to last me several life times. I can tolerate them, but I don't like needles. I'm glad I'm not a diabetic because when I had the Hep C, one of the medications was a self injection once a week which I did not enjoy at all... so no, I wasn't about to go poking around my arms, legs, in between my toes or whatever to inject drugs into my body. Oh, speaking of impulsivity and fighting... I just remembered this one time in grade 10 this fellow pulled out a needle in the boy's room and asked me if I had wanted some. "NO way, man you stay away from me with that shit." But he wouldn't and was teasing me with it. I said "okay, I'll try it" and stuck it into his shoulder and took off. I hope he enjoyed that.

The only other substance I was on were pain killers, I went from T-3's to Oxy and they always gave me a shot of Toradol in the hospital when I went in with back trauma. A few times a year I'd faked a back injury to receive a shot in the butt. Sometimes I'd go to the MIR faking an injury just to get a refill on the Oxy. When I couldn't get a script, I'd get some off of the street. However, I kicked those and barely use anything more than an extra-strength Tylenol for the headaches, and I rarely reach for those anymore. I just live with the headaches and the back pain. My daughter and brother swear by medical Maryjane so I just might look into it... Ya, right, that would go over well and it would bring an entirely different meaning to 'holy roller' now wouldn't it? LOL When I broke my ribs last summer they gave me about 50 tablets of T-3's, I've taken them sparingly because I'm afraid of becoming addicted again. So, that's it for the substances.

Here comes perhaps the toughest question of them all... Those with Bipolar Disorder may find themselves in promiscuous situations. Multiple partners at one time, or various one-night stands, or mistresses on the side or many relationships over the years. Can you tell us about your intimacy history?

Well, I had mentioned about having multiple girlfriends past the age of 13 and I had mentioned that one time in the hotel when I met a lady in the elevator. That was weird but interesting at the same time for some reason. Obviously maniac cycling? I don't know. Nothing like that had ever happened again, but there were a couple of times when it was 2 and 2 and we'd switch or there would be 1 of me and 2 ladies, that was always fun. I've also mentioned other stuff above but there is more... there's always more insanity to this merry-go-round. Now, I'm not sure if some of these exploits have anything to do with the bipolar disorder or if it's normal guy stuff... or perverted guy stuff, or twisted sex stuff and I really have no idea to be honest with you but these are just some of the situations that I have found myself to have been in over the years... so I'll let you figure out which category to fit them into. Oh, and I'm not letting you in on this to brag, really, there isn't anything to brag about here, believe me. I'm only filling in the blanks here because they keep saying its one of the symptoms and I wasn't a Saint. Please believe me when I say: "I'm not proud of this stuff", it too, like a lot of other stuff in my life just happened and I couldn't say "NO!"

I had mention that there were skeletons in the closet and every man has his darkest secrets, jumbled up with guilt, remorse, shame, embarrassment, awkwardness, shyness, insecurities and what have you. I feel as though I probably shouldn't but this too is probably apart of the healing process as well, getting this sick shit out and burying it once and for all I suppose is necessary. Not to mention letting you know how revolting the people were who raised me. I've been carrying this around too for over 50 years now. I suppose that's a long time to keep a secret, but secrets are not meant to be told... that's why they're called a "secret!" Perhaps it was just her sick perversion, I don't know but I do know that either way it went down, it wasn't my fault. The problem is though, sometimes I enjoyed it, most of the time, I was indifferent to the actions. I was just being a dutiful son I suppose. Does that make me a bad person? I don't know, you tell me. No, I would have to say that it does not, I was an innocent victim and then carried that on into life as well as all the other garbage.

Well, when my siblings called me 'momma's boy', I wondered if they knew what she would have me do for and to her. When she was a little girl, she fell into a hot scalding tub of water. It scared up her back something terrible and she ended up with arthritis and would often have me massage her back for her. I think I was about 7 when this all started, I don't remember exactly but we would go into her bedroom and she would take her off her top and her bra and lay face down on the bed. I'd stand off to the side and massage her back and shoulders with various sorts of lotions. This went on for a year or so and then one day she rolled over and had me massage her upper shoulders and then work my way down to her breasts. This went on for a couple of years and I think I was about 10 years old when one day she called me to her room for a massage, I had arrived and she was totally naked. Of course, I didn't know what was going on I was so young. After massaging her back she had me work on the back of her legs. Then she rolled over and I massaged her shoulders and breasts as usual. Then she had me massaging her upper thighs and while doing so, she guided my hand to massage her vagina then her clitoris. Looking back now, I suppose she was especially horny [all the time apparently] because she'd have me massage her just about once a week after that day. I guess I was a good student or something because she made some strange noises. It's no wonder I experienced an erection when I saw my sister that day when I was 12. Shortly after that, I experienced my first climax.

I was massaging her when I felt this wonderful feeling and my underwear became hot and wet. I told mom about it because I didn't know what had just happened [come to think of it, it was probably shortly after that was when the old man threw "the" book at me]. Mom kind of chuckled and told me she'd teach me what to do about that the next time it occurred. I was forced, coerced, and bribed or whatever to have intercourse with her off and on over the next couple of years. Along with the messages of course. So, thanks old man for throwing that Doctor's book my way… I had already known what was going on. Nice try though, asshole. If you were more loving to your wife and pleased her more often, perhaps others wouldn't have had to do your job for you… So, yes, this is another thing I blame YOU for… Our "time" together had abruptly stopped when I was about 13… "I understand that you have a girlfriend now, so you don't need me anymore" she said. "Huh? I don't think that I needed you in the first place, it was more like the other way around if you ask me." And that was that. I just figured she found someone else to meet her needs, nor did I care because I didn't have to do that to her anymore. I didn't really enjoy doing that with my mom anyway. There was just something wrong about that but I didn't know what. However; the back massages continued but she kept her bra on from that day forward.

I mentioned that my parents had people over all the time. I was about 9 and this one night I woke up in the middle of the night [when wasn't I waking up in the middle of the night?] I went downstairs because the lights were on but I didn't hear the television or anything. I thought that the monster had fallen asleep in his chair like he had done 1,000 times before. But instead of the old guy in his chair, I found a naked lady asleep on our couch. I reached out and started playing with her to 'wake her up' [because that's what mom said it did for her] but it hadn't, she just made funny noises and rolled over. So, I covered her up with a blanket and went back to bed. When I got up in the morning she was gone. I always wondered what type of parties my parents had. I guess I had to wait until I was a little older before I'd figure that one out.

I had a few girlfriends along the way that I was sexually active with during my high school years. As well as some who I wasn't active with, had to mix it up right? This one time when I was 15, I went calling on a girlfriend [we didn't have plans of getting together, I just went over] she had gone out to the movies with some of her girl friends and wouldn't be back for awhile. Her mom invited me in. Okay... I thought she was just allowing me to watch t.v. or something while I waited for my girlfriend to return home. We went into the kitchen and she poured us a glass of wine [oh, what's this?] Then she made her moves on me..."I can give you something that I don't want my daughter giving up just yet" Oh, okay... that was fun and exciting, you have to like these single moms. We did it a few times after that until my girlfriend came home unexpectedly one day. Oh well... shit happens, right?

I went out with this one girl for a while. One day out of the blue, she puts my hand up her top while we were kissing. But then breaks up with me because she couldn't give me what I needed she said... wait a minute here, you started this, I was just going with the flow. Next thing I knew, her best friend calls me up wanting to get together. We had hung out a few times in a group so of course I knew who she was. I hadn't realized that she liked me though. I was invited over one Saturday afternoon and when I arrived she answered the door in her birthday suite... oh my? Need I say more? What's with these girls opening the door naked? The next week she called me up and when I arrive at her house, I stepped into the foyer only to discover her and her mother were both naked... Oh dear, whatever is a young guy to do? Hmmm? I suppose I could think of a few things. I went out with her for sometime, had fun with her and her mother both together and separately. The fondest memory though was Christmas time. Her mother poured us some rum and eggnog. She then closed the drapes and spread a blanket on the floor in front of the Christmas tree and took off all of her clothes while dancing to the music. My girlfriend followed suit and we made out by the light of the tree... ho, ho, ho! Merry Christmas! I know, the Bible says we're not to do that but what did I know at 16?

My parents had a friend who had rental cottages at a favourite beach resort town in Ontario and while on vacation there the son's girlfriend was frustrated or something because he got drunk and passed out in front of the fire. Awe, we were sitting around the campfire, drinking and smoking dope when she got frisky and led me off into one of the cabins. Who was I to disappoint? Of course, she was a couple of years older, so what?

I liked to sleep over at this one friend's house because his mom was cute and we'd have a roll between the sheets just about every time I was there. I mean at 15 and 16, who'd say no? Again, I aimed to please and you have to love these single moms, eh? Yes, this went on for a about a year and a half until I left home. Yes, I had a couple of steady girlfriends at the same time who were my age, what's your point?

When we were in grade 10, several of us were drinking at our house while the folks were out and my younger brother had dozed off without satisfying his girlfriend I guess... I walked into the bedroom not realizing they were in there. She held out her hand for me to help her out from underneath the bottom bunk... she kissed me as she soon as she stood upright so we went into my sister's room and did the nasty in there... oh well, sucked to be him, didn't it?

When I was in Borden in the mid 1970's I had a girlfriend back home, my friend and I were invited to a party [yes the same friend I had the Bermuda experience with]. I didn't arrive alone, I hadn't stayed all night with the one I arrived with nor did I leave alone, if you know what I mean... gee, how many times can a guy do it in one night? And I thought the 60's was the era of free love, who knew it would spill over into the 70's?

Well, they say that a true sailor has a girl in every port... I don't know about every port, but there were several of them where I wasn't alone while visiting. I had 2 lady friends in home port, but I was only intimate with one of them. I had one back home in the K-W area, and I was still fooling around in some of these foreign ports. Such is life! Oh, did I mention that we went to Bermuda on 4 separate occasions that year? Well, needless to say, on my first trip [the day after the bartender experience] I met up with a group of American Navy personnel stationed there who offered to show me the sites... they took me to a footie match where I hooked up with a young lady and didn't see much of the game... I visited with her each time we went to Bermuda that year. Of course, that's the one I went to see when I jumped the plane from Halifax a couple of times as well.

This next part is sick in my opinion but it was part of my life that I wanted nothing to do with... I'm not gay! I never been and never will I be with a man in the same respects as I've been with a woman. So, other than goofing around with that guy in Bermuda, and no, I never let him kiss me or anything... ew! There were a few guys along the way that attempted to pick me up. There were a couple of guys in Bermuda, 1 in Liverpool England, 1 in London Ontario, another 1 in Toronto, a couple in Halifax and 1 in Montreal. I was walking downtown Halifax this one particular warm summer evening by myself, but then when wasn't I by myself? Oh, right, when I wasn't with a lady. I heard music coming from this upper lounge. I wanted to just check it out but the doorman said that there was a $5.00 cover charge... I thought that was expensive so I said "I just want to see if there's a couple of my friends in there." "Nope, sorry, can't let you do that." This fellow who was standing beside me took my hand and said, "I'll pay the cover sweetheart" ah, no, thanks... then I realized what kind of place that was and went down the block to another bar for a drink. Another time I was hitch hiking when I was picked up outside of Montreal. The guy offered to take me out to dinner than invited me back to his place to spend the night because it was after 8:00 p.m. Meanwhile, when he extended his invitation, he put his hand on my leg... okay, I'm getting out at the next interchange please. This one group I met at a bar in Bermuda had invited me to a party. I went along with this one fellow because he knew the address. When I arrived, I quickly realized it was a party for '2', again... No thank you! I knew I was good looking but to be appealing to both sexes... yuck! Oh ya, and there's that time at the Pickle Park I told you about.

That redhead over yonder who's looking at me is looking prettier and prettier with each passing second.

I worked at Ho Jo's as a waiter when I was about 22 or 23? I had a group of 30ish aged women who were regular customers. This one particular Friday night it was only two of them... as they paid their check, one of them pinches my butt, the other one slips their room key into my shirt pocket... needless to say I made up some excuse and punched out immediately. It was pretty close to the end of my shift anyway and the place was particularly dead... this happened a few times.

I was at a country bar dancing one time with a young lady my age when out of nowhere, this older pretty woman in her early 40's cuts in. "You want an experienced woman" she said, "not some little tart" Oh my, oh okay, that was rather forward and direct. It hadn't been my first rodeo with an older woman so, why not? I saw her for from time to time for about 3 months... That's when I learned what a <u>cougar</u> was.

<u>Cougar</u>: An older woman who frequents clubs in order to score with a much younger man. The cougar can be a real hottie or milf. Cougars are gaining in popularity -- particularly the true hotties -- as young men find not only a sexual high, but many times a chick with her shit together.

When I was working as a bartender... this lady about 10 years older than I [yes, another cougar] asks if she could have a piece of paper and to borrow my pen... I naturally obliged, and continued to pour drinks for the waiters. She folded the piece of paper in ½ and signals me to the end of the bar… now we're standing face to face only a couple of feet apart when says: "If you want your pen back, you'll have to come and get it." With that, she puts my pen down her top and off to one side into her bra… I had never seen that approach before, so I smiled and said; "Interesting, but I'm not shy" and reached down to retrieve my pen from it's hiding place, and yes, I had a good feel thank you… while doing so she buckles on and pulls me in for a kiss. Then she hands me the piece of paper with her phone number… to which I said: "I get off at 11:00, why don't you stick around?" She does, I buy her a couple of drinks… well, okay, the boss buys her a couple of drinks and we leave together… another Rodeo that went on for several month.

Oh, right… that time in North Bay when I rented a room downtown. Oh my. What I didn't realize when I walked into the office and booked my room for the week was that it was a strip bar… it was 10:00am, no one was around yet. So, I find my room and get acquainted with the upstairs. I found what I hadn't realized was the 'shared' bathroom facilities but I hadn't noticed any signs that read "Male" and/or "Female" it just said "Bathroom" my curiosity was peaked but hadn't asked about it. As I investigated further… I noticed that there were urinals and stalls in the bathroom, nothing out of the ordinary… there were showers off to the side in another room, so… nothing out of the ordinary. But this is rather peculiar, perhaps the Ladies Bathroom was at the other end of the hall and I hadn't bothered to venture down in that direction to have a look. I went out for a walk around town, grabbed a newspaper because I was contemplating on looking for work there. When I returned to the hotel later that evening for supper, I realized what type of place I was in… I ate, drank, enjoyed a show or two, went off to bed. I got up some time the next morning, shaved, did my business and went into the shower. I wasn't even wet down yet when a couple of the strippers had joined me. Oh… okay, now everything suddenly made sense. Well of course I 'rose' to the occasion to which the girls chuckled… one of them came over, took me in her hand and said "let me take care of that for you" "oh, okay" what was I suppose to do?

Oh, this one is funny…. Do you know what a **'pickle park'** is?

No, I have no idea.

Well, I didn't know either but my very first trip into the US, the guys at the barn were telling me to be aware of the pickle parks, but they laughed and wouldn't tell me what a pickle park was... other than to say that I would find out soon enough. I pulled my rig into a rest area. I went into the washroom, thinking nothing of the other guys coming and going because it was the men's room after all. Besides, who pays any attention other than to the business at hand? I washed up, walked out heading back to my vehicle and just like in the movies... this telephone rings just as I was passing by a public telephone... huh? Being the curious sort that I am... I picked up the phone...

Me: "Hello?"
Voice: "I saw your dick in the men's room and it turned me on"
Me: "oh, really?"
Voice: "Yes, and I'll pay you $10.00 if you let me suck it for you"
Me: "Oh, really?" I had no idea what to say...
Voice: "Yes, really. If you're interested, take off your ball cap and I'll tell you which vehicle I'm in"

Suddenly it dawned on me... a pickle park was a pick-up spot for homosexuals...

Gross!

Me: "I don't think so!" and I hung up the phone quickly looking around trying to find out who was making the call.

<u>Pickle Park</u>: A trucker's term for a roadside rest area where homosexual activity and prostitution occur.

I have often wondered over the years though if I were addicted to sex as I regularly felt as though I was never satisfied. Or is that just a 'normal' healthy male thing?

My current wife and I have our moments like any normal couple but were doing okay in that department. I've managed to curb my sexual urges and situations during this marriage, but it hasn't been easy, in fact it's been very damn difficult to be honest with you! That's probably why I've stayed home more over the years and drank at home so that I wouldn't get into 'that' sort of trouble. I can find enough other excitement to get myself into without adding sexual encounters into the mix.

I will say... that I am currently dealing with a pest though. No, a trawler? A stalker? A crazy person... I have no idea what to call her but she is definitely obsessive and compulsive. We've been friends for a few years now. She's single and my wife and I have helped her out on numerous occasions with one thing or another. We've even had her over for dinner because she was my step-son's girlfriend and she ended up having his baby... oops! Then she'd proceed to tell me that she is madly in love with me and has been ever since she first laid eyes on me. She needs me in her bed, in her shower, or wherever else she can get her hands on me. Seriously? She's a younger woman [aged 33] and as an older guy, naturally I was flattered but hold your horses here little lady! Okay, I looked it up in the Urban dictionary... a younger lady who goes after an older guy is called a <u>Gerbil</u>... Funny or what? I know you're probably laughing right about now because it may be funny to you, and maybe you've experienced the same thing but... OMG, the texts... non-stop, never ending... all day and sometimes in the middle of the night. I swear, she must wake up, think of me and shoot off a text message. "I'm horny, can you sneak away?" "NO!" "But I need you!" "NO! what part about my being married don't you understand?" "Oh, that doesn't bother me" she says. I 'm not kidding... she's bold, and I'd have to turn my phone off. I'd often be rude to her and I don't like to be but rude to anyone but I don't know how to get rid of her. When she was emailing, I'd write back "FUCK YOU, leave me alone!" She'd write back... "That's exactly what I'd like to do to you and I won't leave you alone until I do." With a winky face... I wouldn't respond to the texts but they kept coming. I wouldn't respond to her emails but they'd keep coming, I'd hang up the phone on her and she'd keep calling. I blocked her number but some how she'd get through and fill up my voice mail... "Oh, please come over and stay in my bed all night long. I'm horny, come take me in my shower... Come cuddle with me, we don't have to have sex, we can just cuddle together on the couch... I just want to be with you. Why don't you want me?" and shit like that. The communication was never ending! REALLY? I don't know how many times I've told her it was inappropriate and to stop.

I don't know how many times I've said NO! "What part of the word NO! Do you not understand?" The N or the O? Or the entire word? I often wondered if she's ever been told no in her life because she just keeps it up. One time I sent her this long email explaining to her how 'we' wouldn't work out, how so very wrong that would be on so many levels mostly because of the fact that I'm married, the age difference and the family dynamics and stuff like that. I even told her that she had to muster the courage and just 'walk' away. I went to the police to find out what could be done about her. "Has she threatened you in anyway sir?" "No" "Sorry, there isn't anything we can do to help." Oh boy... what am I to do? I had to change my phone number and I've changed my email address. I suppose if she see's a copy of this book, she'll have that again as well... oh well, I'll deal with that should the time come.

Gerbil: noun; Term originating from Saturday Night Live meaning the opposite of a cougar; a younger woman who likes older men the way an older woman (cougar) likes younger men.... Oh my! Interesting to say the least, but still, NO!

Bartender: "Here you go gentlemen, two shots of tequila
Me: "We didn't order these"
Bartender: "They're from the two ladies over there", pointing to the two 20 something year old at the end of the bar
Buddy: "Dude, nice! Thank you, ladies"
Bartender: "Watch out boys... they're gerbils"
Me: "Gerbils?"
Bartender: "Yeah, The opposite of cougars"

Buddy: "Nothing wrong with that, lets go say hello!"

You keep saying that no one IS or WAS listening, tells us about your counseling experiences over the years.

Yes please, let's change the subject.

Okay, but there isn't really much to tell.

I remember speaking with some nurses and social workers after the various times when I was hospitalized after my attempted suicides when I was a child but I hadn't gone for therapy on a regular basis. I was never given any meds as far as I knew except for my AIHA. As was previously mentioned, I was prescribed antidepressants when I was 16, but the old man wouldn't pay for them because I was working so I hadn't filled the prescription and I wasn't in counseling then either. However; I don't remember being 'diagnosed' with anything... other than the depression. I was diagnosed with clinical depression when I was in my 20's and ordered by the judge to go for counseling... 'clinical depression' he said, we already knew that. I do remember attending sessions about how to take care of myself, who to call when I was feeling down and/or had thoughts of suicide but that was about it. If we had any 1-800-help lines back in the 70's, I don't remember, but I never called any of them because most of my crazy shit was just that, crazy spur of the moment impulsive stuff... remember; without forethought or just attention seeking stuff. I didn't receive any regular counseling the first time in the military either and if I had, perhaps they may have caught something there, other than the fact that I didn't want to be on board ship. I do remember being diagnosed with "chronic sea-sickness" and an "anxiety disorder" though. Right... so, what did they do? I saw a shrink once for all of 45 minutes... and they started a psych evaluation to kick me out of the Service, that's what. No, meds, and no counselling and I was released about ten months later... Thank you for your Service, but your services are no longer required and I was discharged on a 3B medical release.

Let's Pause there for a moment...

Yes?

If you were medically released back in 1979, how did you get accepted in 2002? I thought these 'medical' categories followed you for life?

Being 'medically' released, my category was a 3B... meaning I was considered to be 'unfit' for Service and this title or category should have followed me for the rest of my life. I showed them my high school and college certificates, they let me redo the entrance exam which I passed with flying colours but they required that I undergo a psych evaluation...

if I passed that, they would reenrol me. Piece of cake really… you have to remember, I'm a smart guy who doesn't often get credit for it… I think they thought that I would never pass and they'd have nothing to worry about. This evaluation cost us $250.00 for full testing… did you know you can manipulate those things to have any desired outcome if you know what you're looking for and can see the patterns? You have to read the questions two or three ahead or even sometimes five or six ahead to get your desired results. Easy-peasy… my scores were very high, above average intelligence, above average problem solving but average on the math scores… I never did like math. Along with high scores on attitude and aptitude and stuff like that… I still have the tests to prove it. Nothing to it really. So, I presented those scores to them and they enrolled me… sucks to be them, now didn't it? In some sense, I knew I was batshit but no one else did so, what did I have to lose? It was a steady job, steady pay check, benefits, etc., etc.

Back to the Counseling…

The first time I went for counselling was to a Christian psychologist, he was a help with the depression for a while. But, as previously mentioned, I couldn't afford to see him on a regular basis nor could I afford the medication which he recommended to my family doctor and then we moved again. So, no meds, no counseling once again, I was on my own. I've proven over and over that doesn't turn out very well now, does it? So, I went from the age of 20 something, to 40 something without any regular therapy… just little conversations here and there after another attempted suicide. Family physicians were never of any help either. Nor had I burdened any of my pastors with any of my family or personal life. During my second run in the military, I did receive some counseling from a Padre, but sorry, he was a nice guy, but he wasn't much help at all. It was more for depression and 'not fitting in' if you will. The biggest problem was that my Sgt. Supervisor was an ass and I intimidated him because even though I hadn't known his job, I proved that I was more than capable of learning it in a matter of months. That and the fact a little miss nobody didn't like me because I 'put her in her place' for yelling at me one time for making a mistake and 'she' ran the orderly room and not the Sgt. Needless to say, I was finished and I found myself being kicked out the second time. I submitted a 93-page redress of grievance that went all the way up to the Chief of Defence Staff's office. I won my case and returned to wearing the uniform ten months later.

My wife and I went for a few visits for couple's counseling because we were having difficulty with the 'blended family thing' and with communication, I'm sure my depression and drinking were in the mix there somewhere as well. But, no diagnosis or medications or follow-ups. We had our 8 or 10 sessions [can't remember] and that was about it. Really, how much can you accomplish in 10 sessions? Not much I'd say. Not to mention me cycling through from my highs to lows but some of it appeared to be stress on the job.

My third go-round, after a suicide attempt in Winnipeg, I met with this lady Mary, for some time... probably about a year. She was nice, we worked on a fair bit of stuff and was of some help but without the proper meds I required, I was still cycling through the bipolar disorder that she failed to pick up on. She did send me to see the shrink and he was the ass that had me write my autobiography the first time, but didn't read it... If he had done that, we would be playing a different ball game now wouldn't we?

We moved to Cold Lake and I found myself having difficulties with my back, with drinking, attitude, some anger and stuff that I wasn't sure where it was all coming from. I visited mental health on somewhat of a regular basis but it wasn't regular enough if you ask me. I submitted some reports below for the hell of it. I did have a couple of people helped me remain somewhat level and eventually got me into rehab, but they all missed the bipolar thing, because no one was putting 2 + 2 together nor were they asking the appropriate questions apparently. No one really dug into my history, except for the psychiatrist who read my autobiography because a copy was in my file. Huh? He came up with the PTSD from my childhood and I do believe the Cluster 'B' personalities. It wasn't until I was released that I acquired the notes they had on me which I've shared with mental health professionals and my family doctor. Visits to the 'Mental Health' folks here in Cold Lake started around February of 2015... I arrived here in April 2014 = 10 months later. I was given meds from my Nurse Practitioner and sent up stairs to the Mental Health department... a narrative report indicated that I mentioned that I had been 'less volatile' and does not 'react' to the environment (both personal and events) with the same 'quickness' and 'negativity.' That I felt 'less moody' and was able to 'organize my thinking.' Well of course I was, I was on some meds, which was better than nothing, and I had been going for some counseling, which was better than nothing, or was it? It sounded as though I were being misdiagnosed once again.

2nd Note: The use of an antidepressant is warranted because of the <u>dysphoria</u> (Chronic) and negative self-image which has a way of modulating his values for the life he perceives around him. Also mentioned… suicide attempts.

Red Flag #1.

Diagnosis: (1) PTSD (Chronic) Non-operational and related to multiple, pervasive childhood and adolescent trauma (Physical, Sexual, Emotional)

Red Flag #2

(2) Persistent Depressive Disorder (Dysthymia): Co-morbid with the PTSD

Red Flag #3

(3) <u>Cluster B Personality Traits</u>.

Cluster B is called the dramatic, emotional, and erratic cluster which includes:

- Borderline Personality Disorder.
- Narcissistic Personality Disorder.
- Histrionic Personality Disorder.
- Antisocial Personality Disorder.

<u>Antisocial Personality Disorder</u>: is characterized by a pervasive pattern of disregard for the rights of other people that often manifests as hostility and/or aggression. Deceit and manipulation are also central features.

Histrionic Personality Disorder: is characterized by a pattern of excessive emotionality and attention seeking. Their lives are full of drama (so-called "drama queens"). They are uncomfortable in situations where they are not the center of attention.

Narcissistic Personality Disorder: have significant problems with their sense of self-worth stemming from a powerful sense of entitlement. This leads them to believe they deserve special treatment, and to assume they have special powers, are uniquely talented, or that they are especially brilliant or attractive. Their sense of entitlement can lead them to act in ways that fundamentally disregard and disrespect the worth of those around them. Sounds like the maniac phase of bipolar disorder if you ask me.

Borderline Personality Disorder: is one of the most widely studied personality disorders. People with Borderline Personality Disorder tend to experience intense and unstable emotions and moods that can shift fairly quickly.

They generally have a hard time calming down once they have become upset. [I can relate to that]. As a result, they frequently have angry outbursts and engage in impulsive behaviors such as substance abuse, risky sexual liaisons, self-injury, overspending, or binge eating. These behaviors often function to sooth them in the short-term, but harm them in the longer term. Gee, and what have I been describing all along?

How could these folks have missed the mark, how could they not put 2 + 2 together and come up with bipolar disorder? And, how do these traits go away... oh, I know... during a maniac phase of course, now why didn't I think of that?

https://www.mentalhelp.net/articles/dsm-5-the-ten-personality-disorders-cluster-b/

(4) Chronic Pain Syndrome (Multiple Orthopedic Problems)

Red Flag #4

3rd **Note:** Cpl Driver appears to be his normal 'intense' self but his demeanor was 'contained' and was not 'explosive' but complained that he had not benefited from the anger and anxiety seminars we placed him on. Complained that the current medications do not appear to be effective and wonders whether he might have a change. He continues in isolation as he maintains that he does not need friends, nor does he want any and he prefers to work by himself to avoid his more difficult moments.

Red Flag #5

4th **Note:** Complains of constant lower back pain and uses a cane for mobility. He reports 'no enjoyment in life' (anhedonia), had no interests in his usual pursuits, feels bored and tends to isolate himself, has a poor to no appetite, is unable to sleep consistently even with the Melatonin. Complained about feelings of being 'useless', he remains confrontational, and easily argumentative, and doesn't tolerate mistakes at any level, especially his own… has reported episodes of road rage,

Red Flag #6

Does anyone see the Bipolar Symptoms here besides me? How could they have missed them? I have no fucking idea… **QUACK!**

Anhedonia refers to a diverse array of deficits in hedonic function, including reduced motivation or ability to experience pleasure. While earlier definitions of anhedonia emphasized the inability to experience pleasure, anhedonia is used by researchers to refer to reduced motivation, reduced anticipatory pleasure, reduced consummatory pleasure, and deficits in reinforcement learning. In the DSM-V, anhedonia is a component of depressive disorders, substance related disorders, psychotic disorders, and personality disorders, where it is defined by either a reduced ability to experience pleasure, or a diminished interest in engaging in pleasurable activities. While the ICD-10 does not explicitly mention anhedonia, the depressive symptom analogous to anhedonia as described in the DSM-V is a loss of interest or pleasure. **OMG!**

Red Flag #7

5th Note: Appears to be more relaxed and engages easily. Feels that his mood as of late has improved and perhaps the medications might be having some affect. He endorses a use of alcohol in an analgesic role, as sedation, and as a relaxant. Has reported the use of alcohol in the middle of the work day. He admits to being able to have a bottle of wine a night or several beers and a few shots of Scotch in an evening. I feel the problem is serious.

Diagnosis: Added: Substance Abuse Disorder (Alcohol) **Oops!**

Red Flag #8

6th Note: Cpl Driver appeared to be 'relaxed' (even mellow) and was easily spontaneous. There were no pathological cognitive symptoms in either thought form or content. Mood was <u>euthymic</u> for the most part, but has complained of episodes of chest pains, difficulty breathing to the point of having depleted oxygen levels to the point of feeling faint [sounds like a panic attack to me].

Red Flag #9

How many flags do we need on the field to call the play?

Wayne would benefit an admission to a Rehabilitation Centre for his difficulties with alcohol. He reports that his 'outbursts' have been minimalized, and the most salient feature of Wayne's presentation over recent times is the lack of 'explosiveness' and anger.

<u>Euthymia</u> is defined as a normal, tranquil mental state or mood. It is often used to describe a stable mental state or mood in those affected with **bipolar disorder** [Did You Catch That?] that is neither manic nor depressive [like I explained... coasting in between] yet is distinguishable from healthy controls. Euthymia is also used to describe the "baseline" of other cyclical mood disorders like major depressive disorder (MDD) and narcissistic personality disorder (NPD). This state is the goal of psychiatric and psychological interventions

7th **Note**: Quite relaxed, spontaneous, and easily interactive, very coherent and able to reflect on his chosen path which led him to be an inpatient at the Rehabilitation Centre. No issues of cognitive pathology, no reports on mood variations, appears to be in 'high spirits', still suffers from sleep disturbances. Reports being bored at work and is not being utilized to the best of his abilities and training.

Red Flag #10

New Diagnosis: Cluster B Traits: Now quite 'muted' hmm? I don't have a degree in phycology but that sounds fishy even to me.

Red Flag #11

Side Note from Nurse Practitioner: 23-09-2015

Cpl Driver presented calmly (so much different that a year ago!) was engaged easily, normal reactivity in conversation. Does not demonstrated any pathology cognitively in either thought form or content. No experiences of sustained anxiety, mood is mostly euthymic. Patterns of sustainable episodes of interrupted sleep on a nightly basis.

Red Flag #12

of course, I'm cycling through… Good Lord, I'm not a psychiatrist but I see Bipolar all over this.

Diagnosis: (1) Persistent Depressive Disorder

(2) PTSD – Non-operational (same as above)

(3) Substance Abuse Disorder (Alcohol)

(4) Cluster B Traits: Now Muted [like what, they're going away, of course they are… I'm not maniac and I'm not depressed, Hello!]

Side Note from Nurse Practitioner: 25-11-2015

Almost a mirror image of the note above... 'Relaxed', 'Easily Conversant', Reports of 'feeling fine'. No pathological symptoms in either thought form or content. This Service Member has made a manifest transformation over the past year; he no longer exhibits a sense of dysphoria or irritability.

New Diagnoses: Cluster B Traits: No Longer Applicable...

Apparently, all was well... Medication reduced to Cymbalta 60 mg and Abilify 5mg

For some reason I wasn't given the notes between 01-08-2015 and 30-07-2016

There is an entire year of notes missing because I wasn't released until July of 2016. Huh?

Cymbalta = Duloxetine HCL... Duloxetine is a selective serotonin and norepinephrine reuptake inhibitor antidepressant (SSNRI). Duloxetine affects chemicals in the brain that may become unbalanced and cause depression. It is also used to treat major depressive disorder and general anxiety disorder. Well, one of the side effects is causing trouble sleeping... I already have enough trouble with that... dry mouth; drowsiness; tired feeling; mild nausea or loss of appetite [I have no appetite as it is]; or constipation, [no problem here].

Abilify did help somewhat... but I don't think I was prescribed a high enough dose. Aripiprazole is used to treat certain mental/mood disorders (such as bipolar disorder, [there you go] schizophrenia, Tourette's disorder, and irritability associated with autistic disorder). It may also be used in combination with other medication to treat depression. Aripiprazole is known as an antipsychotic drug (atypical type). It works by helping to restore the balance of certain natural chemicals in the brain (neurotransmitters).

Amitriptyline 25 mgs: Suicidality and Antidepressant Drugs. For the relief of symptoms of depression. Endogenous depression is more likely to be alleviated than are other depressive states. Although amitriptyline is only licensed for use in depression, it is commonly prescribed 'off-licence' to help ease certain types of <u>nerve pain</u>, and also to help <u>prevent migraines</u>. Current medical practice supports the use of amitriptyline for these reasons, but if you have any questions about your treatment, it is important that you ask your doctor.

<u>Zoloft</u> 50 mg: Sertraline is used to treat <u>depression, panic attacks, obsessive compulsive disorder, post-traumatic stress disorder, social anxiety disorder</u> (social phobia), and a severe form of premenstrual syndrome (premenstrual dysphoric disorder).

TAKE YOUR PICK HERE… as to why it was prescribed.

This medication may improve your mood, sleep, appetite, and energy level and may help restore your interest in daily living. It may decrease fear, anxiety, unwanted thoughts, and the number of panic attacks. It may also reduce the urge to perform repeated tasks (compulsions such as hand-washing, counting, and checking) that interfere with daily living. Sertraline is known as a selective serotonin reuptake inhibitor (SSRI). It works by helping to restore the balance of a certain natural substance (serotonin) in the brain.

<u>Risperdal</u> 0.5 mg: is used to treat certain mental/<u>mood disorders</u> (such as schizophrenia, **bipolar disorder**, irritability associated with autistic disorder). This medication can help you to think clearly and take part in everyday life. Risperidone belongs to a class of drugs called atypical antipsychotics. It works by helping to restore the balance of certain natural substances in the brain.

He may have been onto something here, but he discontinued use when I reported that I was feeling better… dah! Bad move if you ask me.

<u>Sertraline</u> 50 mg: is used to treat <u>depression</u>, <u>panic attacks</u>, <u>obsessive compulsive disorder</u>, <u>post-traumatic stress disorder</u>, <u>social anxiety disorder</u> (social phobia), and a severe form of premenstrual syndrome (premenstrual dysphoric disorder).

This medication <u>may improve</u> your <u>mood</u>, <u>sleep</u>, <u>appetite</u>, and <u>energy level</u> and <u>may help restore your interest in daily living</u>. It <u>may decrease</u>

fear, anxiety, unwanted thoughts, and the number of panic attacks. It may also reduce the urge to perform repeated tasks (compulsions such as hand-washing, counting, and checking) that interfere with daily living. Sertraline is known as a selective serotonin reuptake inhibitor (SSRI). It works by helping to restore the balance of a certain natural substance (serotonin) in the brain.

He may also have been onto something here, but again, he stopped the meds when I reported that I was feeling better... another dumb move if you ask me and where did that get me?

Aripiprazole: It appears as though I may have been taking some of the right stuff... This medication can decrease hallucination and improve your concentration. It helps you to think more clearly and positively about yourself, feel less nervous, and take a more active part in everyday life. Aripiprazole can treat severe mood swings and decrease how often mood swings occur. Some side effects: Dizziness, light-headedness, drowsiness, nausea, vomiting, tiredness, excess saliva/drooling, blurred vision, weight gain, constipation, blurred vision, headache, and trouble sleeping may occur. If any of these effects persist or worsen, tell your doctor or pharmacist promptly.

This might explain the weight gain, the headaches and the trouble sleeping. However, I've always had problems with those already. Then of course when I retired, there wasn't anything... the medications ran out, I had no doctor, no counselors, nothing. Well, we all know how that ended up, now don't we?

I was on my own once again and we all know how far that got me. I eventually found a doctor but I was 'fine', I didn't need the medications, so I never asked for any. I didn't tell her what my problems were because I didn't have any problems. Euphoric stage of mania obviously. Then my son was killed, I thought I handled that very well, moved on a few months down the road then the depression kicked in again, then the drinking and I sunk lower and lower until I found myself back into a full-blown cyclone of a shit storm. Meanwhile the family physician had changed and I had not yet seen the new one.

What is the biggest issue about your bipolar disorder you feel may be plaguing you today?

What part isn't? I mean, seriously? I think that's an odd question that I don't even know where it came from.

I'm still cleaning up from the last depressive episode. If I had to narrow it down to what is going on it would be more the way people are treating me... like I'm some kind of stupid ass [like the old man always said I was] or something. They're treating me that way without probable cause and I haven't done any thing to them for them to treat me like this. Falling into the pit of despair, severe depression, trying to and wanting to kill myself again and now, an attitude of "I JUST DON'T CARE!" What part of 'Just leave my alone' don't people understand? The second biggest thing would have to be the insomnia. It's tough going for many days or weeks on end with little to no sleep. I took a new sleeping pill last night, it's supposed to be faster acting and not as long lasting... well, it didn't work... I was awake most of the night and I do believe I maybe had 3 hours of sleep? Adjusting to new medication is never easy either. These past few days as I've been writing [its 16-Jul-2018 today] it's been tough just staying in my chair. I feel like I'm bouncing off of the walls inside for some reason. I'm actually vibrating and my mind is racing 1,000 kms an hour. Mario Andre and his top speeds have nothing on me today. I'm regretting from impulsively resigning from yet another position. I have regret and remorse all jumbled up with a mixture of fuck-it-all. Some days I just don't have the energy to do anything, so I don't.

The idea of wanting to kill myself returns again, and again, the boredom of being unemployed, wanting to just walk away but yet the yearning to stay all at the same time. It's really exhausting, and so very damned confusing all at the same time. I shave every other day just to stay in some sort of routine, but I spend most of the day in my lounge wear unless I have to go out. As soon as I return, I'm changing back again. Actually, all I have been doing this past 4 days now is being held up in front of this computer knocking off this book... doing research along the way, drinking coffee... both regular and decafe and I'm only leaving to use the washroom, and to retrieve more beverages and to take Jake for his walks... I even forgot to eat all day yesterday again. Damn, nothing makes sense again... it's this or that or nothing at all! Why do I have to choose? Go away, leave me alone... "What do you want for supper?" "Anything, nothing, I don't know, I don't care! I don't even want to eat." "But you have to eat" "says who?" Did I say that already? I ate dinner the other night about 1830 and not again until about 10:00 or something this morning, but that's normal for me. Damn these decisions yet indecisions are killing me. I'm irritable, I can't sleep, I don't want to eat, see, I'm repeating myself. I don't want to do anything or go anywhere... Why can't I just sleep the rest of my life away like Rip Van Winkle?

Rip Van Winkle: is a short story by the American author Washington Irving first published in 1819. It follows a Dutch-American villager in colonial America named Rip Van Winkle who falls asleep in the Catskill Mountains and wakes up 20 years later, having missed the American Revolution.

https://en.wikipedia.org/wiki/Rip_Van_Winkle

I've recently been prescribed Teva-Quetiapine XR for sleep and whatever else it's for. It's slow acting and long lasting so I'm still trying to figure out when to take it during the evening so that when I'm ready to go to bed I can go right to sleep. I didn't take it last night because I may have to take a friend into Edmonton Airport [which is a 4 hour drive one-way from here]. If I take the sleep aide there is no way I'll be able to get up at 6:00am. But if I don't take it then I won't sleep at all... again, decisions, decisions... So, I didn't take it. I went to bed at 2330 and you guessed it, I couldn't sleep and finally got out of bed at 1:34 and here I am at 2:15 am, still clicking away on the key board. I hate this not sleeping. I'm hoping he doesn't require me to take him to the airport so I can just go back to bed and sleep the morning away.

Interjection: 4:35-29-06-2018; Needless to say, I didn't take it and I didn't sleep. I was up for 31 hours straight. At the end of the 31 hours I took the pill and went to bed and I think I slept for 14 hours. I took the sleeping pill last night about 1800 [probably too early]. I was in bed by 2015 but only slept until 0120. Laid awake until 02:30 and finally got out of bed.

Interjection: 1105-16—07-2018: We changed things up: Quetiapine Fumarate 25mg. I took it about an hour before going to be and I was awake most of the night... are we going to get this sorted out or what?

Interjection: 2251-18-07-2018: I took the slow reacting, long lasting sleeping pill last night at about 1900hrs. I went to bed at 2305, last time I saw the clock was 0230 because I hadn't fallen asleep as of yet. I woke up this morning at 0900hrs and didn't want to get out of bed. I ran several errands today only because the Mrs. said that I hadn't a choice. I'm back at the computer and still feel restless. I want to go for a drive. Where too? I don't know, just to be anywhere but here.

The part about having to attend all of these meetings with various 'professionals' is extremely annoying though, but, it is something that I've been asking for so I won't really complain too much about them. I just get tired of repeating myself over and over, and over... and are they going to do anything this time? Why can't we just set up a conference meeting and we'll all get together in one location at the same time? Is all of this or any of this going to amount to anything? Please tell me that I'm not just wasting my time once again. Then there is the present state of mind in which I find myself, and that is having an "I don't give a shit attitude" why won't it just go away already? To put it mildly is extremely frustrating. I know I keep repeating myself but that's how it is... I don't know what to do, what to say, what to do? I have to take this medication that takes away the craving for alcohol but I can't take it as prescribed because it makes the insomnia worse, if that's possible... well, it is okay! I have to go to these AA meetings. Nice bunch of people, I've read the literature a few times, but it's like the other stuff... I don't care, really, I just don't care... but I keep going and I share... perhaps something they say may help me and something I share, someone else might be able to relate too. I don't have cravings for a drink but I had thoughts today about how nice it would be to have one. For some reason, I can't seem to get a sponsor. I couldn't get one the other times either, may-be that's why I wasn't successful or it could have been the fact that I really didn't want to stop drinking or just figured I couldn't stop so, why bother trying? I can control it, that's the ticket... look how far that got me... not very, I can assure you. Again, Eeyore wins and I went out and bought some beer and Bourbon. I'm by myself so there's no harm in having a drink. I started this book by writing my notes in the evening by the camp fire. A week or so later, I can't even read my own writing. Typical. For the most part it's really confusing and most assuredly a living hell. So, NO, my Wall does NOT have a Window today either, Okay?

You've mentioned that you've earned a doctorate in Ministry.

Where does religion come in to play for you?

To be polite… It doesn't. I don't like and never have liked the term/word 'Religion' because to me it is nothing more than a bunch of man-made rules with feeble attempts to get us into heaven, that is, if we're good enough. Well, if anyone has even read the Book of John or the Epistles of Paul, they would know that we can never be 'good enough' because the only thing that we can do is accept Christ as our Saviour… beyond that, it was all up to him and God. Many 'Denominations' today are no better than the Pharisees in Christ's day. My earliest days of church attendance was when I was about 6, I think. Looking back, it was just exactly that; 'Religion'. I was forced to go to an Anglican Church down the block because monster was forced out to church as a kid so, I suppose he thought it would be good for me as well… yet he couldn't tell me what he did/not believes, but he forced me to go to church anyway. If he had any faith [which I doubt] he never shared it nor had he lived it, that's for sure.

Religion is a fundamental set of beliefs and practices generally agreed upon by a group of people. [Right there… Man Made Rules!] These set of beliefs concern the cause, nature, and purpose of the universe, and involve devotional and ritual observances. They also often contain a moral code governing the conduct of human affairs. Ever since the world began, man has demonstrated a natural inclination towards faith and worship of anything he considered superior/difficult to understand. His religion consisted of trying to appease and get favors from the supreme being he feared. This resulted in performing rituals (some of them barbaric) and keeping traditions or laws to earn goodness and/or everlasting life.

Christianity has always stressed a personal relationship with God as the touchstone of religion. When God created Adam and Eve, He walked with them in the Garden of Eden, in the cool of the day, and enjoyed their fellowship. Religion was, and still is, a close, personal, and satisfying relationship with the creator God. No… no, it isn't… RELATIONSHIP and RELIGION are two separate things.

A brief definition of the meaning of Religion: All About. . . www. allaboutreligion.org/meaning-of-religion-faq.htm

So, religion as it is defined here has never really played a big part in my life. Many would say that they are 'spiritual' but not religious. Meaning that they believe in God, and perhaps even Christ but they do not hold to any religious values or practice their faith on a regular basis. As further expressed in our definition above, I don't look at my faith as being 'Religious' because religion is full of man-made rules, rituals and man's poor attempt to reconnect with God and we shall always fall short of the mark in our feeble attempts, won't we? Christ is God's attempt to reconnect with man but many do not accept him as the only begotten of the heavenly father… why? Mostly because they don't or can't believe in miracles and the fact that Christ was raised from the dead or that a loving God would permit so much evil in the world. Not to mention that we are fighting an invisible war with the Devil and his minions and… how can a 'loving' God send people to hell, they ask. In short: Christ came to fulfill the laws and prophecies of God and since he was the sacrificial lamb, we don't need the blood sacrifices as found in the Book of Leviticus any longer. He was also our high priest so what need of we of a Catholic Priest to hear our confessions when we have direct access to the throne of Grace through Christ? Simply put… Christians prefer to look at it as having a relationship with Christ as it is laid out in the Bible. Well, that's the way I prefer to look at it. It is possible to be Spiritual without being 'religious' as some people would put it… and still practice their faith on a regular basis.

I personally have accepted Christ as my Saviour and become one with him and the Heavenly Father… I become a son and therefore an heir to the throne in heaven and can call Christ my brother. Even at the level of Education for which I have studied I have a lot to learn about 'heart knowledge' and how to treat people in a kind manner because Christ compels me too do so, no matter how people treat me. But, being one in Christ means I have become a big happy family with other believers, even if they don't see it that way and don't treat me very nice. And, as mentioned at the beginning of this book, what family is without difficulties? I could spout off all kinds of Bible Verses, passages and doctrine here, but I won't but simply offer you this… if you are struggling with life's questions, Christianity, may have many of the answers you are seeking. If you are not sure about all of this 'God' and 'Jesus' stuff… I would suggest that you start with an open mind, an open heart, whisper a little prayer for guidance and read the Book of John. Then I would invite you to check out: **AllAboutGOD.com**

www.allaboutgod.com/all-subjects.htm

There are a lot of websites out there but I believe this one does a very good job of breaking the tough questions down into solid practical answers. In fact; I challenge you to ask questions and read their answers and email me. I'd love to hear from you. While you're asking your questions, dig into the book of Acts and then the letters of Paul. Like everyone, I had to work out my salvation for myself.

I have both head and heart knowledge but have struggled with EVERYTING in life, why should Christianity be any different? Remember, I'm not playing with a full deck so with this bipolar stuff, there is often a disconnect between head and heart and I, for the lack of a better term… don't know any better, or can't logically see my way through a tough situation. I can and have been the sweetest guy you'd ever want to know, but when crossed, I can and have become someone's worse nightmare. I realize it isn't supposed to be like that as I am supposed to turn the other cheek. I'm supposed to treat people with love and kindness despite how they treat me, just as Christ had… I'm working on it. But like I said; there is often a disconnect. Oh, I may let you get away with it the first few times but then you've shown a pattern of a lifestyle, so why should I continue to subject myself to your abuse? I may not treat you as you treat me, but I may not give you my attention either. I just don't understand why people treat others the way they wouldn't want to be treated in the first place? I just pray that we undergo a transformation and not only take on the love of Christ but extend his love to our fellow man. There really is no need to be mean or discourteous to each other.

Along life's journey I went through what I refer to as my own 'Judges' cycle. Read the book of Judges and you'll understand more of what I'm referring too. The books of the Kings and Chronicles are more of the same to I believe. Through my life it would appear that I walked with God, I walked without him and I walked with him again. Not that I'm anything special or bragging or anything, but the last time I checked, I had not done anything for which God would not forgive me for. I will have to answer for my actions, but I can not change the past. However; I can learn from it and by the Grace of God, change my future so my past does not continue to repeat itself. Sometimes Jesus would be near, other times afar off while other times he is nowhere to be found, yet he has promised to never leave me nor to forsake me [Deuteronomy 31:6 (NIV), 6 Be strong and courageous. Do not be afraid or terrified because of them, for the Lord your God goes with you; he will never leave you nor forsake you." Hebrews 13:5 (NIV), 5 Keep your lives free from the love of money and be content with what you have, because God has said, "Never will I leave you; never will I forsake you." but yet I can not find him. Whether I'm up, down or sometimes in between, I often feel that I truly am alone. But that is a problem with me, not him, isn't it? Funny? Odd? Crazy thing is though, for all the time I have spent alone, I'm never really lonely because I have been accustomed to my own company. I've helped a fair number of people over the years and I generally can hold my own in a conversation but more often than not, looking back, I have been alone. But God says that his Son has also been there with me whether I saw him or not. Being an associate Pastor has helped me to discover though that I prefer to work with small groups, or one on one. I'm not sure if I was meant to be a Pastor but God could change that.

That's probably the reason for the farming and trucking positions all of those years, I suppose. I worked in the office environment for many years while in the military. Sure, I was around other people, I had personnel coming to see me for one thing or another but for the most part, I was left to myself to accomplish my own tasks... which is probably why I lasted so long. But then I got tired of that, plus I found myself in and out of trouble because of the close proximity of being with other people that I found myself to be back to wanting to rip people's heads off instead of working with them. But again, that was the symptoms of the bipolar, not necessarily me. I do so enjoy helping people, I enjoy being around people, sometimes it just has to be on MY terms, not theirs. I'll help anyone in a crisis, I'll come running if you call, don't get me wrong. Not to offend anyone, but if I'm working around the yard and you just drop in' be ready to pitch in and help or, I'll have to see you later. Speaking of reaching out to others... as I have mentioned: I've reached out to aide total strangers who have been down and out or on the streets, and in need of a hot meal, a hot shower, clean clothes, or a bed for the night, or a helping hand of some sort. I've even given some of them temporary jobs and put them on to others who require assistance on the farm... I've even offered some full-time positions only to discover they are unable to fulfill their commitments. But then again, that's probably why they're on the street, isn't it?

However; more often than not, I feel like David in his Psalms... why have you forsaken me?

Some of Psalm 22:

¹ My God, my God, why have you forsaken me?
  Why are you so far from saving me,
    so far from my cries of anguish?
² My God, I cry out by day, but you do not answer,
    by night, but I find no rest.
⁶ But I am a worm and not a man,
    scorned by everyone, despised by the people.
⁷ All who see me mock me;
    they hurl insults, shaking their heads....

Now of course this Psalm points to what Christ would endure upon the Cross... but I can whole heartedly identify with most of it. I'm am taken for granted, I am perceived to be smarter than the average person and have intimidated a fair number of people over the years. I come across as being too helpful that they wonder what my ulterior motive is... there isn't one... it is only because Christ compels me, that's all. But they are suspicious nonetheless to the point where I don't get hired or am over looked. While I was a kid, I was mocked, called names, beat up... as an adult, the insults came in other ways and I called out to my God only to be met with silence. So, I can definitely understand this Psalm.

I'm not saying that I am without heart knowledge, but I am more of an intellectual who enjoys analyzing deep things of his nature before I put it into practice, and then I want to do the best darn job I can at it. But then that impulsivity factor kicks in and it's a whole new ball game. Am I doing it for the accolades of man or praise of my heavenly Father? I have to remember to check my ulterior motives every time I do something. Or when I'm maniac or depressed, we're in 2 different leagues altogether. I never know what game I'm playing until I step out onto the field and I never know how you're going to react until I throw the ball your way. Not to mention having people verbally pummelling me because I've dropped the ball. Then when I was a kid, I could never trust any boy to be my 'friend' because I never knew when they would turn on me for whatever reason. I could never trust the kids in grade school, the ones in the hood were always picking on me, so who was I suppose to make friends with? It was hard to show Christ's love to kids who picked on you… and several of them sat right next to me in Sunday School.

What do you mean you were "forced" to go to church?"

I mean exactly that… if he got up and I was home without a Current Sunday school paper, he would know that I hadn't attended Sunday School and he'd beat me for disobeying. There was no way I'd bring a paper home for my brother and he wouldn't bring one home for me… we had the attitude that, if I have to suffer through this, so do you! Mom later wanted me to go to confirmation classes. But during my first meeting the minister asked everyone why they were there. I was honest with him so I told him that "I was here because my mom wanted me to be here."

Minister: "You mean, you don't want to be here?"
Me: "No, Sir"
Minister: "Well, you go home and tell your mother that I don't want you here until you are ready to be here"
Me: "Okay, see Ya"

I went home, told mom that the minister didn't want me in the classes… "did he say why?" she asked, "nope, probably because I was too young… I was the youngest one there." I never went back to that church again, not even on Sundays. When we moved though, there was a large brand-new Pentecostal Church right next door, and I knew exactly what the meant… the old man didn't care what denomination it was, I was attending unless they were the JW's or LDS that is. There was a family of JW's who lived in the neighbourhood that we weren't allowed to play with because they would brain wash me… but yet he wouldn't share any of his beliefs with me either… I supposed that was because he didn't have any. Well, according to his life style it was quite evident. So, I went to church faithfully over the next two or maybe three years I think, while we lived in that town house. I remember a lot of mornings, I would get my youngest sister ready for church as well. My older brother kept regular attendance at the Anglican Church, so my little sister became my responsibility. Heaven forbid mom should get her lazy drunken ass out of bed to feed and dress her kids. He of course was sleeping off a drunk as usual and we had to be as quiet as church mice so as not to wake him up. God forbid we should make a noise because the monster ate children remember. I also remember going to summer camp a couple of years and at one of those camps I accepted the Lord as my Saviour but I wasn't allowed to talk about that 'shit' [he called it] at home. Hmmm? Naturally, I was confused.

Then on the flip side of the coin… picture this: Bible Camp run by "goodie two-shoes," well, that's what monster called them [who obviously wouldn't say "shit" if they had a mouthful] and Summer Camp for under privileged kids run by the Psych department from the University of Waterloo in the 60's… [where folks couldn't put a sentence together without some form of a swear word in it] he, he, he… it was like Woodstock for Children… naked body panting, sleeping in the same sleeping bag with the girls or with female counselors, swimming naked, smoking dope, eating whatever, including magic mushrooms, dancing naked around the camp fire, showering and sleeping with the girls [no sex though, we were too young to even know what that was]. I think they were running a nudist colony or something because it seemed like we were always naked. Hippie music playing all of the time. It was a blast!

Either way, both the camps were free for him, and it got me out of the house for a couple of weeks during the summer.

The Woodstock Music & Art Fair—informally, the Woodstock Festival or simply Woodstock—was a music festival in the United States in 1969 which attracted an audience of more than 400,000. Scheduled for August 15–17 on a dairy farm in the Catskill Mountains of southern New York State, northwest of New York City, it ran over to Monday, August 18.

So, it's no wonder I was confused. I didn't understand why we had to go church in the first place, why we had to say grace and why we had to say our prayers at night. I knew who Jesus was but I wasn't sure about this loving Invisible 'Heavenly Father' called 'God' as I explained earlier. If we couldn't see this God fellow, why did we have to pray to him? And why didn't he save me from all of those beatings? Especially the ones where I didn't do anything wrong… or the ones where the monster came close to killing me? Or the ones where I didn't stop my younger brother from doing something stupid and I was punished for it as well… Besides, this 'God' never answered any of my prayers either so why bother praying to Him? I may as well have been talking to the four walls for all the difference it made. Simple logic for a kid, right?

So, when we moved again, I stopped going to church and never looked back until after I was married and in my late 20's I think? I only went to church the few times in the military because attendance was mandatory. I was working at Sears warehouse later on when I came across a group of Bible College students who also worked there. I was told to be aware of the Popes! We have Catholics working here or what? No! JWs? LDS? Yes, both of those but these guys are way worse and they'll get you if you aren't careful. "What the hell are you guys talking about?" "Bible College Students, that's what" "O, okay…?" I had no idea what the hell the guys were talking about. I soon found out that they all grouped together and would have biblical discussions around the dinner table. That was a time when 'free speech' was actually free and one could discuss anything in public without fear of some sort of persecution for 'offending' someone… now a days, we can't say this or that because we might 'offend' some pansy ass. One day I asked if I could join in… they let me of course, so I started hanging out with these guys. And, Another One Bites the Dust! One evening God got a hold of me and I rededicated my life to Christ. My late wife rededicated that next day and we started attending a Baptist church down the block and 3 months later we were baptised. Turns out that she grew up in the Free Methodist Church where we were married, and I knew that, but we never discussed this 'God' stuff when we were dating. We became like most people and only went to church for weddings and funerals. Remember there was this 'disconnect' thing and the bipolar thing mixed together so our Church attendance was hit and miss over the next 15 years depending on where we lived, what my work schedule was like and what my demeanour was at any particular moment. The last time we were active together, she ended up dying and I was ostracized.

After remarrying, my wife and I attended on a regular basis which did help keep me somewhat on an even playing field, but it was tricky. Coming and going on various training Exercises, moving, etc. While in Winnipeg we were attending Church of the Rock and really enjoyed it. Moving to Cold Lake we visited a few churches and we were led to a local church. It was during my transition from the Military that I was sure I heard God say "what about me?" But, because of the way things have gone, I suppose now looking back, I must have been delusional.

Over the years though, I hadn't stayed away completely and you could say, I did my best, even though my mental state wasn't the greatest. I've assisted with youth, children's ministry, baptisms, weddings, funerals, communions, baby dedications, I've done some mentoring, discipling, street ministry, lead men's groups as well as bible studies, I've taught Sunday School to adults and youth groups, and I was an usher and a greeter and I've preached on many occasions. I was a Cub Leader a Scout Leader and a Cadet Instructor. I've volunteered at Church functions, food banks, soup kitchens and have lead worship services at the Extended Care facility for Seniors. I've prayed for healing many times over what ailed me [and for others] but so far, my answer has been NO. Like I said; I'm not proud of the things I've done but all the prayer in the world didn't seem to matter or help when I was either high in a maniac phase or low in a depressive state... except to save my sorry ass from killing myself or being killed... but that in and of itself is quite a lot when you look at it.

The saddest thing of all is that all the education, whether biblical or otherwise never came into play during a crisis on either end. When I get some stupid-ass thing in my head, **I just do it!** No forethought required, no second thought and that is part of my never-ending situation. It's scary as hell I know, but there are/were never any warning bells, no red flags, no red lights, no sirens going off to wake me the hell up and get me to take a second look at what I was doing or what I was about to do... "I Just Do it" no matter what it was I was going to do! It is/was and always has been a **Green Light** which means GO! I appear to be its slave and it my master or something. The biggest shameful part of all of this are the sexual exploits of my past, especially when I was married the first time. Plus, the fact that I'm educated now... I know that I'm not a medical doctor but the phrase: "Physician heal thyself" comes to mind many times when I'm in the 'coasting' phase I talked about earlier but, how can I? I'm okay during this phase and all is right with the world but for how long? I'm not saying that I have all of the answers, but I have many of them and more than most to be sure, but where are they when I have need them? They are nowhere to be found, that's where. I've written many papers, sermons and Bible studies, but I just can't seem to find the answers when I need them for myself. It's like a doctor who knows all about the facts and the effects of smoking, he tells his patients to quit but he can't bring himself to drop the habit. When I'm in a crisis... I don't know how or why, and more often than not, who gives a shit? There are no thoughts of the damages or any repercussions or questions as to how I'm going to clean up the mess once the storm passes. Does a Tornado worry about the wake of destruction it is about to leave behind? No, of course not! So, why should I? But I'm not a tornado I know, but I may as well be because after the wind moves on or ceases to blow... it is only after the storm do I come up out of my fall out shelter and see the devastation and wonder what the hell have I done and how am I going to clean up this mess once again? If I could get insurance against my stupidity, they'd make a fortune off of me I'm sure. Over the years I have attended anger management, suicide and leadership seminars, anxiety classes, holy spirit encounters, couple's and men's retreat and who knows how many Bible study classes, not to mention my own personal devotions and both formal and informal studies. But where or what does all this get me when shit hits the fan? **NOWHERE** and **NOTHING!** A big fat ZERO! And further into trouble and/or deeper in debt and sometimes both. It's like I'm a different person, mostly standing on the outside looking in as if this were some sort of a spectator's sport. In a maniac phase I become my own cheering squad, in a depressive state… who cares? And I want to die.

Therefore; **I TRULY AM MY OWN WORST ENEMY,
I TRULY AM LIVING A HELLISH NIGHTMARE!
AND NO ONE HAS TRULY CARED TO LISTENING!
I TRULY AM ALONE!**

You've mentioned AA, which of course is short for Alcoholics Anonymous… How's that working for you?

In a nut shell, it's like everything else in my life: hit and miss. When I first starting going back in my late 20's, I went because my wife thought that I had a problem with alcohol. I'm sure she was right so I calmed down and even quit for a while but I had nothing in common with those folks. Besides, I can't 'give up' something/anything for someone else, I had to do it for myself. Well, I wasn't ready to do it for myself. Oh, sure I saw myself getting into situations I probably wouldn't have found myself in if I weren't drinking, but I couldn't relate… I didn't have a house to lose, but I still had a wife, I still had my kids, I did have various employment situations but I was sure they weren't because of my drinking… I knew something was wrong with me but I didn't have a clue what that was but I knew it wasn't alcohol. I was only clinically depressed remember, so it had nothing to do with alcohol. I hadn't thought that I had lost any of my employment positions because of my drinking… well, except those 2 part-time ones that is. I stayed long enough to get a 30-day coin and didn't go back. I attended a few meetings somewhere in my mid 30s, still there was no connection. I went again in my 40's somewhere, but, besides, I didn't want to quit drinking. I liked my Guinness, my Scotch, my Bourbon and my wine. Now I'm sure if she had of said it was the booze or me, I would have chosen her, but there was nothing of that sort. So, I didn't have to make a choice. I attended a few meetings after

I was released from rehab, but I had a handle on the not drinking thing, so, why attend the meetings? I never got anything out of them anyway. I could never get a sponsor and had no one who'd be there should I ever find myself in trouble? NO ONE! So, once again, it is me against the world because it doesn't matter what situation I find myself to be... I AM ALONE!

Besides, I'm an intellectual, aren't I? Why yes, I am, thank you for noticing. I have a bunch of literature, I have digested it to the point where I could even find loopholes in the program... I could even rewrite some of it too for that matter and I can quite anytime I want to... I just haven't found that right reason for wanting to. So, is this time any different? I know that I have a situation going on that I have to fight to overcome all of this. So, for now, I'm going regularly, am finding very little to no 'comfort' in the meetings as I had before. I suppose one could call it that. But then again, over the years I've attended suicide prevention courses and yet look at how many times I tried to kill myself or thought of killing myself? Is there hope this time? I don't know and don't really care. It is truly 'one day at a time' no matter if we're talking, feelings, alcohol, medications, mania or depression. Today, 16-07-2018... I can't say that I'm 'feeling' anything right now... nope, nothing really. I'm just coasting, but when I interact with people, I get angry easily, so I suppose I'm still very irritated and don't know what to do with this irritation or how to handle it so that I don't blow up at anyone. Oh, yes, I do... keep to myself, but then they say that, that isn't good for me either. Perhaps not, but it's best for everyone else right now, isn't it?

That incident at Timmies last week really put me over the edge and fast... I just wanted to verbally rip that young ladies head off for some stupid reason. I didn't but, I wanted to and that's just as bad. I was fuming so much so that I submitted an online complaint. What I really wanted to do was ask her how fucking stupid she was and then continue on telling her how stupid I thought she was. Today in fact, at the same Tim Hortons, I get a donut and coffee to go through the drive-thru... yet another reason why I hate drive-thru. The young lady hadn't given me napkins with my order. I asked the young lady for a 'serviette'.... she looks at me like I had 3 heads or something and froze-right there on the spot and she stared at me for a moment completely out of it. She had no idea what the hell I was asking for and it was quite evident. I repeated my question… still frozen, she didn't know what to do; "A fucking napkin you moron, they're right there beside your right hand…" she finally comes out of her trance and hands me several napkins. Good Greif! She didn't know what a serviette was. Good God what's wrong with these young people today, do they not have a vocabulary beyond emojis and LOL shortcuts and crap like that? Get your face into a book or something and put your damn phones, tablets and what have you down already. Get out and actually socialize with people instead of these stupid online social media sites and you might expand your horizons in life, not to mention your vocabulary.

See, can't even stay on track… I have no idea how I wandered to Timmies.

Um, ya, so, I'm going to these AA meetings regularly and I'll receive my 2-month sobriety coin… big deal! Well, I made it to my 3rd month and opened another bottle for no other reason than because I want to. I'm here by myself, there isn't anyone going to get hurt by it and I took my time with it… so what?

Oh, this one time… when I was up and feeling on top of the world and more talkative than usual. We had this new Med-tech who was about to give me an allergy shot… well, I winked at the other Med-tech who knew me quite well, and as soon as she got close to me with that thing, I 'fainted' on her. This of course after informing her that I had no problems with needles. She panicked, I laughed, the other Med-tech called me an asshole, she was furious, called me a bugger… "hey, that's what mom always called me" while picking myself up off of the floor. She threatened me of course should I ever pull another stunt like that one her… she then jabbed that thing into my arm so that it would hurt. "ouch", "well, you deserved it" she said… I suppose I had, but that was fun.

You mentioned that you think they're starting to listen to you now… what is it that you want out of all of this and from them?

I WANT MY HELLISH NIGHTMARE TO BE OVER!

If that is at all possible. Well, at the very least to be somewhat manageable because I don't believe it will ever be over.

Is it too much to ask to want to live what we can not define as a 'normal' life?

Is it too much to actually know what 'happiness' is and be able to live it instead of just being in pursuit of it?

I want the valleys depth to be raised and the mountain peaks to be leveled off to more of an even playing field. Or at the very least, with little wave instead of a tsunami.

I realize that life isn't smooth sailing for anyone but not everyone experiences mount Everest one month and then walks through the depts of hell the next. Or experiences a blissful day one moment and then wants to rip someone out of their car and beat the crap out of them the next either.

I want to wake up to know who Wayne is.

I want to wake up and know that I'm not cleaning up after another shit storm.

I want to know who I'm waking up to the next morning.

I want to know that I don't have to be afraid of myself.

I want people not to be afraid of me.

I want the voices in my head to stop!

I want the music to be silenced!

I want the visions to disappear!

I want the hallucinations to stop!

I want to be on the right medication that will allow all of this crap... to stop!

I want to sleep and wake up on somewhat of a normal schedule without being draggy or wanting to go 1,000 miles per second.

I want to stop chasing my tail and never catching it.

I want to know what it is to be content.

I don't want to be talking to the darkness as if it's my old friend.

It would appear that I WANT a lot of things, doesn't?

I know, some may say that I'm asking a lot, but I don't think that I am.

Am I?

Do you thinking I'm asking too much?

Or is this another pipe dream?

I just want some relief, some balance… some sense of normality.

Is that too much to ask for?

Is It?

How Is Bipolar Disorder Treated?

Because bipolar disorder is a lifelong disease with <u>NO CURE</u>, [**well isn't that just Jim-dandily-andy?**] treatment must be long term [**I can handle that but get me on some sort of treatment that will help**]. In most cases, that means combining medications with psychotherapy ("talk" therapy) [**which I'm not seeing advantageous at all**] and lifestyle changes to help maintain stable moods. Cognitive behavior therapy, psycho-education, family therapy, and interpersonal and social rhythm therapy work well for some with bipolar disorder [**so, a life in therapy,** cool! Well, if it helps I suppose and it's better than what I have been getting... which has been nothing]. Treatment depends on the severity of the symptoms and whether the illness is in an acute highly symptomatic phase or in a quieter chronic phase of remission [**remission, that's funny. How do the symptoms calm to a 'quieter chronic phase of remission'?**] The cornerstone treatment for bipolar disorder is mood stabilizers, which may be combined with anti-psychotic medication. Anti-depressants have little role in the treatment of bipolar disorder and may actually make it worse [**interesting... and what did they prescribe for the clinical depression? Yup, you got it! So, they've actually been an accessory to my misery. Fan-fucking-tastic!**] This is why proper diagnosis is critical since antidepressants are the primary treatment for unipolar depression [**again, you've got the wrong number!**] In some cases – for example, if medicines can't be used or depression or mania is very severe – electroconvulsive therapy (ECT) is a treatment option [**Ya? NO! That Ain't happening!**]

How Do I Make Sure My Bipolar Disorder Is Managed Well? [**Please, do tell**]

By adopting regular habits, people with bipolar disorder may help avoid manic and depressive episodes.

+ Establish a regular routine - go to bed and get up at the same time, eat meals at a regular time, exercise at the same time each day. [**Um? Ya, right... like that's going to happen. And how do we accomplish this?**]

   Have you ever heard Bill Cosby laugh, well that's how I'm laughing now, no seriously... how do I manage to accomplish this? I can't sleep, I don't want to eat and why bother exercising when all it does is aggravate my back to the point where it's difficult to walk, sit, or lay down?

+ Try to avoid stress. [**Oh, another good one, can I just avoid people all together?**] Know what causes you stress and have a plan for relieving it [**as of late, I realize that people, in multiple numbers,** cause me stress. Again, living as a hermit in a cabin in the woods sounds like an even better idea right about now].

+ Recognize your early warning signs for manic and depressive episodes. Talk to your doctor as soon as you notice changes [**I'm just beginning to put 2 and 2 together here so that's going to take some time, but I'm working on this one**]

+ Consider keeping a diary of your daily symptoms, treatment, sleep patterns and events in your life [**tried that diary stuff, many times and it only lasts for a short time, then I forget or get high or low and who gives a shit then? But I've decided to give it another go**]

This may help you better understand the illness and assist your doctor in treating you most effectively.

+ Take medication as prescribed for your bipolar disorder. Keep your doctor informed of any other drugs you take.

+ Avoid caffeine and alcohol [**my 'drinking' is hit and miss, I drink herbal teas without caffeine, I've even switched to decafe coffee later in the day, so I'm not about to give my 'high test' in the mornings too!**]

+ Consider joining a support group [**I've joined AA, but there aren't any other support groups around here that would pertain to people with bipolar disorder and I'm not driving anywhere out of town to find one either. I just might have to start my own group. To get anywhere, I'd have to join a group for depression, another one for anxiety disorders, another one for impulsivity disorder… etc., etc. I don't really know**]

To back up a bit: After that last suicide attempt I went to see the new family Doctor… very nice lady. I spoke with her as to why I was in the hospital, why I tried to commit suicide, she asked a little bit about my background by asking a few of the 8 questions listed above and she asked if I had ever been diagnosed with Bipolar Disorder. I had informed her that I had not and suspected that, that was what my problem has been all along and she had her suspicions as well. I like this one, she's got it all together. Where have you been all my life? Why do you ask? Because, she took the time to listen to me, that's why, and she asked all of the right questions and figured it out within the first ten minutes of our meeting. But then I later found out that her mother is a fellow sufferer so she knew the symptoms and knew all the right questions to ask. Perhaps I have finally found one who is listening. She had referred me to a psychiatrist and I had a teleconference with him at the end of July 2018... Finally, I think someone is listening!

Interjection: 0803-23-08-2018

I have their attention now... [7 or 8 labels later] we are beginning to properly treat the bi-polar disorder. My meds have been steadily increasing and I'm feeling pretty 'steady' which is good. The meds make me feel tired though so, I either have to take them earlier in the evening before I retire for the night or I end up sleeping in a little later in the morning. I'm not sure if this is a repeat, and it probably is... but the psychiatrist said that I have all the classic symptoms of PTSD, Oppositional Defiance Disorder, Anxiety Disorder, Mood Disorders, Clinical Depression, Clinical Insomnia, Borderline Personality Disorder, Bipolar Disorder... so that's what? Eight disorders of varying sorts and some of them have the same symptoms. In other words, folks, I'm completely Batshit! And there isn't anything anyone can do about it. Oh Joy! I'm sure she would have concurred in grade school! After the interview on the 25th of July, **FINALLY**! I've been heard... I've been on some new meds, they've been adjusted a couple of times, no more hearing voices, the music for the most part has stopped. I 'm still seeing things, but perhaps they'll go away as well and I'm finally sleeping again... too much so, but I'm sure we'll sort that out. I'm having some stupid dreams mind you, but at least, I'm dreaming again.

He has me on Divalproex 1,000mgs... Divalproex sodium is also used to treat the manic phase of bipolar disorder (manic-depressive illness), and helps prevent migraine headaches.

And, Quetiapine 150mgs... is used to treat certain mental/mood conditions (such as schizophrenia, bipolar disorder, sudden episodes of mania or depression associated with bipolar disorder). Quetiapine is known as an anti-psychotic drug (atypical type). It works by helping to restore the balance of certain natural substances (neurotransmitters) in the brain.

This medication can decrease hallucinations and improve your concentration. It helps you to think more clearly and positively about yourself, feel less nervous, and take a more active part in everyday life. It may also improve your mood, sleep, appetite, and energy level. Quetiapine can help prevent severe mood swings or decrease how often mood swings occur.

Interjection: 2004-02-09-2018; we've been increasing the two medications that I'm on, on a weekly basis but I'm extremely tired the next day. I'm on 1500mg of Divalproex and 150mg of Quetiapine a day. I've been speaking with an associate and a therapist who have both mentioned this <u>EMDR</u>, to assist with my complex PTSD. Huh? It's been around for some time so why is it that I'm just hearing about it now?

<u>EMDR</u> (Eye Movement Desensitization and Reprocessing) is a psychotherapy that enables people to heal from the symptoms and emotional distress that are the result of disturbing life experiences. Repeated studies show that by using EMDR therapy people can experience the benefits of psychotherapy that once took years to make a difference. It is widely assumed that severe emotional pain requires a long time to heal. EMDR therapy shows that the mind can in fact heal from psychological trauma much as the body recovers from physical trauma. When you cut your hand, your body works to close the wound. If a foreign object or repeated injury irritates the wound, it festers and causes pain. Once the block is removed, healing resumes. EMDR therapy demonstrates that a similar sequence of events occurs with mental processes. The brain's information processing system naturally moves toward mental health. If the system is blocked or imbalanced by the impact of a disturbing event, the emotional wound festers and can cause intense suffering. Once the block is removed, healing resumes. Using the detailed protocols and procedures learned in EMDR therapy training sessions, clinicians help clients activate their natural healing processes.

http://www.emdr.com/what-is-emdr/

Interjection: 1824-09-09-2018: they've adjusted my meds a couple of times now. The Quetiapine is still at 150mgs but the Divalproex is at 1500mgs per day. I'm beginning to feel better, I have clearer thoughts, I'm am in somewhat of a normal sleeping pattern but still feeling tired. I still find myself getting a little impatient but I have to talk to myself to steady that.

I hadn't wanted to submit this at the beginning because it would have been a Spoiler Alert!

BECAUSE OF A COUPLE OF SPECIAL PEOPLE:

I JUST MIGHT DIMLY SEE A WINDOW IN MY WALL!

Special Thanks go out to my Nurse Practitioner and the Couple's therapist who said that "I can fix the two of you until Wayne is treated for bipolar disorder." The therapist was the second person who picked up on it right away... not five minutes into 'our' history and she asks me if I've ever been treated for Bipolar Disorder. My NP, who immediately picked up on the Bipolar Disorder and set the wheels in motion for me for an official diagnosis. I finally had a Psych consult and was awarded the following labels: Bipolar Disorder, PTSD (Post Traumatic Stress Disorder), ODD (Oppositional Defiance Disorder), Mood Disorder, Anxiety Disorder, Clinical Depression, Borderline Personality Disorder, Chronic Insomnia, and Type B Personalities... oh what joy? But then, I knew about most of them, hadn't I? I have more labels on me than a piece of clothing on the sales rack at Macie's for Pete's sake. Oh well! I guess I truly am BATSHIT after all! But that's what I've been trying to tell them my entire life.

Seroquel is to be increased; this medication is used to treat certain mental/mood conditions (such as schizophrenia, bipolar disorder, sudden episodes of mania or depression associated with bipolar disorder). Quetiapine is known as an anti-psychotic drug (atypical type). It works by helping to restore the balance of certain natural substances (neurotransmitters) in the brain. This medication can decrease hallucinations and improve your concentration. It helps you to think more clearly and positively about yourself, feel less nervous, and take a more active part in everyday life. It may also improve your mood, sleep, appetite, and energy level. Quetiapine can help prevent severe mood swings or decrease how often mood swings occur.

….. added: DIVALPROEX SODIUM ENTERIC-COATED TABLETS 500mg 1x per day to start. I have to go in for blood work, then once a month to check the levels of this new medication. So far, I think it's working for the 'maniac' phase of bipolar disorder because I don't feel as if I'm on the rise, but I think I'll need something else for this irritability.

This medication is used to treat seizure disorders, certain psychiatric conditions (manic phase of bipolar disorder), and to prevent migraine headaches. It works by restoring the balance of certain natural substances (neurotransmitters) in the brain.

The problem though is that 'Counseling' has been stalled for now. They did some restructuring up at the Mental Health Unit and there really isn't anyone in town qualified to handle the complexities of Bipolar Disorder… and I'm not going to multiple therapy groups for 'depression', 'anxiety', 'AA', and what have you.

SECTION THREE

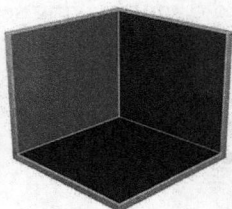

HOW TO HELP SOMEONE WITH BIPOLAR DISORDER

Again; there are over eleven million websites on how to help someone suffering from Bipolar Disorder. The best thing you can do for yourself and your family member or friend is to Educate Yourself so that you can be of assistance to them! This is just a small sample of what I've found to assist you in the right direction.

<u>A person requires immediate help when they</u>:

+ Have deliberately hurt themselves
+ Talks about suicide or harming someone else
+ Is disoriented (don't know who/where or what time of day it is)
+ Is experiencing hallucinations (hearing/seeing things that aren't there)
+ May be delusional (have very strange beliefs, often based on the content of the hallucinations
+ May-be confused or not making sense
+ Makes unrealistic plans.

It is also helpful if you could stay in contact with their mental/medical care provider, with their consent of course.

Have a plan of action when the person shows signs of mania or depression.

Be prepared to make attempts to stop a person from making important decisions that may risk losing money, their job, or friends while displaying manic symptoms. They aren't thinking clearly and you will need to reassure them that you are on their side whether they can see that or not. (My latest episode has caused a major financial shit-storm that could take months to get out of).

<u>What does not help</u>

Taking what they say and do personally during a manic episode. They aren't thinking clearly and they need your patience and understanding. ry to avoid these common reactions:

- blaming the person for their actions when they are not able to judge correctly
- telling the person to change their behaviour or act normally – instead, explain how their actions affect you.

<u>What happens if the person doesn't want help?</u>

Folks who display symptoms of hypomania or mania, often don't realize their behavior is out of the ordinary and are enjoying the 'high' and don't want it to end. They may have stopped taking their medications, or they may have hidden them because they feel better or somehow that they've been cured. Trying to get someone in this position to take their medications regularly may/does cause difficulties between family members and friends. The best thing for you to do is talk them through the past situations that have occurred during this phase. It may also help if you kept a journal with them and tracked their moods, habits and behaviors so that you have something tangible in front of you to support your cause. Reassure them that you have their best interest at heart. When I was talking about going down to the US to live out the winter no one really tried talking me out of it and it probably wouldn't have done them any good. But the thing is, they didn't try. It turned out to be a dumb plan and put me in a financial crisis. What's that old saying? "If at first you don't succeed, try, and try again?" Try to talk them out of doing something silly, like going into the car dealership and purchasing two brand new vehicles.

<u>The Bottom Line</u>: this from the web psychology website:

https://www.webpsychology.com/news/2015/06/10/top-10-things-you-can-do-support-someone-bipolar-disorder-220031

<u>The Top 10 Things You Can Do To Support Someone with Bipolar Disorder</u>

1. Educate Yourself
2. Don't try to give advice
3. Offer physical comfort during Depression
4. Understand the Manic cycle

5. Protect yourself
6. Don't shame them after an episode
7. Understand the struggle of medication
8. Know the triggers
9. Facilitate treatment
10. Take suicide talk seriously
11. Take care of yourself (I guess they can't count).

There are over twelve million websites on the Google Search Engine alone on this topic. Here are just a few of the many websites that I had visited to glean my information from… with today's modern technology; there really is no excuse.

Then there is the underlying question: do I or don't I inform my employer? Google research came up with 1, 250,000 websites on this question. Some websites say Yes, others suggest not doing so, while others let you weigh your options and go from there. Either way, having a mental disease in some countries does protect you under the 'Disabilities Act' but the ultimate choice is of course yours and yours alone to make. After I resigned from my position, I informed my area coach of my situation and he pulled my credentials… looking at the research, now I'm wondering if he had a right to do that? I'm going to have to dig a little further into this dilemma.

If you have just been diagnosed with Bipolar Disorder; check out this website, it suggests 20 tips from folks who've been there: https://www.elementsbehavioralhealth.com/mood-disorders/just-diagnosed-with-bipolar-disorder-20-tips-from-those-whove-been-there/

WE'RE NOT ALONE!

Just when we who suffer with bipolar disorder thought that we were alone… according to mental health today.com; we're not!

http://www.mental-health-today.com/bp/famous_people.htm

Famous People with Bipolar Disorder

Much of this list was obtained from the Internet.

Actors & Actresses

Ned Beatty
Maurice Bernard, soap opera
Jeremy Brett
Jim Carey
Lisa Nicole Carson
Rosemary Clooney, singer
Lindsay Crosby
Eric Douglas
Robert Downey Jr.
Patty Duke
Carrie Fisher
Connie Francis, singer and actress
Shecky Greene, comedian
Linda Hamilton
Moss Hart, actor, director, playwright
Mariette Hartley
Margot Kidder
Vivien Leigh
Kevin McDonald, comedian
Kristy McNichols
Burgess Meredith, actor, director
Spike Milligan, actor, writer
Nicola Pagett
Ben Stiller, actor, director, writer
David Strickland

Lili Taylor
Tracy Ullman
Jean-Claude Van Damme
Robin Williams
Jonathon Winters, comedian

Artists

Alvin Alley, dancer, choreographer
Ludwig Von Beethoven
Tim Burton, artist, director
Francis Ford Coppola, director
George Fredrick Handel, composer
Bill Lichtenstein, producer
Joshua Logan, Broadway director, producer
Vincent Van Gogh, painter
Gustav Mahier, composer
Francesco Scavullo, artist, photographer
Robert Schumann, composer
Don Simpson, movie producer
Norman Wexler, screenwriter, playwright

Entrepreneurs

Robert Campeau
Pierre Peladeau
Heinz C. Prechter
Ted Turner, media giant

Financiers

John Mulheren
Murray Pezim
Scientists
Karl Paul Link, chemist
Dimitri Mihalas

Miscellaneous

Buzz Aldrin, astronaut
Clifford Beers, humanitarian
Garnet Coleman, legislator (Texas)
Larry Flynt, publisher and activist
Kit Gingrich, Newt's mom
Phil Graham, owner of Washington Post
Peter Gregg, team owner and manager, race car driver
Susan Panico (Susan Dime-Meenan), business executive
Sol Wachtier, former New York State Chief Judge

Musicians

Ludwig van Beethoven, composer
Alohe Jean Burke, musician, vocalist
Rosemary Clooney, singer
DMX Earl Simmons, rapper and actor
Ray Davies
Lenny Dee
Gaetano Donizetti, opera singer
Peter Gabriel
Jimi Hendrix
Kristen Hersh (Throwing Muses)
Phyllis Hyman
Jack Irons
Daniel Johnston
Otto Klemperer, musician, conductor
Oscar Levant, pianist, composer, television
Phil Ochs, musician, political activist, poet
John Ogden, composer, musician
Jaco Pastorius
Charley Pride
Mac Rebennack (Dr. John)
Jeannie C. Riley
Alys Robi, vocalist in Canada
Axl Rose
Nick Traina

Del Shannon
Phil Spector, musician and producer
Sting, Gordon Sumner, musician, composer
Tom Waits, musician, composer
Brian Wilson, musician, composer, arranger
Townes Van Zandt, musician, composer

Poets

John Berryman
C.E. Chaffin, writer, poet
Hart Crane
Randall Jarrell
Jane Kenyon
Robert Lowell
Sylvia Plath
Robert Schumann
Delmore Schwartz

Political

Robert Boorstin, special assistant to President Clinton
L. Brent Bozell, political scientist, attorney, writer
Bob Bullock, ex secretary of state, state comptroller and lieutenant governor
Winston Churchill, British Prime minister
Kitty Dukasis, former First Lady of Massachusetts
Thomas Eagleton, lawyer, former U.S. Senator
Lynne Rivers, U.S. Congress
Theodore Roosevelt, President of the United States

Scholars

John Strugnell, biblical scholar

Sports

Shelley Beattie, bodybuilding, sailing
John Daly, golf

Muffin Spencer-Devlin, pro golf
Ilie Nastase, tennis
Jimmy Piersail, baseball player, Boston Red Sox, sports announcer
Barret Robbins, football
Wyatt Sexton, football
Alonzo Spellman, football
Darryl Strawberry, baseball
Dimitrius Underwood, football
Luther Wright, basketball
Bert Yancey, athlete

TV & Radio

Dick Cavett
Jay Marvin, radio, writer
Jane Pauley, NBC Journalist

Writers

Louis Althusser, philosopher, writer
Honors de Balzac
Art Buchwald, writer, humorist
Neal Cassady
Patricia Cornwell
Margot Early
Kaye Gibbons
Johann Goethe
Graham Greene
Abbie Hoffman, writer, political activist
Kay Redfield Jamison, writer, psychologist
Peter Nolan Lawrence
Frances Lear, writer, editor, women's rights activist
Rika Lesser, writer, translator
Kate Millet
Robert Munsch
Margo Orum
Edgar Allen Poe
Theodore Roethke

Lori Schiller, writer, educator
Frances Sherwood
Scott Simmie, writer, journalist
August Strindberg
Mark Twain
Joseph Vasquez, writer, movie director
Mark Vonnegut, doctor, writer
Sol Wachtler, writer, judge
Mary Jane Ward
Virginia Woolf

Recognize anyone? I sure do. Here's another famous person for us Canadians...

Margaret Trudeau has so many stories... After going **undiagnosed for decades,** [sound familiar?] she was eventually found to have bipolar disorder, which causes depression and mania, you don't say? I do believe that, that is what this book is all about.

Read her full story: https://www.goodhousekeeping.com/health/a46206/margaret-trudeau/

And I'm sure there are a host of other well know folks, if they know or would care to admit to it, that is...

Here is a list of a few of the many websites I visited to glean my information from:

Canadian Mental Health Association:

https://cmha.ca/mental-health/understanding-mental-illness/bipolar-disorder

Government of Canada:

https://www.canada.ca/en/public-health/services/chronic-diseases/mental-illness/what-should-know-about-bipolar-disorder-manic-depression.html

Health Link BC:

https://www.healthlinkbc.ca/health-topics/hw148751

Mood Disorder Society of Canada:

https://mdsc.ca/educate/what-is-bipolar-disorder/

Mayo Clinic:

https://www.mayoclinic.org/diseases-conditions/bipolar-disorder/symptoms-causes/syc-20355955

National Institute of Mental Health:

https://www.nimh.nih.gov/health/topics/bipolar-disorder/index.shtml

WebMD:

https://www.webmd.com/bipolar-disorder/default.htm

https://www.webmd.com/bipolar-disorder/bipolar-life-17/slideshow-help-someone-with-bipolar

Health Line:

https://www.healthline.com/health/could-it-be-bipolar-signs-to-look-for

Mental Health America:

http://www.mentalhealthamerica.net/conditions/bipolar-disorder

HELPGUIDE.ORG:

https://www.helpguide.org/articles/bipolar-disorder/helping-someone-with-bipolar-disorder.htm

Bp Hope: Hope & Harmony for people with bipolar disorder

https://www.bphope.com/the-big-payoff-of-well-chosen-words/

Your Health in Mind:

https://www.yourhealthinmind.org/mental-illnesses-disorders/bipolar-disorder/helping-someone

A final word: I guess I should have researched a little deeper because apparently there are a number of books available for sale on Amazon about living with Bipolar Disorder, etc. However; this book is not intended to be a 'self help' guide in anyway, it is an autobiography. As was previously mentioned; there are over 12, million websites on the subject of Bipolar Disorder. Over 2, million on how to help yourself. Over 9, million on how to help a friend. Over 1, million as to whether or not you inform your employer on the Google Search Engine alone. My final question is: With all this information out there, how are people still being misdiagnosed and permitted to live a life time in a living hell?

I believe that I have finally come to realize that:
"God isn't finished with me yet!"
Thanks Mom

And Now I have come to realize that:
"Wayne Mustn't be Finished with Wayne!"
Thanks, AZ!

I hope you have found this book to have been somewhat inspirational, educational and entertaining as well as a blessing to you all.

Let me know if there is anyway I can be of assistance to you:

wayne_driver@outlook.com

Good Bye, and Godspeed

Hope to see you, on the other side!

THE END, or IS IT?

CPSIA information can be obtained
at www.ICGtesting.com
Printed in the USA
LVHW111042040619
620091LV00004B/6/P